T0362354

Contemporary Management of Acute and Chronic Venous Disease

With a focus on evidence-based, contemporary, and clinically relevant information, this practical new resource provides a concise, clinical, and techniques-focused guide to the medical, endovenous, and surgical management of patients with acute and chronic venous disease.

Internationally recognized chapter authors cover the general principles of the pathophysiology, diagnosis, indications, and decision-making around the management of acute and chronic venous disease. The text emphasizes endovenous and surgical techniques where applicable and also addresses symptomatic peripheral venous insufficiency, deep venous thrombosis, and the care of patients with symptomatic central venous disease.

Vascular surgeons will find this a valuable guide, providing insights into key techniques and approaches to the treatment of acute and chronic venous disorders. This book is an invaluable resource for vascular trainees preparing for examinations and for physicians in other specialities looking to expand their knowledge base.

Contemporary Management of Acute and Chronic Venous Disease

Edited by

Juan Carlos Jimenez, MD, MBA, FACS

Professor of Surgery
Director, Gonda (Goldschmied) Vascular Center
Division of Vascular Surgery
David Geffen School of Medicine at UCLA
Los Angeles, California

Samuel Eric Wilson, MD, FACS

Distinguished Professor of Surgery and Chair Emeritus
University of California Irvine
Irvine, California

CRC Press
Taylor & Francis Group
Boca Raton London New York

CRC Press is an imprint of the
Taylor & Francis Group, an **informa** business

First edition published 2024
by CRC Press
6000 Broken Sound Parkway NW, Suite 300, Boca Raton, FL 33487-2742

and by CRC Press
4 Park Square, Milton Park, Abingdon, Oxon, OX14 4RN

CRC Press is an imprint of Taylor & Francis Group, LLC

ISBN: 9781032327747 (hbk)
ISBN: 9781032327020 (pbk)
ISBN: 9781003316626 (ebk)

DOI: 10.1201/9781003316626

Typeset in Sabon
by Apex CoVantage, LLC

Juan Carlos Jimenez: "For Daniel and Christian, my inspirations!"

Samuel Eric Wilson: "This one's for Sandy."

Contents

Preface

From the first description of varicose veins in the papyrus of Ebers in 1550 BCE to Keller's saphenous vein stripper in 1905, and on to the beginning of the 21st century, treatment of superficial venous disease remained limited to often ineffective pressure bandages, sclerosants, and a few surgical techniques. Since then, the rapid progression in evidence-based technologies to treat patients with venous disease cannot be overstated. Over the last 20 years, multiple endovenous therapies have emerged with equal to improved outcomes over open surgery, decreased patient morbidity, and increased safety.

This comprehensive overview of the contemporary management of venous disorders focuses on clinical diagnosis, imaging modalities, decision-making, medical management, and descriptions of endovenous and open surgical techniques. Results of evidence-based methods, along with analysis of current clinical practice guidelines issued by international societies are discussed. Our goal for this collection is to improve working knowledge and overall ability to provide up-to-date care for patients suffering from venous disease.

Sincerely,
Juan Carlos Jimenez
Samuel Eric Wilson

Contributors

Jose I. Almeida, MD, FACS
University of Miami
Miami, FL, USA

Samuel P. Arnot
Pitzer College
Claremont, CA, USA

Charles A. Banks, MD
University of Alabama at Birmingham
Birmingham, AL, USA

Paola Batarseh, MD
Yale School of Medicine
New Haven, CT, USA

Mary A. Binko, MS
University of Pittsburgh
Pittsburgh, PA, USA

Tyler Callese, MD
University of California Los Angeles
Los Angeles, CA, USA

Drayson Campbell, BS
Ohio State University
Columbus, OH, USA

John G. Carson, MD
Maine Medical Center
Portland, ME, USA

Ankur Chandra, MD, RPVI
Scripps Clinic
La Jolla, CA, USA

Amanda L. Chin, MD, MBA
University of California Los Angeles
Los Angeles, CA, USA

Christopher Chow, MD
University of Miami
Miami, FL, USA

Lucas Cusumano, MD
University of California Los Angeles
Los Angeles, CA, USA

Leo Daab, MD
Oregon Health & Science University
Portland, OR, USA

Fachreza Aryo Damara, MD
Cleveland Clinic
Cleveland, OH, USA

Steven M. Dean, DO, FSVM, RPVI
Ohio State University
Columbus, OH, USA

Benjamin J. DiPardo, MD
University of California Los Angeles
Los Angeles, CA, USA

William Duong, MD
University of California Los Angeles
Los Angeles, CA, USA

Young Erben, MD
Mayo Clinic
Jacksonville, FL, USA

Steven M. Farley, MD
University of California Los Angeles
Los Angeles, CA, USA

Savannah Fletcher, MD
University of California Los Angeles
Los Angeles, CA, USA

Ana Fuentes
Mayo Clinic
Jacksonville, FL, USA

Hugh A. Gelabert, MD
University of California Los Angeles
Los Angeles, CA, USA

Roberta Lozano Gonzalez, MD
Mayo Clinic
Jacksonville, FL, USA

Eric S. Hager, MD, FACS
University of Pittsburgh
Pittsburgh, PA, USA

Antalya Jano, BA
University of Pittsburgh
Pittsburgh, PA, USA

Juan Carlos Jimenez, MD, MBA, FACS
University of California, Los Angeles
Los Angeles, CA, USA

Aniket Joglekar, MD
University of California Los Angeles
Los Angeles, CA, USA

Nii-Kabu Kabutey, MD
University of California, Irvine
Irvine, CA, USA

Manju Kalra
Mayo Clinic
Rochester, MN, USA

Misaki M. Kiguchi, MD, MBA, FACS
MedStar Washington Hospital Center
Washington DC, USA

Ducksoo Kim, MD
Boston VA Healthcare System
Boston, MA, USA

Peter F. Lawrence, MD
University of California Los Angeles
Los Angeles, CA, USA

Reid C. Mahoney, MD
Oregon Health & Science University
Portland, OR, USA

Justin McWilliams, MD
University of California Los Angeles
Los Angeles, CA, USA

Gregory Moneta, MD
Oregon Health & Science University
Portland, OR, USA

Christopher Montoya, MD
University of Miami
Miami, FL, USA

Oscar Y. Moreno-Rocha, MD
University of Michigan
Ann Arbor, MI, USA

John Moriarty, MD
University of California Los Angeles
Los Angeles, CA, USA

Andrea T. Obi, MD
University of Michigan
Ann Arbor, MI, USA

Cassius Iyad Ochoa Chaar, MD, MPH, MS
Yale School of Medicine
New Haven, CT, USA

Marc A. Passman, MD
University of Alabama at Birmingham
Birmingham, AL, USA

Neeraj Rastogi, MD
Boston, MA, USA

David Rigberg, MD
University of California Los Angeles
Los Angeles, CA, USA

Johnathon C. Rollo, MD
University of California Los Angeles
Los Angeles, CA, USA

Indrani Sen
Mayo Clinic Health Systems
Eau Claire, WI, USA

Jacob W. Soucy, MSI
Pennsylvania State College of Medicine
Hershey, PA, USA

Jordan F. Stafford, MD
Ohio State University
Columbus, OH, USA

Emily Swafford, BS
University of Miami
Miami, FL, USA

Jesus G. Ulloa, MD, MBA, MSHPM
University of California Los Angeles
Los Angeles, CA, USA

Thomas W. Wakefield, MD
University of Michigan
Ann Arbor, MI, USA

Samuel E. Wilson, MD, FACS
University of California Irvine
Irvine, CA, USA

Section I

General Principles

Chapter 1

Non-Invasive Imaging of the Venous System

Ankur Chandra

INTRODUCTION

Appropriate diagnosis of venous disease without proper imaging is a challenge for clinicians. Venography, through the introduction of an intravenous catheter and administration of contrast, was the initial invasive imaging modality used to diagnose venous pathology including thrombotic and insufficiency disorders. Unfortunately, this modality was painful and would result in complications such as venous thrombosis and embolism. The application of continuous wave Doppler by Strandness and Sigel[1,2] throughout the 1960s provided the first non-invasive assessment of venous flow. Prior to the development and validation of duplex scanning and pulse wave Doppler principles, there was widespread use of physiologic methods such as impedance phlebography in the 1970s–1980s. However, since that time, duplex scanning has been the predominant non-invasive imaging used to diagnose disorders of the venous system. In this chapter we will begin by discussing the principles that underlie duplex ultrasound. Then we will describe the targeted application of both continuous wave Doppler as well as pulse wave Doppler/duplex ultrasound in the diagnosis of common venous conditions including thrombotic events, venous insufficiency, anatomic assessment of superficial veins, and clinical follow-up after treatment of venous reflux.

PRINCIPLES OF DUPLEX ULTRASOUND

The application of ultrasound to the development of vascular imaging and Doppler-based measurements has enabled the clinical study of normal and pathologic venous hemodynamics. Beginning in the 1960s, a continuous wave Doppler was first applied to assess blood flow in battlefield scenarios and then transitioned to routine clinical care. The application of piezoelectric crystals to transmit ultrasonic waves into tissue was then modified by varying the pulse frequency of these waves with more sophisticated algorithms to generate visual images of the underlying tissue. Dr. Eugene Strandness and his vascular surgery colleagues at the University of Washington are credited with the further development of the application of Doppler principles to existing B-mode ultrasound to create duplex imaging. This discovery enabled modern day non-invasive vascular imaging. This section will cover the concepts of ultrasound physics and instrumentation, Doppler shift, and duplex imaging.

Ultrasound Instrumentation and Physics

A clinical ultrasound machine involves three components: the probe (or transducer), a signal translation algorithm, and a display. The probe serves as the interface with the patient to send and receive sound waves, the signal translation algorithm converts the received sound wave from the probe to functional clinical data, and the display is used to present this data. An ultrasound probe is composed of a small array of piezoelectric crystals. A piezoelectric crystal

DOI: 10.1201/9781003316626-2

$$\Delta f = \frac{2\,fV\ \cos\theta}{C}$$

Figure 1.1 Doppler equation showing the Doppler frequency shift (Δf) is equal to the product of frequency of the insonent sound wave (f), the velocity of the object in motion (V), and the cosine of the angle of insonation (Θ) divided by the speed of sound in tissue (C = 1540m/sec).

changes its shape when an electric current is applied across it. The new shape of the crystal holds the stored mechanical energy and, when a variable current is applied, the transducer produces sound waves at precise frequencies transmitted in the direction of probe. This concept also holds in reverse, in that, if a force such as a sound wave is applied to the piezoelectric crystal, the crystal will create voltage that can be measured. This is the mechanism in which piezoelectric crystals on an ultrasound transducer both transmit sound waves and measure the reflected sound wave that returns from tissue.

A continuous wave Doppler is an ultrasound probe that continuously transmits and receives soundwaves. A pulse wave Doppler is a probe that transmits sound waves in packets of varying lengths and frequencies and varies the window during which it receives them. The continuous wave Doppler sacrifices the ability to distinguish location or depth in tissue in exchange for requiring far less computational effort in its signal translation algorithm. These probes traditionally use a speaker as its display to produce an audible Doppler signal. An example of a continuous wave Doppler is the bedside Doppler "pencil" or probe. A pulse wave Doppler generates a visual result on a video display of both tissue structure (grayscale or brightness ["B"] mode imaging) and blood velocity (Doppler effect) through the decoding of the ultrasound pulses. The combination of B-mode imaging and doppler effect is called duplex ultrasound. The standard clinical ultrasound machine used in vascular labs is a pulse wave machine which produces duplex imaging.

The use of pulse wave imaging to generate a velocity versus time waveform occurs through the application of a fast Fourier transform (FFT). This process allows the binning of discrete frequency data over time to generate a spectral waveform. The frequencies in the spectral waveform are converted to velocities through the Doppler equation (Figure 1.1). This is how the clinical velocity over time waveform used in duplex interpretation is generated. There are unique waveforms for each venous segment based on the location and presence of thrombotic or reflux disease.

Doppler Shift and Duplex Imaging

Through the measurement of the frequency shift of a reflected sound wave, the velocity of blood can be noninvasively measured within a vein. The velocity of blood is derived using the Doppler equation (Figure 1.1). The Doppler effect represents a phenomenon when an insonant sound wave reflects off an object in motion and its frequency predictably changes based on the velocity of the reflecting object. The Doppler equation shows that the velocity of the reflector is directly proportional to the speed of sound in a given medium (c) and the difference in the transmitted frequency (F_T) and retuned frequency (F_R). This velocity is inversely proportional to the transmitted frequency (F_T) and the cosine of the angle theta. Theta is the "angle of insonation" or the angle at which the sound contacts the blood vessel.

For very superficial veins, it is frequently impossible to interrogate velocities perpendicular to the flow direction, as this would result in theta equal to 90 degrees for which the cosine of 90 degrees is zero. To measure the accurate velocity of blood, the ideal angle of insonation is

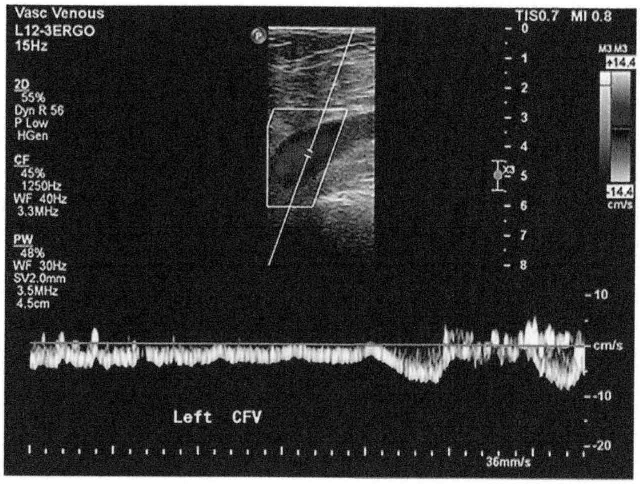

Figure 1.2 Duplex exam of the common femoral vein with flow heading away from the probe in a cephalad direction shown in blue and represented on the color bar as negative (away from probe). This also corresponds to flow waveform below the baseline which is normal for most venous scanning.

as close to 60 degrees as possible. This produces a cosine value of 0.5. As theta approaches zero degrees and the vessel is interrogated nearly parallel to flow, the cosine would approach 1 resulting in artificially elevated results. In venous duplex imaging, velocity direction is displayed as color flow with a legend corresponding the velocity and the direction of flow relative to the ultrasound probe (Figure 1.2).

CLINICAL APPLICATIONS

Acute Deep Venous Thrombosis

A physical exam is often inadequate in the diagnosis of acute DVT of the leg. As a result, the sensitivity and specificity of the non-invasive diagnosis of acute thrombotic occlusion has significantly improved with the application of duplex ultrasound. The continuous wave device was previously a crucial tool for assessing acute DVT in the leg. However, it has been replaced by more advanced imaging techniques using pulsed wave Doppler/duplex. Duplex scanning is now the primary method for diagnosing acute DVT, with alternative imaging studies reserved for cases with inconclusive results or when a scan is unattainable. This practice has been justified by the high accuracy achieved by different investigators.[3–6] Scanning offers significant benefits, including pinpointing the exact location of disease, particularly when multiple thrombi are present. It also detects partially obstructing thrombi, overcoming a major drawback of earlier physiological methods. Scanning not only helps confirm the initial diagnosis but also tracks changes and improvement during treatment.

Continuous Wave Doppler Exam

Occluded segments can be identified by the absence of flow on Doppler examination. The patient lies supine with their head slightly raised, and deep veins are located near the corresponding arteries. Healthy veins exhibit spontaneous flow with respiratory-related fluctuations. Breath-holding or a Valsalva maneuver reduces or halts flow, while its release leads to a brief increase in the signal. Briefly compressing the extremity below the probe results in flow enhancement, often followed by a short decrease upon release. Applying pressure on the upper abdomen or leg diminishes or stops the flow signal, which then increases upon release. Doppler examination detects changes in venous flow patterns, and various types of external compression can cause similar alterations. Abnormal results may stem from venous issues or external compression due to large hematomas, severe edema, or ruptured popliteal cysts. False-positive tests can also occur in cases of advanced pregnancy, ascites, extreme obesity, or abdominal masses that compress the inferior vena cava.

Pulse Wave Doppler/Duplex Exam

Duplex scanners' high resolution enables visualization of venous thrombosis, with a focus on imaging. Thrombus appears within the vein lumen with varying echogenicity levels (Figure 1.3). Sometimes fresh thrombus may resemble flowing blood, necessitating further evaluation by compressing the vein using the probe. Normally, gentle pressure completely flattens the vein (Figure 1.3). However, a partially or fully occluding thrombus inhibits collapse under external pressure. Compression is carried out in the transverse mode to ensure accurate assessment. During longitudinal examination, it is possible to misalign the ultrasound beam, causing the vein to appear collapsed when it is not. Doppler velocity signal abnormalities at rest or during augmentation maneuvers suggest lesions that may not be visible through imaging. Color-coded Doppler is particularly useful for detecting partially occluding thrombi. The color scanner also enhances the examination of calf veins, which are more challenging to visualize without color flow due to their location alongside arteries. Most centers conduct a thorough examination from the inguinal ligament to the calf veins, including imaging of superficial veins. The primary challenge in many exams is tracing the vein through the adductor canal. The common femoral and femoral veins are assessed in the supine position with moderate leg dependency (the deep femoral vein is typically not examined beyond its origin). The popliteal vein is best imaged with the patient in a lateral or prone position. Infrapopliteal

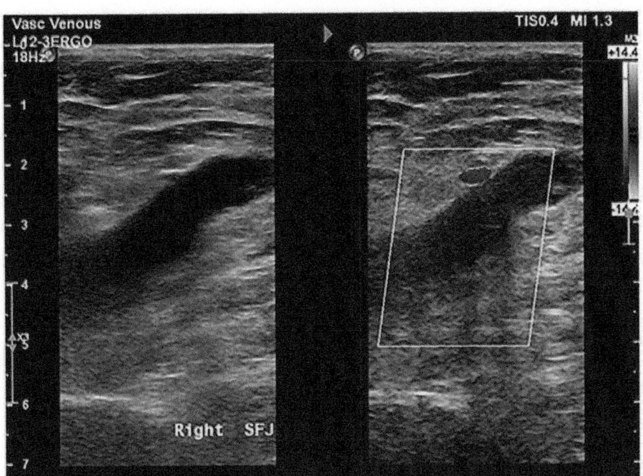

Figure 1.3 Acute DVT of the saphenofemoral junction, which appears echolucent on the noncompressed window (left) but is noncompressible when compression is applied (right), which is diagnostic for occlusive thrombus. Age is estimated as acute by presence of echolucency, whereas thrombus would appear more echogenic for subacute or chronic thrombus.

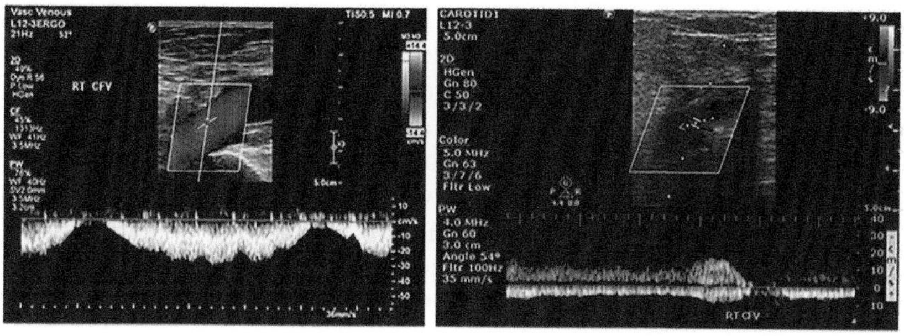

Figure 1.4 Unobstructed venous flow through the proximal iliac veins and IVC has respiratory variation as seen in normal scan on left. When proximal venous obstruction in iliocaval system is present, the flow waveform becomes continuous (right) and is diagnostic for proximal venous obstruction from thrombus or compression even if direct visualization of DVT is not possible.

branches can be challenging to fully evaluate, but extra attention should be given to these if the patient has focal calf symptoms.

Another problematic area is detecting thrombus in the common or external iliac veins. Imaging these veins is difficult, so indirect evidence from the common femoral vein flow signal is often relied upon. Proximal occlusion results in a loss of respiratory phasic variation and limited or no change with the Valsalva maneuver (Figure 1.4). Vogel and colleagues suggested using the change in common femoral vein diameter during the Valsalva maneuver, with an increase of less than 10% indicating suspicion of iliofemoral thrombosis.[3]

Recurrent/Chronic Deep Venous Thrombosis

Diagnosing recurrent DVT in patients with post-thrombotic syndrome poses a significant challenge for clinicians. Worsening symptoms can resemble the original thrombosis, often leading to anticoagulant administration without objective evidence of recurrence. Non-invasive testing can provide objective diagnosis, and comparing a new study with a previous one can help determine if a new thrombus has formed. Duplex scanning can also identify residual chronic thrombus due to its high echogenicity. Other features include thickened vein walls, fibrosed segments of occluded veins, and valvular insufficiency with reverse flow on Doppler examination. These characteristics enable examiners to differentiate recent from chronic clots using a duplex scan, unlike venograms, which display all lesions as filling defects.

Continuous Wave Doppler Exam

In a chronically thrombosed vein segment, there is no flow, and nearby collateral veins exhibit a high-pitched signal. The unobstructed part of the vein beyond the blockage presents continuous flow without respiratory variation, and the Valsalva maneuver causes no alterations. Limb compression may result in limited augmentation, but it is noticeably less than in a healthy vein. The vein segment before the occlusion may display phasic flow, akin to a normal leg, but compressing the distal region induces minimal change.

Pulse Wave Doppler/Duplex Exam

Duplex scanning of deep leg veins for thrombus is technically challenging and demands significant experience for accurate diagnosis. Skilled investigators have reported sensitivities and specificities around 95% for thrombus detection.[3–6] Although most studies focus on acute thrombosis, Rollins et al. demonstrated similar accuracy in identifying chronic disease, with 89% accuracy for calf veins and 93% for proximal veins.[6] Clinicians often want to know the thrombus duration. Currently, no specific method determines its age, but acute thrombus usually appears hypoechoic and homogeneous on grayscale imaging, with a distended vein lumen and a possible "floating tail" at the thrombus' upper end. In the chronic phase, the lesion appears more echoic and heterogeneous, with a smaller-than-normal vein diameter and potential venous collaterals. If direct visualization of the iliocaval segments is not possible, examining the common femoral vein as a reference for proximal venous thrombosis (iliac/IVC) reveals continuous flow without respiratory variation (Figure 1.4).

Venous Insufficiency

Chronic venous stasis complications are often evident, but assessing the relative contributions of outflow obstruction and reflux can be challenging. While initial conservative management is similar, further surgical treatment targets the specific cause. Doppler examination can detect venous reflux and measuring reverse blood flow lasting over 500 msec provides quantitative assessment unavailable with simpler tests.[7,8] Duplex ultrasound of the superficial, perforator, and deep veins can identify the most probable site and cause of venous insufficiency, aiding in the selection of targeted interventions.

Continuous Wave Doppler Exam

Doppler venous examination can also identify venous valvular insufficiency. Under normal conditions, compression proximal to the probe or a Valsalva maneuver should not generate flow, as valves prevent flow toward the probe. However, with incompetent valves, proximal compression or a Valsalva maneuver causes augmentation due to retrograde flow.

Pulse Wave Doppler/Duplex Exam

Ultrasound is utilized to assess reflux in specific venous segments as well. Many labs perform this evaluation with patients in a recumbent position. However, Van Bemmelen et al. stressed the importance of examining patients in the standing position to maximize reflux stimulus.[7] They also highlighted the significance of sufficient compression. A reverse velocity of 30 cm/s is required for consistent valvular closure.[9] Displaying significant reverse flow lasting over 500 msec is evidence of venous insufficiency and valvular incompetence. Inadequate compression may lead to incomplete closure, allowing slow reverse flow through a normal valve and potentially misinterpreting a segment as abnormal.

Preoperative Vein Mapping

When utilizing the great saphenous vein as a surgical conduit, understanding the patient's specific anatomy is crucial. Shah et al. found through contrast venograms that only 65% of thighs and 45% of calves had a single saphenous trunk, with the remainder displaying double systems and cross-connections.[8] Due to the risks associated with contrast venography, duplex scanning has become the standard method for mapping superficial veins in both arms and legs.[10,11] The high-resolution images allow for determining size, course, double segments, and varicosities, closely correlating with the superficial venous anatomy observed during surgery.

Follow-Up of Endovenous Ablation

Endovenous closure has become the primary treatment for significant reflux in the great saphenous vein. Initial experiences with closure techniques demonstrated high vein closure rates, but concerns arose about potential thrombosis extension into the deep system and subsequent pulmonary embolization risk. Most practitioners perform a duplex scan within the first week post-procedure to check for proximal extension. Figure 1.5 displays thrombus extending from the saphenofemoral junction, adhering to the common femoral vein's anterior wall without occluding the vein. Lawrence et al. have developed a classification system for thrombosis levels following ablation procedures.[12]

CONCLUSIONS

The development of non-invasive vascular laboratory devices and techniques has expanded the amount of objective venous data that can be gathered noninvasively. However, it's crucial to remember that these tests should complement, not replace, the information obtained from a thorough history and physical examination. Unfortunately, some physicians increasingly rely on vascular laboratory test results without correlating them with symptoms and physical findings.

For optimal use of non-invasive test results, understanding the value and limitations of specific exams is essential. Non-invasive test selection should depend on the clinical questions to answer, as some questions cannot be addressed by these techniques. Errors, including false-positives and false-negatives, can occur in all diagnostic studies, so being aware of the tests' accuracy is important. Published studies often represent the best achievable results, while newly established laboratories may not attain optimal outcomes. To appropriately apply non-invasive results, it's vital to know the accuracy of the laboratory performing the test.

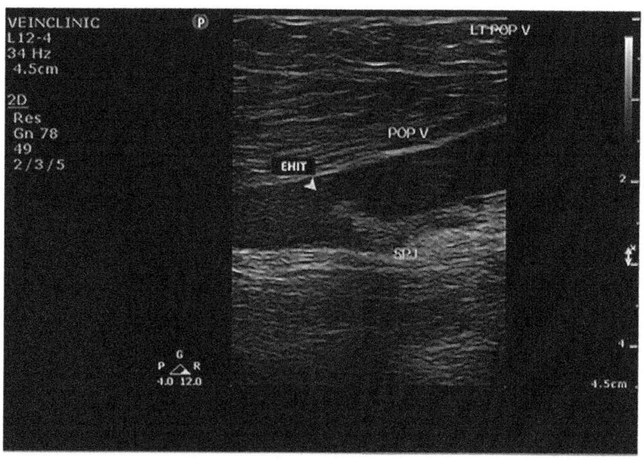

Figure 1.5 Presence of endovenous heat induced thrombus (EHIT) Lawrence level 4 at the saphenopopliteal junction, which involves the lumen of the adjacent popliteal vein as well as adherent to the adjacent wall.

REFERENCES

1. Strandness DE, Schultz RD, Summer DS, et al: Ultrasonic flow detection – a useful technique in the evaluation of peripheral vascular disease. Am J Surg 113:311–320, 1967.
2. Sigel B, Popky GL, Wagner DK, et al: A doppler ultrasound method for diagnosing lower extremity venous disease. Surg Gynecol Obstet 127:339–350, 1968.
3. Vogel P, Laing FC, Jeffrey RB, et al: Deep venous thrombosis of the lower extremity: US evaluation. Radiology 163:747–751, 1987.
4. Cronan JJ, Dorfman GS, Scola FH, et al: Deep venous thrombosis: US assessment using venous compression. Radiology 162:191–194, 1987.
5. Rollins DL, Semrow CM, Friedell ML, et al: Progress in the diagnosis of deep venous thrombosis: The efficacy of real-time B-mode ultrasonic imaging. J Vasc Surg 7:638–641, 1988.
6. Sullivan ED, Peter DJ, Cranley JJ: Real-time B-mode venous ultrasound. J Vasc Surg 1:465–471, 1984.
7. van Bemmelen PS, Bedford G, Beach K, et al: The mechanism of venous valve closure. Arch Surg 125:617–619, 1990.
8. Shah DM, Chang BB, Leopold PW, et al: The anatomy of the greater saphenous vein system. J Vasc Surg 3:273–283, 1986.
9. Vasdekis SN, Clarke GH, Nicolaides AN: Quantification of venous reflux by means of duplex scanning. J Vasc Surg 10:670–677, 1989.
10. Ruoff BA, Cranley JJ, Haannan LA, et al: Real-time duplex ultrasound mapping of the greater saphenous vein before in situ infrainguinal revascularization. J Vasc Surg 6:107–113, 1987.
11. Salles-Cunha SX, Andros G, Harris RW, et al: Preoperative noninvasive assessment of arm veins to be used as bypass grafts in the lower extremities. J Vasc Surg 3:813–816, 1986.
12. Lawrence PF, Chandra A, Wu M, et al: Classification of proximal endovenous closure levels and treatment algorithm. J Vasc Surg 52:388–393, 2010.

Chapter 2

Venography and Intravascular Ultrasound (IVUS) in Venous Imaging

Emily Swafford, Christopher Chow, Christopher Montoya, and Jose I. Almeida

INTRODUCTION

Historically, catheter-directed venography, also known as phlebography or simply venography, served as the primary diagnostic tool for evaluating deep venous obstruction. However, with the prevalence of non-invasive imaging modalities such as duplex ultrasound (DUS), computed tomographic venography (CTV), and magnetic resonance venography (MRV), venography became a secondary imaging modality, primarily used for assessment of post-procedural completion or for iliocaval obstruction; recently, intravascular ultrasound (IVUS) has challenged even these applications. This chapter offers an overview of venography and IVUS and aims to provide clinically focused, evidence-based information surrounding their roles in the diagnosis and management of venous disease.

VENOGRAPHY

Catheter-directed venography involves intravenous injection of contrast material through a catheter with concomitant fluoroscopic X-ray examination. Benefits include visualization of the selected venous segment and qualitative analysis of venous hemodynamics, including flow directionality and valve competency. There are two main techniques: ascending and descending venography.

Ascending Venography

Ascending venography is performed through distal injection of contrast media and relies on antegrade venous blood flow for proximal contrast delivery. The difference in density of contrast media versus blood allows for visualization of many venous segments within each vein. Traditionally, contrast material was injected into the superficial veins of the foot, but this method frequently failed to highlight the vessels of the deep venous system. Supplemental contrast was injected into the femoral vein, with superficial venous compression using an ankle-level tourniquet. For further visualization, a second knee-level tourniquet can be applied or foot movements can be utilized to increase blood flow. In competent deep veins, tourniquet application prevents contrast from entering the superficial system. Therefore, the appearance of contrast material in the superficial system aided by proper tourniquet use indirectly suggests venous incompetence.[1] Large deep venous incompetence can affect this technique by causing the pressures of the superficial and deep systems to equilibrate swiftly and potentially prevent the visualization of other venous abnormalities.

Gravitational force, in concert with the venous system's complex geometry and variations in venous segment resistance, can negatively affect contrast distribution and by extension, venographic results.[2] Therefore, patient positioning is important in regard to contrast

DOI: 10.1201/9781003316626-3

distribution and venous opacification. For optimal ascending venography results, the patient should be placed in a near upright position. Despite proper positioning, imbalances in contrast dissemination will persist, with preferential distal distribution most markedly seen in large veins with slow venous flow.[3] To improve contrast distribution, manual compression of the extremity or muscle contraction maneuvers may be applied. Both constrict select venous segments and fill others more proportionately. However, muscle contraction introduces blood without contrast from intramuscular veins into the deep venous vasculature. Thus, the appearance of a partial venous obstruction secondary to dilution of contrast material may result from these maneuvers and yield a false-positive diagnosis.[4]

Similarly, another potential cause of diagnostic inaccuracy is uneven venous blood flow due to physiological variations in venous segment resistance, such as those seen with venous tone modifications, muscle contraction, and positional compression. These differences in resistance may result in uneven flow – or even halted flow – in certain segments for brief periods. If a venographic study is performed during one of these periods, only a portion of the venous system will be visualized and may lead to overdiagnosis of venous disease. The effect of varying venous segment resistance on ascending venography is exemplified by duplicated veins, which often receive little to no contrast material and frequently remain undetected. This finding is exacerbated in the setting of forced contrast injection or when implementing compression maneuvers.[5]

Additionally, the invasive nature of ascending venography imparts risks, including potential damage to the vasculature or surrounding structures, bleeding or bruising at the puncture site, and infection. Notably, catheter-direct venography is associated with greater patient discomfort, radiation exposure, and nephropathy.

Descending Venography

Descending venography shares many similarities with ascending venography but involves proximal contrast injection and is typically performed by advancing a catheter from the contralateral extremity, often the common femoral vein (CFV). Descending venography mainly functions to evaluate for venous valve incompetency but may also be useful in rare cases of deep valve reconstructive surgery. This technique requires that the patient assume a semi-erect position and engage in a reflux provoking maneuver, such as Valsalva, during contrast injection.[6,7] Of note, when specifically evaluating for saphenous valve reflux, one should inject additional contrast after the catheter is positioned distal to the saphenofemoral junction, and when evaluating for distal femoral or popliteal valve reflux, the catheter should be advanced to a location immediately proximal to the target segment.[8]

Anatomic findings of deep venous reflux from descending venography can be described using the Kistner classification, a five-point grading scale with 0 representing no reflux and 4 representing reflux from the CFV to below the popliteal vein.[6] The disadvantages of descending venography are similar to those seen in ascending venography, although descending venography requires greater radiation exposure as fluoroscopy is near continuously necessary.

Technique

In current practice, catheter-directed venography is generally performed via the femoral vein at the mid-thigh or through the popliteal vein via the popliteal fossa with intent-to-treat a lesion if identified. After positioning, prepping, and draping the patient in the typical fashion, venous access is obtained under ultrasound guidance with a micropuncture kit. The sheath can then be upsized to an 8 French (Fr) for femoral access or 5–6 Fr for popliteal access. A wire and catheter system of choice is advanced to the desired venous segment (i.e., femoral-deep femoral confluence, CFV, EIV, CIV, adjacent IVC, etc.). Contrast material is then injected to delineate the venous anatomy. A pigtail catheter with a pressure injector may be used to bolus contrast for caval lesions, and hand-injected venography may be effective for more distal lesions. Venography should be performed with at least two orthogonal views (i.e., right or left anterior oblique) in addition to the standard anteroposterior view.

Utility

Although catheter-based venography has almost been entirely replaced by more modern imaging modalities, it still important in the diagnosis and management of iliac vein obstruction.[9–11] There are four main venographic signs indicative of an iliac lesion: visual stenosis, decreased opacification, collateral vessels bypassing a segment, and "pancaking" or flattening of the vein. The presence or absence of each sign affects diagnostic sensitivity. When all present, the sensitivity ranges from 97.1% if located in the CIV, 57.7% if in the EIV, or 48.1% in the CFV. Incomplete filling is the sign associated with the highest sensitivity and has been found to be more sensitive if identified on the left side as compared to the right. If visualized in the left CIV (Figure 2.1), incomplete filling is associated with a sensitivity of 92.9%.[12]

Nevertheless, the overall sensitivity of single-plane venography for venous stenosis above 70% remains low (~45%).[13] Multi-plane venography has been shown to improve diagnostic properties when compared to single-plane venography, with the downside of significantly increased radiation exposure and contrast use. Additionally, both single-plane and multi-plane venography lack an internal scale and have demonstrated limited ability in accurately measuring vein diameter. Currently, neither are recommended as the sole imaging modality.[14,15]

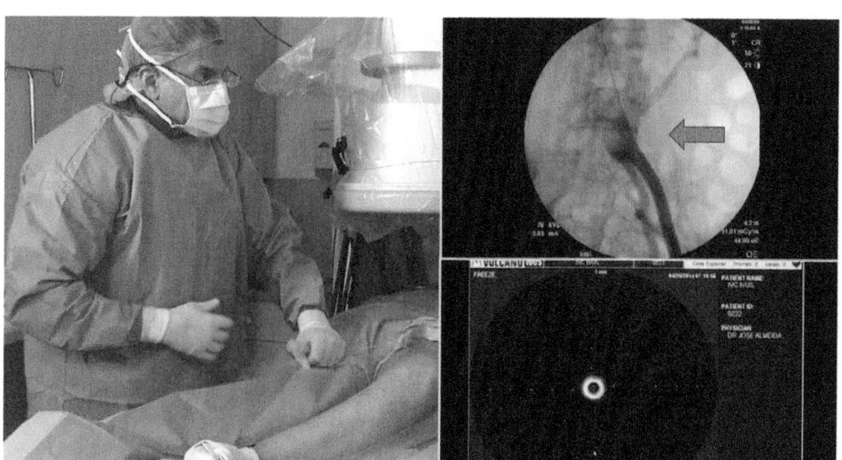

Figure 2.1 Left panel: Contrast injection via femoral vein sheath. Upper right panel: Blue arrow demonstrates left common iliac vein occlusion with visualization of ascending lumbar and hypogastric vein collaterals.

INTRAVASCULAR ULTRASOUND (IVUS)

IVUS utilizes a special catheter with a miniature ultrasound probe connected to an external visualization system to precisely assesses the lumen and vessel wall major axial veins.[16] Using ultrasound waves to characterize endoluminal information, the software creates images that are perpendicular to the long axis of the catheter.[17]

There are two main types of IVUS transducers: mechanical and solid-state. Mechanical transducers utilize a rotating ultrasound crystal with a short, rigid catheter tip. The guidewire angles the transducer and produces images slightly more forward than the intended area, known as wire artifact. To offset this artifact, dual-purpose channels have since been installed into the catheter of mechanical IVUS systems to permit wire removal. Additionally proximal and distal movement inside the vessel may be employed to best view area of interest.

Alternatively, solid-state transducers image the vasculature without rotation and therefore require a more complex system of elements and electrical signals. As a result, this system possesses a longer rigid catheter tip that allows for greater elemental control, and consequently, it is a more expensive device. Of note, there is a third, less utilized transducer type used in the electronic IVUS system. This transducer operates via a circular array of up to 64 elements that each produce images in rapid sequence.[18]

Technique

Similar to traditional venography, IVUS begins by obtaining venous access with a guidewire and catheter. Upon selecting the vessel of choice, the access sheath is upsized to an 8 Fr sheath accommodate the IVUS catheter. The transducer of choice (i.e., 10 MHz transducer, Volcano, Philips Healthcare, Netherlands) is then inserted over the guidewire and connected to the ultrasound system (i.e., Volcano S5). The lesion(s) should be overviewed by performing a preliminary pullback scan, starting proximally and moving distally. This allows for the nature, degree, and extent of the stenosis/thrombus to be recorded and characterized. Upon completion, the catheter should be reintroduced and the cross-sectional areas of interest (i.e., the distal IVC; bilateral CFVs; proximal, mid, and distal CIV; and proximal, mid, and distal EIV) should be measured (Figure 2.2). During insonation of the IVC and iliac veins, other critical landmarks to be identified include visualization of the right atrium, right renal artery, renal veins, common iliac vein bifurcation, right common iliac artery, and external/internal iliac vein confluence.[18]

Utility

With high probe frequency and close luminal distance, IVUS transmits high-resolution images capable of accurately estimating the severity and extent of venous lesions and venous diameters.[9] The direct endoluminal visualization achieved by IVUS provides valuable information that improves diagnostic capacity. For example, directly visualizing a deep vein thrombosis (DVT) via IVUS not only confirms the diagnosis but provides a measurement of its echogenicity, which aids in estimating the duration of the DVT's presence and further classifies it as acute or chronic. Of note, chronic thrombi are associated with high echogenicity due to their highly organized fibrin.[16] IVUS also accurately diagnoses finer endoluminal lesions, such as webs, trabeculations, or spur morphologies that are frequently missed by less precise imaging modalities.[13] Additionally, IVUS allows for examination of the structures surrounding the venous abnormality and provides critical information in the setting of external venous compression. Identification of the source of venous compression (i.e., tumors, arterial aneurysms, ligaments, etc.) often confirms the diagnosis and underlying etiology of venous disease,

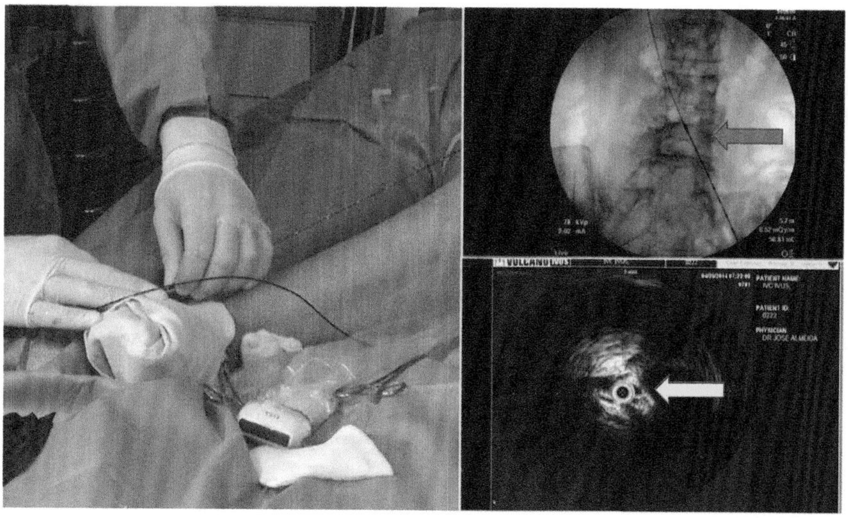

Figure 2.2 Left panel: IVUS catheter withdrawal. Upper right panel: IVUS catheter visualized under fluoroscopy, blue arrow. Lower right panel: IVUS catheter inside compressed left iliac vein, yellow arrow.

such as in the case of May-Thurner syndrome, when compression of left common iliac vein by the right common iliac artery is visualized.[18]

Calcification, IVC filters, and stent struts may limit the visibility of IVUS due to acoustic shadowing in all transducer types. Reverberation can also occur when the transducer reflects a returned ultrasound beam. Given the user-dependent nature of IVUS, awareness of its functionality and restrictions will improve operation and application.[16] Of note, color, 3D, and virtual histology imaging modalities arose due to IVUS technology; however, their application in the venous system has been limited thus far.[19–21]

COMPUTED TOMOGRAPHIC VENOGRAPHY (CTV)

Computed tomography (CT) scanners employ a rotating X-ray tube and multiple rows of detectors to acquire images measuring the attenuation of different tissues inside the body from multiple different angles.

CTV vs Venography

The non-invasive nature of CTV decreases the risk associated with catheter insertion required. Contrast CTV additionally offers cross-sectional imaging, providing an internal scale with calipers, allowing for measurement of venous segment diameters.

CTV vs IVUS

When compared to IVUS, advantages to CTV include its non-invasive nature as well as its ability to remove structures not of interest during 3D reconstruction. Indirect CTV has the additional advantage of allowing for bilateral venous imaging with a single-contrast bolus. In a systematic review by Saleem et al. comparing CTV to IVUS in characterizing chronic occlusive iliofemoral venous disease, CTV was found to precisely determine the point of compression when compared with IVUS as well as predict the stent diameter used at intervention within 2 mm for over 90% of patients.[15] When compared to IVUS in assessing for iliac vein stenosis, the sensitivity of CTV was found to be ~80% for single-segment calibers (83% in CIV and 73% in EIV) but increased to 97% for two-segment caliber measurements if stenosis was seen in at least one of the two segments (CIV and EIV).[15,22] Another study investigating the power of CTV in identifying and characterizing iliac vein obstruction (IVO) in highly symptomatic patients with chronic venous disease found that CTV detected an IVO of 50% of greater (groups II and III) with a sensitivity and specificity of 94% and 79.2%, respectively.[15]

Nevertheless, CTV falls short in identifying venous compressions, and initial CTV misses up to 1/3rd of venous compressions seen on IVUS.[10,14] Additionally, while CTV possesses a centering mechanism, the axial images seen on CTV are centered to the centerline of the body – not the vein.[22] Thus, a CTV axial image, especially of a complex, spiraled vein such as the iliac, may depict an oval section of the vein, larger than the true orthogonal cross-section, and IVUS has been found to more accurately measure the cross-sectional area and diameter of a stenosed vein.[14,23]

MAGNETIC RESONANCE VENOGRAPHY (MRV)

Magnetic resonance imaging utilizes a magnetic field to provide radiofrequency energy for absorption by protons. The resultant proton spin polarization is subsequently detected by radiofrequency coil to produce imagery. While non-contrast MRI may provide anatomical information for large- and medium-sized vessels, contrast use is preferred in magnetic resonance venography (MRV) with blood-pool agents being best suited for venous imaging.[24] Blood-pool agents allow for longer retainment in intravascular space compared to gadolinium-based agents, allowing for higher venous concentration and superior imaging. The best use of MRI for investigating venous hemodynamics is phase-contrast MRI (PC-MRI), which provides both visual and quantitative information on flow patterns. In-plane PC-MRI with time-resolved cine sequence is known as four-dimensional (4D) flow MRI and is used clinically to produce retrospective 2D flow measurements for vessels in the 3D acquisition volume.[25] Currently, 4D flow MRI is used exclusively to study cardiac and arterial blood flow, but its utilization in venous hemodynamics is being investigated.[26–28]

Overarchingly, MRV is a suitable imaging technique for the venous system of the chest, abdomen, pelvis, and extremities.[29–33] In fact, one study even concluded that 3D MRV detects thrombus in central venous structures, particularly the superior vena cava (SVC), with 100% sensitivity. For pelvic or other deep venous vasculature, 2D time-of-flight angiography is more commonly used.[29,31]

MRV vs Venography

Similar to CTV, MRV is a non-invasive technique that possesses an internal scale, allowing for decreased risks and more accurate measurements of stenotic vessels when compared with conventional venography. MRV's superior soft tissue resolution allows for visualization of intraluminal webs.[34] However, when compared to digital subtraction contrast venography, MRV overdiagnosis webs and underdiagnosis stenosis in small vessels with a sensitivity and specificity of 99% and 92%, respectively.[35] While studies have advocated for the use of MRV in iliocaval compression diagnosis, a direct comparison to catheter-based venography has yet to be performed.[36,37] Thus, the sensitivity and specificity of MRV for this purpose have yet to be determined, and MRV should not be used in place of venography in this role.

MRV vs IVUS

In addition to possessing the advantages and disadvantages seen when compared to venography (i.e., non-invasive nature, internal scale, and contraindications to ferromagnetic material), a study by Saleem et al. compared MRV to IVUS in diagnosing chronic iliofemoral venous obstruction (CIVO). This work resolved that the sensitivity of MRV for CIV and EIV was 93% and 100%, respectively, and the specificity was 0% and 50%, respectively. The combination of MRV's high sensitivity and low specificity signifies overestimation of the severity of stenosis, and the authors concluded that MRV is not reliable and should not be used to diagnose iliac vein stenosis in patients with CIVO.[38]

VENOGRAPHY VS IVUS

The IVUS for Diagnosing Iliac vein Obstruction (VIDIO) trial, compared the diagnostic efficacy of IVUS with multiplanar venography for iliofemoral vein obstruction.[14] In this trial, 100 patients with suspected iliofemoral vein obstruction were enrolled at 11 U.S. and 2 European sites and underwent imaging of the IVC, CIV, EIV, and CFV with multiplanar venograms (three views: anteroposterior and right and left 30-degree anterior oblique) and IVUS. The venous diameter was measured for both imaging modalities as well as the cross-sectional area for IVUS. Following deidentification and evaluation by core laboratory, a stenosis severity ratio was determined, and significant stenosis was defined as a 50% diameter stenosis by venography or a 50% cross-sectional area reduction by IVUS. The concordance of the imaging modalities was analyzed to determine the impact on the treatment plan. Discordance resulted in changes to the treatment plan in 57 of 100 patients with the most common reason for discordance being failure of lesion identification by venography (72%). Fifty-four patients had stents placed due to IVUS detection of significant lesion undetected on venography, and three patients with significant lesions seen on venography circumvented stent placement due to IVUS findings. These findings revealed that multiplanar venography has limited ability to assess vein diameter and is insufficient in assessing for treatable iliofemoral vein obstruction.

Similar results were found in a recent systematic review by Saleem et al. comparing multidimensional contrast venography to IVUS in guiding vascular intervention for CIVO. In this study, multiplanar venography failed to identify stenosis seen on IVUS in up to 1/3rd of cases and underestimated residual stenosis when assessing for post-procedural completion.[15] Most recently, a 2022 systematic review by Natesan et al. assessed the role of IVUS as an adjunctive imaging modality for peripheral venous intervention. The included studies analyzed IVUS's effectiveness in evaluating the venous vasculature and characterizing lesion severity, in assessing for post-thrombotic disease, and in optimizing stent placement and deployment. The results established robust evidence of a benefit from IVUS use with 73.7% of the included studies receiving an Oxford Centre for Evidence Based Medicine level of evidence grade of 2B. In characterizing venous vasculature and lesion severity, 9 of 11 studies (81.8%) demonstrated high benefit with 2B grade, and in assessing for post-thrombotic disease, 100% (3 of 3) demonstrated high benefit with 2B grade. IVUS's use in optimizing stent placement and deployment was found to be less beneficial with only five of nine studies (40%) receiving a 2B grade. Nevertheless, IVUS was found to be an effective imaging modality for iliofemoral venous disease. It is associated with superior clinical outcomes and should be widely adopted as an adjunct during peripheral intervention.[39]

Additionally, a prospective randomized study led by Ashoura et al. aimed to compare the use of conventional venography with and without adjunct IVUS in the management of iliofemoral chronic venous insufficiency.[51] In this trial, 40 patients with symptomatic chronic venous insufficiency were stratified into two groups: one group would receive multiplanar venography exclusively and the other would receive IVUS in addition to completion venography. Both the procedure length and the contrast usage were found to be significantly higher in the venography group ($P = 0.014$ and $P < 0.0001$, respectively), and a greater mean increase in serum creatinine was also seen in the venography group ($P < 0.0001$). IVUS detected a significantly higher mean number of lesions compared to venography (2.75 in IVUS and 1.6 in venography, $P < 0.001$), and IVUS possessed higher primary-assisted patency rate compared with venography ($P = 0.017$) and even detected stenoses and occlusions more than CTV during follow-up ($P = 0.018$). This study supports the notion that IVUS exists as one of the most effective tools in the management of venous disease. It is more sensitive, accurate, and precise compared to other imaging modalities, especially venography alone. IVUS should be utilized in treatment planning, stent placement, and follow-up interventions.[40]

In detecting subclavian vein stenosis in patients with Paget-Schroetter syndrome (PSS), or spontaneous subclavian vein (SCV) thrombosis, IVUS has been identified as being more sensitive than venography in identifying significant stenosis.[41] Of the patients presenting for evaluation of PSS, venography showed an average percent reduction in SCV diameter of 41.5%, compared to the IVUS diameters of 61.8% (AP), 41.9% (CC), and 74.5% (CSA; $P < .05$) as measured in the anteroposterior (AP) plane, craniocaudal (CC) plane, and cross-sectional area (CSA), respectively. Subgroup analysis revealed that 28% of patients with no identifiable stenosis on venography had identifiable stenosis on IVUS ($P < 0.05$).

CONCLUSIONS

Over the last few decades, the study of venous disease has undergone immense growth and evolution. Despite conventional venography's historical role as the gold standard for diagnosing venous disease, its utility in current clinical practice is limited as the development of IVUS has challenged venography for supremacy. IVUS has been shown to be more sensitive in diagnosing deep venous pathology and in evaluating iliofemoral vein obstruction. Venography as a sole imaging modality is no longer recommended for the study of any venous disease. The combination of multiplanar venography and IVUS, however, has benefited diagnostic accuracy and improved procedural outcomes when evaluating and managing iliocaval obstruction.

The role of cross-sectional imaging with CTV and MRV has also expanded in its use for venous disease in recent years, and these modalities possess unique advantages and disadvantages when compared to conventional venography and IVUS. Advancements in these non-invasive venous imaging modalities are sure to come and may pave the way for the future study of venous disease.

REFERENCES

1. Halliday P. Intra-osseous phlebography of the lower limb. Br J Surg. 1967;54(4):248–57.
2. Greitz T. The technique of ascending phlebography of the lower extremity. Acta Radiol. 1954;42(6):421–41.
3. Coel MN. Adequacy of lower limb venous opacification: Comparison of supine and upright phlebography. AJR Am J Roentgenol. 1980;134(1):163–65.
4. Almen T, Nylander G. Serial phlebography of the normal lower leg during muscular contraction and relaxation. Acta Radiol. 1962;57:264–72.

5. Meissner MH, Moneta G, Burnand K, et al. The hemodynamics and diagnosis of venous disease. J Vasc Surg. 2007;46(Suppl S):4S–24S.
6. Kistner RL, Ferris EB, Randhawa G, et al. A method of performing descending venography. J Vasc Surg. 1986;4(5):464–68.
7. Raju S, Fredericks R. Evaluation of methods for detecting venous reflux. Perspectives in venous insufficiency. Arch Surg. 1990;125(11):1463–67.
8. Khilnani NM, Min RJ. Imaging of venous insufficiency. Semin Intervent Radiol. 2005;22(3):178–84.
9. Toh MR, Tang TY, Lim H, et al. Review of imaging and endovascular intervention of iliocaval venous compression syndrome. World J Radiol. 2020;12(3):18–28.
10. Birn J, Vedantham S. May-Thurner Syndrome and other obstructive iliac vein lesions: Meaning, myth, and mystery. Vasc Med. 2015;20(1):74–83.
11. Oropallo A, Andersen CA. Venous Stenting. Treasure Island, FL: StatPearls, 2022.
12. Lau I, Png CYM, Eswarappa M, et al. Defining the utility of anteroposterior venography in the diagnosis of venous iliofemoral obstruction. J Vasc Surg Venous Lymphat Disord. 2019;7(4):514–21.e4.
13. Neglen P, Raju S. Intravascular ultrasound scan evaluation of the obstructed vein. J Vasc Surg. 2002;35(4):694–700.
14. Gagne PJ, Tahara RW, Fastabend CP, et al. Venography versus intravascular ultrasound for diagnosing and treating iliofemoral vein obstruction. J Vasc Surg Venous Lymphat Disord. 2017;5(5):678–87.
15. Saleem T, Raju S. Comparison of intravascular ultrasound and multidimensional contrast imaging modalities for characterization of chronic occlusive iliofemoral venous disease: A systematic review. J Vasc Surg Venous Lymphat Disord. 2021;9(6):1545–56.e2.
16. McLafferty RB. The role of intravascular ultrasound in venous thromboembolism. Semin Intervent Radiol. 2012;29(1):10–15.
17. Garcia-Garcia HM, Gogas BD, Serruys PW, et al. IVUS-based imaging modalities for tissue characterization: Similarities and differences. Int J Cardiovasc Imaging. 2011;27(2):215–24.
18. Shung KK, Zippuro M. Ultrasonic transducers and arrays. In Diagnostic Ultrasound: Imaging and Blood Flow Measurements (2nd ed., pp. 39–78). Boca Raton, FL: CRC Press, 2015.
19. Irshad K, Reid DB, Miller PH, et al. Early clinical experience with color three-dimensional intravascular ultrasound in peripheral interventions. J Endovasc Ther. 2001;8(4):329–38.
20. Thrush AJ, Bonnett DE, Elliott MR, et al. An evaluation of the potential and limitations of three-dimensional reconstructions from intravascular ultrasound images. Ultrasound Med Biol. 1997;23(3):437–45.
21. Vince DG, Davies SC. Peripheral application of intravascular ultrasound virtual histology. Semin Vasc Surg. 2004;17(2):119–25.
22. Raju S, Walker W, Noel C, et al. The two-segment caliber method of diagnosing iliac vein stenosis on routine computed tomography with contrast enhancement. J Vasc Surg Venous Lymphat Disord. 2020;8(6):970–77.
23. Asciutto G, Mumme A, Marpe B, et al. MR venography in the detection of pelvic venous congestion. Eur J Vasc Endovasc Surg. 2008;36(4):491–96.
24. Nishimura DG. Time-of-flight MR angiography. Magn Reson Med. 1990;14(2):194–201.
25. Azarine A, Garcon P, Stansal A, et al. Four-dimensional flow MRI: Principles and cardiovascular applications. Radiographics. 2019;39(3):632–48.
26. Ordovas K. Invited commentary on "Four-dimensional flow MRI," with response from Dr Azarine et al. Radiographics. 2019;39(3):648–50.
27. Izawa Y, Hishikawa S, Matsumura Y, et al. Blood flow of the venous system during resuscitative endovascular balloon occlusion of the aorta: Noninvasive evaluation using phase contrast magnetic resonance imaging. J Trauma Acute Care Surg. 2020;88(2):305–9.
28. Promelle V, Bouzerar R, Milazzo S, et al. Quantification of blood flow in the superior ophthalmic vein using phase contrast magnetic resonance imaging. Exp Eye Res. 2018;176:40–45.
29. Evans AJ, Sostman HD, Witty LA, et al. Detection of deep venous thrombosis: Prospective comparison of MR imaging and sonography. J Magn Reson Imaging. 1996;6(1):44–51.

30. Kroencke TJ, Taupitz M, Arnold R, et al. Three-dimensional gadolinium-enhanced magnetic resonance venography in suspected thrombo-occlusive disease of the central chest veins. Chest. 2001;120(5):1570–76.
31. Spritzer CE, Arata MA, Freed KS. Isolated pelvic deep venous thrombosis: Relative frequency as detected with MR imaging. Radiology. 2001;219(2):521–25.
32. Stern JB, Abehsera M, Grenet D, et al. Detection of pelvic vein thrombosis by magnetic resonance angiography in patients with acute pulmonary embolism and normal lower limb compression ultrasonography. Chest. 2002;122(1):115–21.
33. Thornton MJ, Ryan R, Varghese JC, et al. A three-dimensional gadolinium-enhanced MR venography technique for imaging central veins. AJR Am J Roentgenol. 1999;173(4):999–1003.
34. Arnoldussen CW, de Graaf R, Wittens CH, et al. Value of magnetic resonance venography and computed tomographic venography in lower extremity chronic venous disease. Phlebology. 2013;28(Suppl 1):169–75.
35. Helyar VG, Gupta Y, Blakeway L, et al. Depiction of lower limb venous anatomy in patients undergoing interventional deep venous reconstruction-the role of balanced steady state free precession MRI. Br J Radiol. 2018;91(1082):20170005.
36. Hurst DR, Forauer AR, Bloom JR, et al. Diagnosis and endovascular treatment of iliocaval compression syndrome. J Vasc Surg. 2001;34(1):106–13.
37. Wolpert LM, Rahmani O, Stein B, et al. Magnetic resonance venography in the diagnosis and management of May-Thurner Syndrome. Vasc Endovascular Surg. 2002;36(1):51–57.
38. Saleem T, Lucas M, Raju S. Comparison of intravascular ultrasound and magnetic resonance venography in the diagnosis of chronic iliac venous disease. J Vasc Surg Venous Lymphat Disord. 2022;10(5):1066–71.e2.
39. Natesan S, Mosarla RC, Parikh SA, et al. Intravascular ultrasound in peripheral venous and arterial interventions: A contemporary systematic review and grading of the quality of evidence. Vasc Med. 2022;27(4):392–400.
40. Ashour M, Ahmed AER, Kamel A, et al. Comparative study between the use of intravascular ultrasound versus conventional venography in management of iliofemoral chronic venous insufficiency. Egypt J Surg. 2021;40(1):140–52.
41. Ulloa JG, Gelabert HA, O'Connell JB, et al. Intravascular ultrasonography provides more sensitive detection of subclavian vein stenosis than venography in patients presenting with Paget-Schroetter syndrome. J Vasc Surg Venous Lymphat Disord. 2021;9(5):1145–50.e1.

Chapter 3

Pathophysiology and Conservative Management of Chronic Venous Insufficiency

Paola Batarseh, Fachreza Aryo Damara, and Cassius Iyad Ochoa Chaar

PATHOPHYSIOLOGY

Definition

Chronic venous insufficiency (CVI) is a common condition affecting the lower extremities. The term CVI encompasses all abnormalities of the venous system from telangiectasia to venous ulcers.[1] Understanding the pathological processes leading to CVI and its progression is important to clinicians and scientists to develop algorithms for diagnosis and treatment. The two predominant processes leading to the development of CVI are valvular reflux and venous obstruction. The CEAP (Clinical-Etiology-Anatomy-Pathophysiology) classification was developed in 1994 and was recently revised as a precise and standardized classification system to categorize patients with CVI. The CEAP classification divides CVI into the components of clinical (C) manifestation, underlying etiology (E) of the disease, anatomic (A) distribution, and underlying venous pathophysiology (P).[2] Within the CEAP classification, pathophysiology is divided into four categories: reflux, obstruction, reflux and obstruction, and no venous pathophysiology identifiable.

Identification of the specific pathological processes in a patient with CVI is crucial to provide the appropriate treatment that can provide relief of symptoms. While complex biochemical and cellular alterations occur in CVI, the common driver is venous hypertension related to factors preventing the return of blood from the lower extremities to the heart against gravity. Even though most patients present with a complaint of leg swelling or varicose veins, patients may have additional associated complaints such as pelvic pain that warrant tailored evaluation. Thus, some patients may have a combination of reflux and obstruction in the lower extremities and in the pelvis that require intervention to provide adequate relief.[3]

Venous Anatomy and Physiology

The peripheral venous system acts as a reservoir for approximately two-thirds of total blood volume and a channel for its return back to the heart. Proper functioning of this system relies on the patency of veins, competence of the valves, and muscular pumps that propel the blood against gravity to return to the heart. The veins of the lower extremities can be extremely variable. They are divided into the superficial, the deep, and the perforating venous systems. The superficial venous system is located between the muscular fascial layer and the dermis. It contains the great saphenous vein (GSV), small saphenous vein (SSV), and several accessory veins that typically run in an independent fascia. The deep venous system is located below the muscular fascial layer and consists of axial veins, which follow the course of the major arteries, and intramuscular veins. The perforating veins are numerous and variable. They connect

DOI: 10.1201/9781003316626-4

the deep and superficial veins as they transverse the fascia separating the compartments and typically direct the blood flow from the superficial to the deep venous network.[4]

Veins are capacitance vessels with compliance approximately thirty times higher than arteries. They are highly distensible and can accommodate large volumes of blood. Postural changes cause redistribution of blood to the peripheral venous system, and high compliance means that large volumes of blood can pool in the venous system. Thus, normal physiological adjustments are needed to maintain flow through the venous circulation.[5] Histologically, veins are made of three layers. The inner layer, or tunica intima, is comprised mainly of endothelial cells. The tunica media is made of vascular smooth muscle cells, collagen, and fibroblasts. The outer layer, or tunica adventitia, is comprised of collagen, elastic fibers, fibroblasts, and longitudinal smooth muscle cells. This outer layer provides support and elasticity to the vessel wall.[6]

Venous Reflux

Venous reflux is due to a combination of inflammation in the vessel wall, incompetence of the valves, and venous hypertension. It is not completely understood if the inflammatory changes seen in the vessel walls and valves precede reflux or if they are a consequence of venous incompetence. Muscular pumps act in coordination with venous valves to coordinate unidirectional flow. Thus, venous insufficiency can be further intensified by dysfunctional muscular or vascular pumps that contribute to venous stasis.[7] Bicuspid valves within the veins are essential in ensuring unidirectional blood flow. These valves have four phases of function including opening, equilibrium, closing, and closed. Axial blood flow ensures opening of the valve. The vertical velocity which increases mural pressure relative to luminal pressure leads to closure of the valves. There is an increased frequency of valves in the distal leg compared to the proximal leg, which helps to prevent increased pressure distally due to gravitational effects. Normal valvular function is defined as a duration of retrograde flow <1.0 seconds for the femoropopliteal veins and <0.5 seconds for superficial veins in the lower extremities.[8] These valves work in coordination with muscle pumps that force blood out of the venous plexus and prevent its return to the lower extremities after muscle relaxation.[9]

Valvular dysfunction allows retrograde flow of blood to the lower extremities due to gravity, also known as reflux.[8, 10] Dysfunction in the superficial system is the most common pathology and can be caused by preexisting weakness of the vessel walls or valve leaflets.[8] It can also be secondary to direct injury, superficial phlebitis, or excessive distention related to high pressure or hormonal effects. Reflux in the deep system is often secondary to prior deep vein thrombosis, which causes luminal narrowing, valvular scarring and adhesion, and inflammation. Damage to the deep valves allows rapid refiling by retrograde flow. It can also limit the volume of blood exiting the limb. The prevalence of deep venous reflux in patients with superficial reflux is estimated to be 20%.[8, 10] Perforating vein incompetence allows blood flow and reflux from the higher pressure deep venous system into the superficial system.[1]

Muscular pump dysfunction can occur with severe reflux and is highly associated with the development of venous ulcers. Due to inefficient emptying of the muscular pumps mainly within the gastrocnemius and soleus, the pressure in the immediate post ambulatory period is elevated to a similar degree as what is seen after prolonged standing.[9] Sedentary lifestyle, muscle/nerve/joint disease, standing for prolonged periods of time, and being overweight prevent proper functioning of these muscular pumps and can worsen the severity of venous insufficiency.[6]

Vessel wall inflammation can develop in response to changes in shear stress and is a hallmark of chronic venous disease. Hemodynamic changes including venous reflux leads to the release of proinflammatory markers. Vasoactive substances are released from the endothelium and give rise to adhesion molecules, chemokines, and inflammatory mediators. They also cause damage to the endothelial glycocalyx, resulting in breakdown of the permeability barrier. Adhesion molecules, like ICAM-1, cause increased leukocyte adhesion and localized inflammatory responses. Patients with CVI are also found to have increased collagen within the vessel wall and decreased amounts of elastin and laminin.(7) Changes in the microcirculation including increased permeability and venous pressure cause the accumulation of fluid, proteins, and blood cells in the interstitial space.(9)

Prolonged hypoxia of the vessel wall also plays a fundamental role in the pathophysiology of venous disease. The vessel wall is mainly supplied by the vasa vasorum in the adventitia and tunica media and diffusion of oxygen from blood in the lumen. There are two mechanisms that contribute to hypoxia in the vein wall. The first is endoluminal hypoxia due to reduced oxygen replenishment in comparison to normal flow as a result of stagnant blood in the endothelium. The second is compression of the vasa vasorum as a result of venous dilation and increased hydrostatic pressure.(11)

Venous Obstruction

Although only 15% of symptomatic CVI cases are caused by obstruction alone, 55% were estimated to be caused by combined reflux and obstruction.(12, 13) The presence of obstruction together with reflux worsens the overall clinical manifestations of CVI. The prevalence of ulcers in patients with obstructive pathophysiology alone was 5% compared to 25% in CVI due to combined reflux and obstruction.(14) In addition, venous leg ulcer (VLU) prognosis was worse in patients with CVI caused by combined reflux and obstruction.(12) This is thought to be related to a higher ambulatory venous pressure caused by the proximal blockage yielding an increase in distal reflux. Venous obstruction is divided into thrombotic and non-thrombotic depending on the presence or absence of deep venous thrombosis (DVT).

Thrombotic Obstruction

Thrombotic obstruction is also considered secondary intravenous CVI. The most common cause of thrombotic obstruction is DVT. This is due to the poor or absence of recanalization following DVT. The relationship between CVI and DVT is bidirectional. DVT confers venous wall injury mediated by inflammatory reactions leading to thickened, non-compliant venous walls, and incompetent valves.(15) Resolution of the thrombus is an active inflammatory process where neutrophils and monocytes are involved and releasing matric metalloproteases (MMPs) and activating plasmin.(16) The alterations of the extracellular matrix from the released proinflammatory cytokines and cellular fractions caused by DVT are also found to be a part of the vein wall remodeling.(17, 18) The formation of a thrombus in DVT could also damage the surrounding valves leading to valvular incompetence and aggravating the reflux.(19)

The overlap of venous obstruction and valvular reflux pathophysiology in thrombosis is also suggested by genetic predisposition to hypercoagulable states, specifically thrombomodulin (THBD) and methylenetetrahydrofolate reductase (MTHFR).(20) Age and sex-matched case-control studies showed a higher prevalence of single and multiple thrombophilias in patients with varicose veins (VV) and with chronic venous ulceration (CVU).(21) Various strategies of thrombus removal combined with optimal anticoagulation are paramount, particularly in the case of iliofemoral DVT, to limit the injury to the venous wall and valves.[22] On the other hand, residual thrombus was significantly associated with recurrent DVT.[23, 24]

Non-Thrombotic Obstruction

The incidence of non-thrombotic obstruction as the primary cause of CVI is likely under appreciated. However, the significance of non-thrombotic iliac vein lesions (NIVLs) without reflux in causing stasis ulcers should not be underestimated despite its lower prevalence relative to reflux disease.[25] Although the prevalence is difficult to be estimated, NIVLs were detected in 15% of all DVT cases evaluated by the emergency department in one study.[26] Nevertheless, NIVL can be an incidental finding in patients without venous symptoms. In fact, 34.1% of patients undergoing MRI of the abdomen and pelvis for various indications were found to have ≥ 50% stenosis of the iliac veins. Understanding the factors associated with the development of pathological NIVL remains a focus of active research.[27, 28] Unlike thrombotic obstruction, NIVLs tend to affect the left side more commonly compared to the right side. Iliac vein compression syndrome or May-Thurner syndrome or Cockett's syndrome has been traditionally described as left common iliac vein compression between the right common iliac artery and the spine, but various configurations has been described.[29–31] Raju and Neglen considered these anatomic "pathologies" as permissive conditions, which are defined as remain silent until additional superimposed mechanisms result in the development of symptoms.[25] Examples of additional pathologies that promote symptom expressions are trauma, cellulitis, distal thrombosis, secondary lymphatic exhaustion, and reflux.[32] The clinical manifestation would also depend on the degree of compression and the extent of collateralization.[33–35] Sustained compression and mechanical forces caused by constant pulsatile of the artery could also damage the intimal layer of the vein resulting in membranes or bands formation in the vascular lumen that further obstructs the blood flow in the vein, yielding to thrombus formation. Other pathologies that can cause compression of the iliac and vena cava resulting in swelling are malignancies, retroperitoneal fibrosis, iatrogenic injury, irradiation, cysts, and aneurysm.[36]

CONSERVATIVE THERAPY

The mainstay of conservative management of CVI is compression. The goals of treatment include control of symptoms, slowing progression, and healing of venous ulcers. Conservative management also relies heavily on risk modification including weight management, smoking cessation, and regular exercise.

Compression Therapy

Compression therapy remains essential for the treatment of CVI in addition to lifestyle modifications such as leg elevation and avoiding prolonged standing. External circumferential compression is directed at lowering venous hypertension, reducing venous stasis, and increasing tissue vascularization.[37, 38] The basic principle of compression therapy applies to the basic physical law in which pressure that is applied on a confined fluid (i.e. muscle group wrapped by the fascia muscularis and compression bandage) will be equally distributed (Pascal's law).[39] Also, the pressure generated by the bandage is directly proportional to bandage tension but inversely proportional to the limb radius (Laplace's law).[40]

The goal of compression therapy is to narrow the superficial vein to ultimately decrease ambulatory venous hypertension.[41] To achieve this goal, the external pressure must exceed the intravenous pressure. The pressure of the leg vein depends mainly on body position in which highest intravenous pressure occurs during standing. Observations using magnetic resonance imaging (MRI) and duplex ultrasound revealed a compression pressure of > 50 mmHg and > 30 to 40 mmHg are required to occlude veins at lower leg and thigh levels, respectively.[42, 43] However, the compression pressure applied to CVI patients should not be excessive. Restoration of the vein valve function should be preferred over occluding the superficial vein.[44] In studies of patients with varicose vein and edema, and VLUs showed improvements in pain, pigmentation, swelling reductions, and ulcers healing with 30–40 mmHg compression pressure.[45, 46] The Society for Vascular Surgery (SVS) and the American Venous Forum (AVF) recommend 20–30 mmHg stocking for simple varicose veins (C2-C3) patients.[47]

A variety of compression devices exist, such as compression bandages, compression stockings, self-adjustable Velcro devices, Unna boots, pneumatic compression devices, and hybrid devices. These forms of compression devices vary in power and elasticity that should be individually given to CVI patients. A small, randomized control trial (RCT) study showed pneumatic compression device, compression stocking, and multilayered bandage have better healing rates and change of the percentage ulcer size compared to two-layer bandage and Unna boots.[48] Despite the difference in performance of these compression devices, each form varies in patient's comfort, and therefore compression device selection should be individualized.[47, 49]

Compliance

One major challenge in compression therapy is poor adherence, especially when patients are planned for a prolonged course. The reported adherence rates range only between 12% to 52%.[50] Common complaints include difficulties during donning (i.e. pulling up) and doffing (i.e. removing) the compression stockings, slipping of the fixed bandages down the leg, and hygiene concerns due to prolonged wearing of the stockings.[51]

The impacts of treatment adherence are multifaceted from VLU healing time, VLU recurrence, patient quality of life, and overall treatment cost. Moffatt et al. in their review noted six studies that indicated half healing rate and double median healing time in patients with VLU who are not compliant with compression therapy.[52] Similarly, a double blind RCT showed nine times higher VLU recurrence in non-adherent patients compared to patients who wear compression stocking regularly.[53] Further, patient compliance was also reported to positively influence patients' psychosocial quality of life from feeling less depressed about their leg appearance and daily activity levels.[46, 54]

Studies have extensively investigated strategies that can improve patient adherence to compression therapy. Primarily, ensuring communication between healthcare professionals (HCP) and patients is required to achieve patient-centered care by considering patients' knowledge, experiences, belief, and practical needs.[55] Moreover, strategy for delivering educational materials should be adequately established. Several RCTs showed that providing information through different media such as brochures and followed by mobile phone text reminders can improve patient knowledge and compliance.[54, 56] In addition, Brooks et al. reported greater compliance rates among patients attended by vascular specialists compared to general practitioners.[57] Ultimately, proper education on the benefits of wearing compression therapy and choosing the appropriate compression device based on individualized patient need should be prioritized to achieve greater compliance and better outcomes.

Medical Treatment

Medical treatment can be considered for the treatment of ulcers, edema, and symptomatic varicose veins primarily through the use of venoactive substances. These venoactive drugs are believed to improve venous tone and capillary permeability. Many substances have been used including saponins like horse chestnut seed extract (HCSE); gamma-benozopyrenes (flavonoids) like rutosides, diosmin, and hesperidin; micronized purified flavonoid fraction (MPFF); other plant extracts like French maritime pink bark extract; and synthetic agents including calcium dobesilate, naftazone, and benzarone.[47]

A Cochrane meta-analysis evaluated the efficacy and safety of venoactive agents, specifically rutosides, hidrosimine and diosmine, calcium dobesilate, *Centella asiatica*, aminaftone, French maritime pine bark extract, and grape seed extract. The authors found moderate-certainty evidence of a beneficial effect on edema compared to placebo. However, there seemed to be little to no difference in quality of life or ulcer healing. The data further demonstrated moderate-certainty evidence of increased adverse events compared to placebo, with gastrointestinal complaints (constipation, epigastric discomfort, nausea, vomiting) as the most common adverse event. The paper concluded that some phlebotonics were effective for certain signs and symptoms, although these findings were uncertain given the limited number of studies and heterogenous results.[58]

Another Cochrane review evaluated the use of HCSE taken as a capsule over 2–16 weeks and found improvement in leg pain, edema, and pruritis when compared to placebo. Adverse events, mainly gastrointestinal complaints, dizziness, nausea, headache, and pruritis, were mild and infrequent.[59] A systemic review and meta-analysis of the use of MPFF found that it significantly improved leg symptoms including swelling, cramps, parasthesias, and pruritis. MPFF was also associated with reduced leg edema and improved skin appearance and quality of life.[60]

Pentoxifylline is another drug used in the treatment of CVI. It is thought to decrease whole blood viscosity, platelet aggregation, and fibrinogen levels. A Cochrane review of the effect of pentoxifylline (400mg oral three times daily) in combination with compression therapy showed improvement in wound healing.[61] The current SVS Practice Guidelines suggest grade 2B evidence for the use of venoactive drugs for patients swelling and pain in combination with compression in countries where they are available. A similar grade 2B evidence is given for the use of pentoxifylline or MPFF in combination with compression to accelerate the healing of venous ulcers.[47]

REFERENCES

1. Gloviczki P. Handbook of Venous and Lymphatic Disorders: Guidelines of the American Venous Forum (4th ed.). CRC Press, 2017.
2. Lurie F, Passman M, Meisner M, Dalsing M, Masuda E, Welch H, et al. The 2020 update of the CEAP classification system and reporting standards. Journal of Vascular Surgery: Venous and Lymphatic Disorders. 2020;8(3):342–52.
3. Ali S, Pinto P, Huber S, Perez-Lozada JC, Attaran R, Ochoa Chaar CI. Complex pathologies in a patient referred for varicose veins. Journal of Vascular Surgery Cases, Innovations and Techniques. 2023;9(1).
4. Caggiati A, Bergan JJ, Gloviczki P, Jantet G, Wendell-Smith CP, Partsch H, et al. Nomenclature of the veins of the lower limbs: An international interdisciplinary consensus statement. Journal of Vascular Surgery. 2002;36(2):416–22.

5. Tansey EA, Montgomery LEA, Quinn JG, Roe SM, Johnson CD. Understanding basic vein physiology and venous blood pressure through simple physical assessments. Advances in Physiology Education. 2019;43(3):423–29.
6. Ortega MA, Fraile-Martinez O, Garcia-Montero C, Alvarez-Mon MA, Chaowen C, Ruiz-Grande F, et al. Understanding chronic venous disease: A critical overview of its pathophysiology and medical management. Journal of Clinical Medicine. 2021;10(15).
7. Santler B, Goerge T. Chronic venous insufficiency – a review of pathophysiology, diagnosis, and treatment. Journal der Deutschen Dermatologischen Gesellschaft. 2017;15(5):538–56.
8. Labropoulos N, Tiongson J, Pryor L, Tassiopoulos AK, Kang SS, Ashraf Mansour M, et al. Definition of venous reflux in lower-extremity veins. Journal of Vascular Surgery. 2003;38(4):793–98.
9. Eberhardt RT, Raffetto JD. Chronic venous insufficiency. Circulation. 2014;130(4):333–46.
10. Satam K, Aurshina A, Zhuo H, Zhang Y, Cardella J, Aboian E, et al. Incidence and significance of deep venous reflux in patients treated with saphenous vein ablation. Annals of Vascular Surgery. 2023;91:182–90.
11. Lim CS, Gohel MS, Shepherd AC, Paleolog E, Davies AH. Venous hypoxia: A poorly studied etiological factor of varicose veins. Journal of Vascular Research. 2011;48(3):185–94.
12. Johnson BF, Manzo RA, Bergelin RO, Strandness DE, Jr. Relationship between changes in the deep venous system and the development of the postthrombotic syndrome after an acute episode of lower limb deep vein thrombosis: A one- to six-year follow-up. Journal of Vascular Surgery. 1995;21(2):307–12; discussion 13.
13. Johnson BF, Manzo RA, Bergelin RO, Strandness DE, Jr. The site of residual abnormalities in the leg veins in long-term follow-up after deep vein thrombosis and their relationship to the development of the post-thrombotic syndrome. International Angiology. 1996;15(1):14–19.
14. Neglen P, Thrasher TL, Raju S. Venous outflow obstruction: An underestimated contributor to chronic venous disease. Journal of Vascular Surgery. 2003;38(5):879–85.
15. Deatrick KB, Eliason JL, Lynch EM, Moore AJ, Dewyer NA, Varma MR, et al. Vein wall remodeling after deep vein thrombosis involves matrix metalloproteinases and late fibrosis in a mouse model. Journal of Vascular Surgery. 2005;42(1):140–48.
16. Mukhopadhyay S, Johnson TA, Duru N, Buzza MS, Pawar NR, Sarkar R, et al. Fibrinolysis and inflammation in venous thrombus resolution. Frontiers in Immunology. 2019;10.
17. Deatrick KB, Elfline M, Baker N, Luke CE, Blackburn S, Stabler C, et al. Postthrombotic vein wall remodeling: Preliminary observations. Journal of Vascular Surgery. 2011;53(1):139–46.
18. Chandrashekar A, Garry J, Gasparis A, Labropoulos N. Vein wall remodeling in patients with acute deep vein thrombosis and chronic postthrombotic changes. Journal of Thrombosis and Haemostasis. 2017;15(10):1989–93.
19. Markel A, Manzo RA, Bergelin RO, Strandness DE. Valvular reflux after deep vein thrombosis: Incidence and time of occurrence. Journal of Vascular Surgery. 1992;15(2):377–84.
20. Fukaya E, Flores AM, Lindholm D, Gustafsson S, Zanetti D, Ingelsson E, et al. Clinical and genetic determinants of varicose veins. Circulation. 2018;138(25):2869–80.
21. Darvall KAL, Sam RC, Adam DJ, Silverman SH, Fegan CD, Bradbury AW. Higher prevalence of thrombophilia in patients with varicose veins and venous ulcers than controls. Journal of Vascular Surgery. 2009;49(5):1235–41.
22. Comerota AJ, Gravett MH. Iliofemoral venous thrombosis. Journal of Vascular Surgery. 2007;46(5):1065–76.
23. Prandoni P. Residual venous thrombosis as a predictive factor of recurrent venous thromboembolism. Annals of Internal Medicine. 2002;137(12).
24. Tan M, Mos ICM, Klok FA, Huisman MV. Residual venous thrombosis as predictive factor for recurrent venous thromboembolim in patients with proximal deep vein thrombosis: A sytematic review. British Journal of Haematology. 2011;153(2):168–78.
25. Raju S, Neglen P. High prevalence of nonthrombotic iliac vein lesions in chronic venous disease: A permissive role in pathogenicity. Journal of Vascular Surgery. 2006;44(1):136–44.
26. Adhikari S, Zeger W. Non-thrombotic abnormalities on lower extremity venous duplex ultrasound examinations. Western Journal of Emergency Medicine. 2015;16(2):250–54.

27. Aurshina A, Huber S, Deng Y, Attaran R, Nassiri N, Dardik A, et al. Correlation of venous symptoms with iliac vein stenosis on magnetic resonance imaging. Journal of Vascular Surgery: Venous and Lymphatic Disorders. 2021;9(5):1291–96.e1.
28. Kibbe MR, Ujiki M, Goodwin AL, Eskandari M, Yao J, Matsumura J. Iliac vein compression in an asymptomatic patient population. Journal of Vascular Surgery. 2004;39(5):937–43.
29. May R, Thurner J. The cause of the predominantly sinistral occurrence of thrombosis of the pelvic veins. Angiology. 1957;8(5):419–27.
30. Cockett FB, Thomas ML. The iliac compression syndrome. British Journal of Surgery. 1965;52(10):816–21.
31. Kaltenmeier CT, Erben Y, Indes J, Lee A, Dardik A, Sarac T, et al. Systematic review of May-Thurner syndrome with emphasis on gender differences. Journal of Vascular Surgery: Venous and Lymphatic Disorders. 2018;6(3):399–407.e4.
32. Raju S, Owen S, Neglen P. Reversal of abnormal lymphoscintigraphy after placement of venous stents for correction of associated venous obstruction. Journal of Vascular Surgery. 2001;34(5):779–84.
33. Ruggeri M, Tosetto A, Castaman G, Rodeghiero F. Congenital absence of the inferior vena cava: A rare risk factor for idiopathic deep-vein thrombosis. Lancet. 2001;357(9254).
34. Antebi E, Shochat I, Sareli P, Geltner D, Deutsch V, Mozes M. A comparison between partial and complete ligation of the inferior vena cava for the prevention of recurrent pulmonary embolism. Israel Medical Association Journal. 1975;11(2–3):294–98.
35. LoGerfo FW, Coburn MW, Ashworth CW, Francis WW, Morin CW, Broukhim MW. Venous stasis complications of the use of the superficial femoral and popliteal veins for lower extremity bypass. Journal of Vascular Surgery. 1993;17(6):1005–9.
36. Ochoa Chaar CI, Aurshina A. Endovascular treatment of duplicated inferior vena cava compression from retroperitoneal fibrosis. Journal of Vascular Surgery Cases, Innovations and Techniques. 2018;4(4):311–14.
37. Bergan JJ, Schmid-Schönbein GW, Smith PDC, Nicolaides AN, Boisseau MR, Eklof B. Chronic venous disease. New England Journal of Medicine. 2006;355(5):488–98.
38. O'Meara S, Cullum N, Nelson EA, Dumville JC. Compression for venous leg ulcers. Cochrane Database of Systematic Reviews. 2012;11(11):CD000265.
39. Schuren J, Mohr K. Pascal's law and the dynamics of compression therapy: A study on healthy volunteers. International Angiology. 2010;29(5):431–35.
40. Garrigues-Ramón M, Julián M, Zaragoza C, Barrios C. Inability of Laplace's law to estimate sub-bandage pressures after applying a compressive bandage: A clinical study. Journal of Wound Care. 2021;30(4):276–82.
41. Staubesand J, Seydewitz V. An ultrastructural study of sclerosed varices. Phlebologie. 1991;44(1):16–22; discussion 33–6.
42. Partsch H, Mosti G. Thigh compression. Phlebology: The Journal of Venous Disease. 2008;23(6):252–58.
43. Partsch B, Partsch H. Calf compression pressure required to achieve venous closure from supine to standing positions. Journal of Vascular Surgery. 2005;42(4):734–38.
44. Sarin S, Scurr JH, Smith PDC. Mechanism of action of external compression on venous function. British Journal of Surgery. 1992;79(6):499–502.
45. Partsch H, Flour M, Smith PC, International Compression C. Indications for compression therapy in venous and lymphatic disease consensus based on experimental data and scientific evidence. Under the auspices of the IUP. International Angiology. 2008;27(3):193–219.
46. Motykie GD, Caprini JA, Arcelus JI, Reyna JJ, Overom E, Mokhtee D. Evaluation of therapeutic compression stockings in the treatment of chronic venous insufficiency. Dermatologic Surgery. 1999;25(2):116–20.
47. Gloviczki P, Comerota AJ, Dalsing MC, Eklof BG, Gillespie DL, Gloviczki ML, et al. The care of patients with varicose veins and associated chronic venous diseases: Clinical practice guidelines of the Society for Vascular Surgery and the American Venous Forum. Journal of Vascular Surgery. 2011;53(5):2S–48S.

48. Dolibog P, Franek A, Taradaj J, Dolibog P, Blaszczak E, Polak A, et al. A comparative clinical study on five types of compression therapy in patients with venous leg ulcers. International Journal of Medical Sciences. 2014;11(1):34–43.
49. Moneta GL, Nicoloff AD, Porter JM. Compression treatment of chronic venous ulceration: A review. Phlebology: The Journal of Venous Disease. 2016;15(3–4):162–68.
50. Finlayson K, Edwards H, Courtney M. The impact of psychosocial factors on adherence to compression therapy to prevent recurrence of venous leg ulcers. Journal of Clinical Nursing. 2010;19(9–10):1289–97.
51. Lurie F, Lal BK, Antignani PL, Blebea J, Bush R, Caprini J, et al. Compression therapy after invasive treatment of superficial veins of the lower extremities: Clinical practice guidelines of the American Venous Forum, Society for Vascular Surgery, American College of Phlebology, Society for Vascular Medicine, and International Union of Phlebology. Journal of Vascular Surgery: Venous and Lymphatic Disorders. 2019;7(1):17–28.
52. Moffatt C, Kommala D, Dourdin N, Choe Y. Venous leg ulcers: Patient concordance with compression therapy and its impact on healing and prevention of recurrence. International Wound Journal. 2009;6(5):386–93.
53. Kapp S, Miller C, Donohue L. The clinical effectiveness of two compression stocking treatments on venous leg ulcer recurrence. The International Journal of Lower Extremity Wounds. 2013;12(3):189–98.
54. Uhl J-F, Benigni J-P, Chahim M, Fréderic D. Prospective randomized controlled study of patient compliance in using a compression stocking: Importance of recommendations of the practitioner as a factor for better compliance. Phlebology: The Journal of Venous Disease. 2016;33(1):36–43.
55. Bar L, Brandis S, Marks D. Improving adherence to wearing compression stockings for chronic venous insufficiency and venous leg ulcers: A scoping review. Patient Preference and Adherence. 2021;15:2085–102.
56. Protz K, Dissemond J, Seifert M, Hintner M, Temme B, Verheyen-Cronau I, et al. Education in people with venous leg ulcers based on a brochure about compression therapy: A quasi-randomised controlled trial. International Wound Journal. 2019;16(6):1252–62.
57. Brooks J, Ersser SJ, Lloyd A, Ryan TJ. Nurse-led education sets out to improve patient concordance and prevent recurrence of leg ulcers. Journal of Wound Care. 2004;13(3):111–16.
58. Martinez-Zapata MJ, Vernooij RW, Simancas-Racines D, Uriona Tuma SM, Stein AT, Moreno Carriles RMM, et al. Phlebotonics for venous insufficiency. Cochrane Database of Systematic Reviews. 2020;11(11):CD003229.
59. Pittler MH, Ernst E. Horse chestnut seed extract for chronic venous insufficiency. Cochrane Database of Systematic Reviews. 2012;11(11):CD003230.
60. Kakkos SK, Nicolaides AN. Efficacy of micronized purified flavonoid fraction (Daflon(R)) on improving individual symptoms, signs and quality of life in patients with chronic venous disease: A systematic review and meta-analysis of randomized double-blind placebo-controlled trials. International Angiology. 2018;37(2):143–54.
61. Jull AB, Arroll B, Parag V, Waters J. Pentoxifylline for treating venous leg ulcers. Cochrane Database of Systematic Reviews. 2012;12(12):CD001733.

Section 2

Management of Symptomatic Peripheral Venous Insufficiency

Chapter 4

Thermal Ablation of Refluxing Superficial Truncal Veins

Jacob W. Soucy and John G. Carson

Venous disease has a very high prevalence among adults ranging from 40% to 80%, and the highest prevalence is in Western countries.[1] In the United States alone, greater than 30% of adults are affected by chronic venous insufficiency and varicose veins. Chronic venous insufficiency can result in pain and loss of workdays, and thereby result in significant morbidity.[2] Treatment includes non-invasive endovenous techniques and invasive surgical methods. Most frequently used minimally invasive techniques include radiofrequency and laser therapy.

Open surgical treatment of refluxing varicose veins with ligation, stripping and excision of large varicosities, had been the standard for venous treatment for many years. In 1999, radiofrequency ablation (RFA) of the saphenous vein was introduced as a new and minimally invasive modality for the treatment of superficial venous insufficiency. The treatment would be performed in the ambulatory setting, eliminate general anesthesia, and allow for a safe, office-based procedure increased ease of recovery. Initial studies in the 1990s mainly used the ClosurePlus (Covidien, Mansfield, MA, USA) continuous pullback catheter. This device has evolved, and the newer version of the ClosureFast (Medtronic, Santa Rosa, Ca, USA) catheter has a longer heating element. This enables operators to heat the target vein segments at a reduced procedural time of 20 second intervals. Endovenous laser ablation (EVLA) was also approved by the Food and Drug Administration (FDA), 3 years later, in 2002. Now, these endothermal ablation procedures have caused a dramatic shift from open, invasive surgery to a minimally invasive, ambulatory procedure.[3]

LASER ABLATION

Laser devices for use in the treatment of saphenous reflux are currently available from several manufacturers, and the lasers differ primarily in their wavelengths. Endovenous laser ablation (EVLA) is a percutaneous technique that uses laser energy to ablate incompetent superficial veins. The axial veins are the primary target for this therapy and include the great saphenous vein (GSV), small saphenous vein (SSV), and accessory saphenous veins (ASVs).

Studies demonstrate a very high initial technical success rate, in the 97–100% range, with patients demonstrating approximately 90% persistence of occlusion of the treated truncal vein after 24 months. Significant pain was present in 67% of patients for approximately 1 week after laser therapy, and up to 10% of patients were noted to have overt thrombophlebitis for 2 weeks after the procedure.[4]

Technique

Full informed consent should be obtained. Performing this procedure without intravenous sedation and only local anesthesia has its advantages. The patient does not have to be fasting. It is important that the patient is relaxed and well hydrated. Relaxing music and conversation

DOI: 10.1201/9781003316626-6

can ease the patient's anxiety. The most common risks associated with EVLA include transient paresthesias and bruising along the ablation track. Deep venous thrombosis (DVT) has been reported but has a relatively low occurrence rate of less than 1%. Skin burns have been reported with both RFA and laser techniques, although the incidence of these is extremely low with the procedural use of tumescent anesthesia.

Equipment needed for the procedure include a duplex ultrasound machine, laser generator, a tilting table, laser kit, and the pump for subcutaneous injection of the tumescent anesthesia. Having a skilled vascular sonographer is preferred. The mixture of tumescent anesthesia is a combination of saline, epinephrine, bicarbonate, and lidocaine. Skin prep, gown, mask, and gloves are needed as meticulous sterile technique should be used. The draping materials are brought to the field. A micropuncture sheath kit and a 10 mL syringe with needles to withdraw and inject medications are placed on the procedural table. A 21 gauge echogenic needle is utilized for initial access and appropriately sized glide wires. Finally, sterile gauze, compression bandages and stockings are needed. The GSV, which has previously been identified as having reflux on diagnostic ultrasound examination, is mapped from the saphenofemoral junction (SFJ) through the below knee segment. Tortuosity, patency, and location with relation to the skin and the fascia are noted. The GSV is accessed utilizing direct ultrasound guidance and micropuncture technique. The ideal point of entry is caudal to the most caudal point of reflux but not more than 10–15 cm below the knee. Below this area, the risk of saphenous nerve injury is increased.

A sheath is introduced into the vein over the wire, utilizing the Seldinger technique. To minimize the risk of DVT or injury to the central veins, it is of critical importance that the tip of the laser fiber be definitively identified with ultrasound and positioned just caudal to the epigastric vein prior to activation, approximately 2–3 cm distal to the SFJ. This position also decreases the risk for future neovascularization. For greatest accuracy, the SFJ, the epigastric vein, and the laser tip should be identified simultaneously with longitudinal ultrasound imaging. If the epigastric vein can be identified, the tip is positioned within the GSV just caudal to the epigastric vein confluence. Tumescent anesthetic is then administered along the entire length of the GSV within the perivenous space. In addition to providing local analgesia, this diluted mixture of lidocaine and saline (0.15–0.20%) acts as a thermal heat sink that provides external compression to improve the transfer of thermal energy to the vein wall. The needle is slowly advanced toward the outer wall of the GSV under direct ultrasound guidance as the tumescent anesthetic is gently injected. Once the perivenous space is entered, the fluid begins to flow freely up the perivenous potential space along the path of the GSV. The infiltration of fluid is followed cephalad until its progress begins to slow at which time the needle is reinserted more cephalad and tumescent anesthetic is readministered in a similar fashion until the SFJ has been reached. Patients rarely may develop a vasovagal or anaphylactoid response to this introduction of anesthesia. Preparatory measures should be in place if this occurs. At this level, additional anesthetic agent should be administered in the soft tissues deep and superficial to the catheter-fiber tip and saphenous vein because of slightly greater innervation in this region.

At this time, the entire course of the GSV is evaluated with ultrasound to confirm that it is surrounded by tumescent fluid at all levels. Transverse orientation is useful in this determination. One should additionally confirm that the superficial aspect of the GSV is at least 1.0 cm deep to the skin surface along its entire length to reduce the likelihood of skin burns. It is necessary with laser treatment to maintain a small volume of blood within the lumen of the vein, as blood is the chromophore for the absorption of the laser energy to transfer heat to the vein wall and cause injury to the vein wall. The rate of pullback with the laser technique is adjusted to maintain an energy transfer of 80–100 joules/cm within the vein. The catheter is slowly pulled back at an initial rate of 1 mm every second for the first 10 cm of treatment length. Thereafter, the catheter can be pulled back 2 to 3 mm every second. A slow, steady pullback provides even heating of the entire vein segment and minimizes the chance of vein perforation.

At the end of the procedure the catheter is removed, the vein is interrogated for absence of flow, and the common femoral vein is also evaluated for compressibility and absence of DVT extension. The sheath is removed, and localized pressure is held. The leg is then wrapped in 20–30 mmHg graduated elastic compression stocking for 2 days to 2 weeks depending on the preference of the venous specialist.[5]

Complications

The most common complications following laser ablation are ecchymosis, pain, nerve injury, skin burn, superficial thrombophlebitis, and deep venous thrombosis.[6] Deep vein thrombosis is a rare complication, resulting in <1% of patients. A DVT may occur from the propagation of a thrombus into the deep system. This phenomenon is referred to as endovenous heat-induced thrombus (EHIT).[7] Recurrence of varicose veins following thermal ablation is rare and comparable to other ablation methods.[8]

Postoperative Care

Pain following the procedure is typically minimal, and non-steriodal anti-inflammatory medications are generally recommended as first-line analgesia.[9] Concerning findings include swelling, skin burns, excessive pain, persistent numbness, tingling, coolness, or discoloration of the toes. The patients should be encouraged to ambulate and avoid prolonged sitting or standing. Tightness and/or slight bruising may be expected. We perform a follow-up ultrasound in 3–7 days to confirm successful venous closure and to rule out extension of thrombus into the adjacent deep vein.[10]

RADIOFREQUENCY ABLATION

Radiofrequency ablation (RFA) is a minimally invasive procedure that similarly uses thermal energy to ablate refluxing veins. The RFA procedure involves using a catheter electrode to deliver a high-frequency alternating radiofrequency current that leads to venous spasm, collagen shrinkage, and physical contraction.[11] Before the development of RFA in the late 1990s, the method of choice for treatment was more invasive surgical vein stripping.[12]

Indications for RFA were formulated from the combined effort of the Society for Vascular Surgery (SVS) and the American Venous Form (AVF). The guidelines do not differ when comparing RFA to other venous ablation procedures. The indications for RFA are similar to those of laser ablation.[3]

Technique

Once significant reflux is identified, patients are scheduled for RFA if otherwise appropriate. Like laser ablation, this procedure is often completed in an office setting with local anesthesia.

The equipment/medication required are duplex ultrasound machine; an experienced sonographer; endovenous radiofrequency generator and catheter; catheter sheath kit; heparinized saline; 10 mL syringe with appropriate needles to draw up/inject anesthetic;

micropuncture needle, wire, and dilator/sheath (5 French); glide wire and dilator/sheath (7 French); roller pump and tubing; table capable of Trendelenburg and reverse Trendelenburg; sterile drapes; sterile gloves and skin antiseptic; local anesthetic (1% lidocaine); tumescent anesthetic (can substitute with saline 0.9% if there is an allergy); and injectable saline (0.9%).

When the patient arrives, consent is obtained, and the correct laterality is confirmed. Oral sedation is sometimes useful depending on the patient's level of anxiety. Like EVLA, intravenous sedation is rarely required. The target vein can be further evaluated on the day of the procedure with an ultrasound to confirm reflux. At this time, the patient will be prepped and draped in the standard surgical fashion. Subcutaneous lidocaine is injected anterior to the vein at the access site. Percutaneous access is gained into the vein with ultrasound guidance and a micropuncture needle. When treating the GSV it should be accessed at the level of the knee. When treating the SSV, the vein is assessed distal to the reflux that is to be treated. A sheath is then placed into the vein using the over-the-wire technique. The RFA catheter is advanced to the saphenofemoral or saphenopopliteal junction. Tip location is then confirmed with ultrasound, and the catheter is pulled back > 2.5 centimeters from the junction to help to avoid propagation into the deep venous system. With the help of ultrasound, tumescent anesthesia is injected with a spinal needle into the perivenous tissue along the length of the vein to avoid thermal injury when ablation is initiated. The radiofrequency current is then delivered, resulting in denaturation of the collagen matrix and endothelial destruction at a temperature of 110–120° C. Venous segments 3–7 cm in length are treated in 20-second cycles.[11] Compression of the vein during ablation is recommended to compress the vein lumen against the catheter. At the end of the procedure, the catheter is removed, and the vein is quickly interrogated for absence of flow. The common femoral vein is also evaluated for compressibility and absence of deep venous thrombosis extension. Following sheath removal and hemostasis at the access site, the leg is then wrapped in 20–30 mmHg graduated elastic compression stocking for 2 days to 2 weeks practice dependent.[5]

Complications

The most common complications following thermal ablation are sensory nerve injury, DVT, recurrence of varicose veins, thrombophlebitis, infection, and bleeding. When treating distal to the knee the GSV, nerve injury can occur due to the saphenous nerve's proximity. Small saphenous vein (SSV) treatment with thermal ablation is associated with sural nerve paresthesia due to proximity. This can result in pain and paresthesias to the lateral ankle and heel. Other non-thermal ablation techniques may be used to avoid this complication when treating reflux in the below knee truncal veins deep vein thrombosis is a rare complication, resulting in <1% of patients. Similar to laser ablation, DVT may occur and is classified based on location of thrombus (EHIT).[7] Recurrence of varicose veins following thermal ablation is rare and comparable to other ablation methods.[8]

Postoperative Care

Ambulation and nonstrenuous activity are encouraged. If there is any discomfort NSAIDs should be trialed.[9] Similar to postoperative care for laser ablation the patient should have a follow-up duplex scan in 3–7 days to confirm for successful ablation and to rule out deep venous thrombosis.[10]

CONCLUSION

Endovenous ablation techniques have revolutionized the treatment of symptomatic venous insufficiency. Thermal ablative techniques are proven to be safe, effective, and quick. Most venous specialists can master these procedures. They have replaced the need for operating room time and general anesthesia or sedation, and they have proven to have excellent results with limited recovery time.

Limitations of thermal ablation include nerve injury and skin burns opening the door for non-thermal techniques in the treatment of venous insufficiency. In summary, thermal ablation is a desirable procedure, which is safe with minimal major complications, effective and time efficient and has a low learning curve. The future may bring new techniques that are virtually painless and may completely avoid the need for thermal energy with equal efficacy.

REFERENCES

1. Davies AH. The seriousness of chronic venous disease: A review of real-world evidence. Adv Ther. 2019;36(Suppl 1):5–12. doi:10.1007/s12325-019-0881-7.
2. Gloviczki P, Comerota AJ, Dalsing MC, et al. The care of patients with varicose veins and associated chronic venous diseases: Clinical practice guidelines of the Society for Vascular Surgery and the American Venous Forum. J Vasc Surg 2011;53:2S.
3. Jones RT, Kabnick LS. Perioperative duplex ultrasound following endothermal ablation of the saphenous vein: Is it worthless? J Invasive Cardiol. 2014;26(10):548–550.
4. Proebstle TM, Lehr HA, Kargl A, et al. Endovenous treatment of the greater saphenous vein with a 940-nm diode laser: Thrombotic occlusion after endoluminal thermal damage by laser-generated steam bubbles. J Vasc Surg. 2002;35(4):729–736.
5. Ayo D, Blumberg SN, Rockman CR, et al. Compression versus no compression after endovenous ablation of the great saphenous vein: A randomized controlled trial. Ann Vasc Surg 2017;38:72.
6. Van Den Bos RR, Neumann M, De Roos KP, et al. Endovenous laser ablation-induced complications: Review of the literature and new cases. Dermatol Surg. 2009 Aug;35(8):1206–1214. doi:10.1111/j.1524-4725.2009.01215.x.
7. Puggioni A, Kalra M, Carmo M, et al. Endovenous laser therapy and radiofrequency ablation of the great saphenous vein: Analysis of early efficacy and complications. J Vasc Surg 2005;42:488.
8. Kheirelseid EAH, Crowe G, Sehgal R, et al. Systematic review and meta-analysis of randomized controlled trials evaluating long-term outcomes of endovenous management of lower extremity varicose veins. J Vasc Surg Venous Lymphat Disord 2018;6:256.
9. Mariano ER, Dickerson DM, Szokol JW, et al. A multisociety organizational consensus process to define guiding principles for acute perioperative pain management. Reg Anesth Pain Med 2022;47:118.
10. Mozes G, Kalra M, Carmo M, et al. Extension of saphenous thrombus into the femoral vein: A potential complication of new endovenous ablation techniques. J Vasc Surg 2005;41:130.
11. Kayssi A, Pope M, Vucemilo I, Werneck C. Endovenous radiofrequency ablation for the treatment of varicose veins. Can J Surg. 2015 Apr;58(2):85–86. doi:10.1503/cjs.014914.
12. Sarin S, Scurr JH, Coleridge-Smith PD. Stripping of the long saphenous vein in the treatment of primary varicose veins. Br J Surg. 1994;81:1455–1458.

Chapter 5

Polidocanol Microfoam Ablation of Refluxing Superficial Veins

Techniques and Results

Juan Carlos Jimenez

BACKGROUND

Until the introduction of thermal ablation for superficial venous insufficiency approximately 20 years ago, mostly surgical options (ie. high ligation and stripping of the saphenous vein, stab phlebectomy, open perforator ligation) were available.[1] Alternatives for treatment have expanded with availability of non-thermal alternatives, which can be added to the armamentarium of the vascular surgeon and venous specialist.

One alternative is commercially manufactured polidocanol microfoam (Varithena, Boston Scientific, Boston MA). This compound is a 1% injectable polidocanol solution comprised of an oxygen to carbon dioxide ratio of 65:35 with a low nitrogen concentration (<0.8%). This microfoam (MF) demonstrates a uniform density, size, and stability with a small bubble size (median diameter <100 uM) relative to physician compounded foam (PCF) using the Tessari method. It was approved by the US Food and Drug Administration (FDA) in 2013 for treatment of incompetent great saphenous veins (GSV), accessory saphenous veins (AASV), and visible varicosities of the GSV system above and below the knee.[2]

Microfoam ablation (MFA) of superficial truncal and tributary veins can be routinely performed in the ambulatory setting with local anesthesia with oral sedation if needed. Varithena is injected directly into refluxing target veins through a small profile (4F) sheath, butterfly needle, or angiocath. The compound adheres to the lipid cell membrane of the venous endothelial lining resulting in interruption of the osmotic barrier and damage to the endothelium with resultant vasospasm[3] (Figure 5.1). The endothelial disruption leads to acute thrombosis and occlusion of the venous lumen. Chronic thrombosis of the vein results in filling of the venous lumen with fibrous connective tissue.

PATIENT SELECTION AND CLINICAL ADVANTAGES

Microfoam ablation of the truncal veins is indicated for patients who present with lifestyle limiting physical signs and symptoms associated with varicose veins. These include but not are not limited to pain, aching, heaviness, fatigue, edema, venous stasis skin changes (lipodermatosclerosis), and both active and healed ulceration. Evidence of failed conservative treatment is usually required for insurance coverage and may include the use of graded compression stockings, leg elevation, avoidance of prolonged standing, exercise, and weight control. Prior to the procedure, we perform a detailed lower extremity venous insufficiency ultrasound mapping the anatomy of the refluxing truncal and tributary veins and confirm the patency of the deep venous system. All patients with venous ulceration are treated concurrently in our ambulatory wound care center and are compliant with weekly dressing changes, offloading,

DOI: 10.1201/9781003316626-7

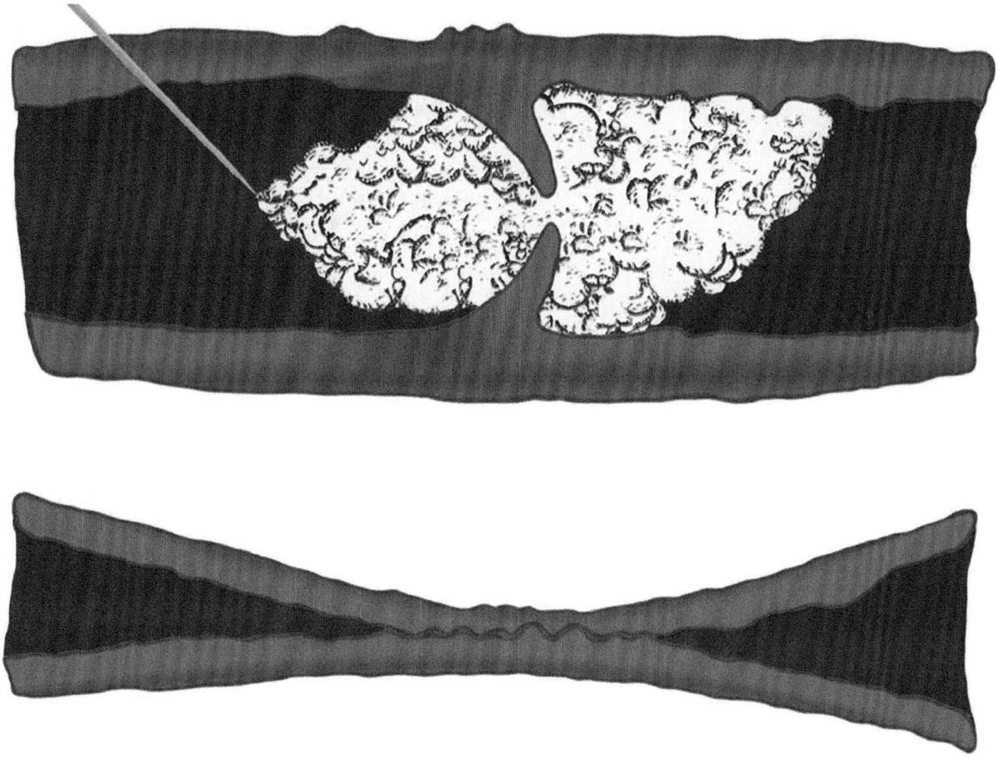

Figure 5.1 Endothelial destruction with resultant vasospasm of the venous lumen following microfoam ablation.

nutritional counseling, and compression. Specific incompetent veins indicated for treatment (and approved by the FDA) include the GSV and AASVs and associated tributaries. We also perform MFA of the small saphenous vein (SSV); however this is still considered "off-label" use for Varithena. Our early reported clinical outcomes with MFA of the SSV have been excellent.[4]

The properties of Varithena provide unique clinical advantages for patients with chronic venous insufficiency and symptomatic varicose veins. It is distinct from traditional PCF because it is commercially manufactured with carbon dioxide gas and not mixed at the bedside using room air, which contains high levels of nitrogen. Polidocanol microfoam results in smaller and more uniform bubble size that is protective against microcirculatory obstruction and cerebral ischemia from potential cerebrovascular gas bubbles embolizing following injection foam sclerotherapy.[5] Evidence suggests microfoam may be safer than PCF due to decreased clinical manifestations from cerebrovascular emboli. In a study by Regan and colleagues, patients with right-to-left intracardiac shunts were monitored with transcranial Doppler surveillance following treatment with low nitrogen polidocanol endovenous microfoam.[5] Although middle cerebral artery emboli were detected in 60 of 82 treated patients, no patients developed magnetic resonance imaging abnormalities, neurological signs, or elevated cardiac troponin levels.

Incompetent tortuous superficial veins are frequently not amenable to the passage of a stiff catheter required for radiofrequency and laser ablation. Because only minimal sheath or

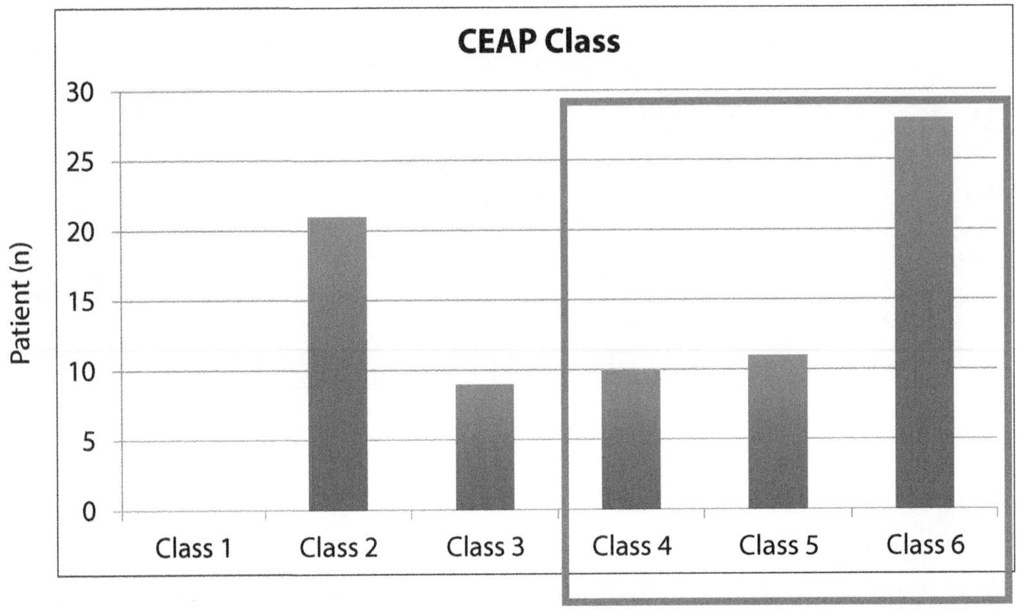

Figure 5.2 Our use of microfoam in below knee truncal veins resulted in excellent outcomes despite a study cohort comprised of mostly patients with advanced CEAP class and chronic, refractory venous insufficiency.

catheter advancement is required for MFA, it can be readily injected with maximal luminal contact in patients with tortuous and redundant venous anatomy.

Non-thermal superficial vein closure with MFA does not require injection of tumescent anesthesia because there is no risk of heat-induced nerve injury or thermal propagation, which can be a source of persistent, postoperative neuropathic pain following thermal ablation. Superficial veins can also be treated without the risk of thermal skin burns. There is usually less pain in sensitive and anxious patients because the multiple subcutaneous perivenous injections required for tumescent administration are not required. Thus, the risk of lidocaine toxicity is also lower because significantly less volumes are used with Varithena.

Microfoam treatment is an ideal choice for superficial vein closure below the knee and in patients with prior above knee truncal vein ablation and stripping.[6] In our recent published experience, MFA of below knee truncal veins has been a safe and effective modality in these patients. We reviewed 68 limbs treated with MFA for superficial truncal vein reflux following prior saphenous ablation or stripping at our institution. The study population was comprised mostly of patients with advanced chronic venous insufficiency (CEAP 4–6, 63%) (Figure 5.2). Overall symptomatic relief was 78% following MFA, and the median preoperative Venous Clinical Severity Score (VCSS) decreased from 12.5 to 10 post-procedure. Good clinical results were demonstrated despite a patient cohort comprised largely of patients with advanced, refractory venous insufficiency (Figure 5.3A and Figure 5.3B). One ablation related thrombus extension (ARTE) occurred and was resolved with anticoagulation and patient with an asymptomatic tibial vein deep vein thrombosis did not require anticoagulation.

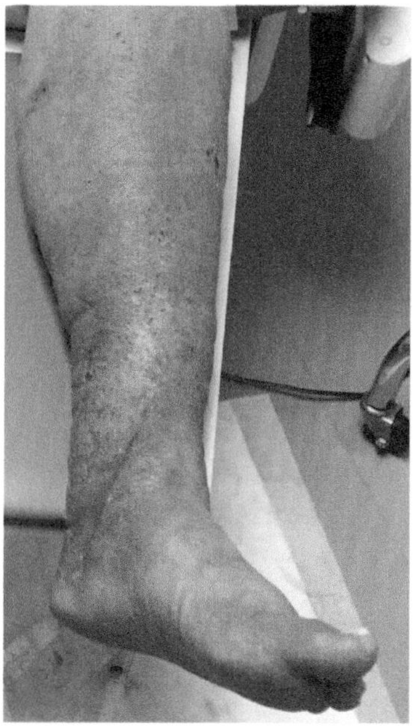

Figure 5.3A A patient with severe, symptomatic chronic venous ulceration prior to Varithena microfoam ablation.

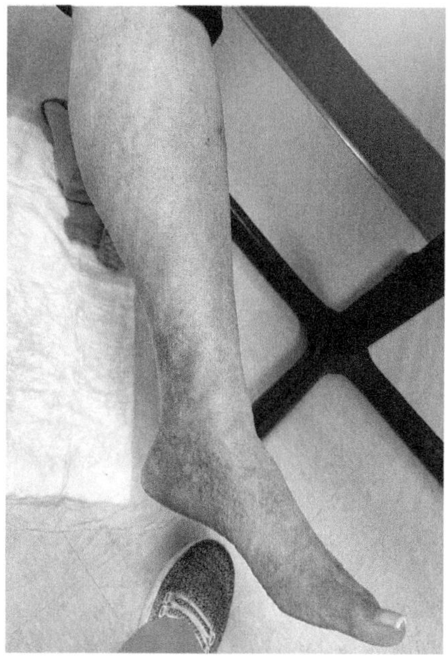

Figure 5.3B The same patient 3 years following microfoam ablation of her left great saphenous vein (GSV). Her GSV remains occluded, and her ulcer healed without recurrence.

TECHNIQUES

All MFA procedures are performed in our ambulatory venous center using local anesthesia and occasionally oral sedation (diazepam 5–10 mg). Patients are positioned supine for GSV and AASV treatment and prone when the SSV is treated. In addition to the initial preprocedure ultrasound performed in the vascular lab, it is important for the venous specialist to carefully map the target vein to confirm location, depth, diameter, anatomic variability, and the presence of associated perforator veins (Figure 5.4). Percutaneous ultrasound-guided access for truncal veins is obtained with a micropuncture needle allowing for guidewire entry into the venous lumen. We prefer to place a 4F sheath over the wire using Seldinger technique whenever possible. A 21G butterfly needle is most often used for direct injection of tributary veins. Once venous access is obtained, the limb is elevated to greater than 45 degrees. We utilize a tilt table that is placed in steep Trendelenburg position for this portion of the procedure.

Two individuals are required to be in the room at the time of microfoam administration. The clinician injects 10 mL of sterile saline solution to flush blood from the venous lumen. At this time, the assistant withdraws MF from the Varithena canister based on the instructions for use. If perforator veins are present in the target vein, the assistant may digitally compress previously marked perforator veins prior to MF injection.

Microfoam is then directly injected in retrograde fashion into the target vein. This should be performed as soon as possible following withdrawal from the proprietary canister to reduce microfoam degradation. For truncal veins, we visualize the target vein 3–5 cm caudal to the saphenofemoral or saphenopopliteal junctions. Varithena is highly echogenic, and when it reaches this level, the vein is then firmly compressed with the ultrasound probe for

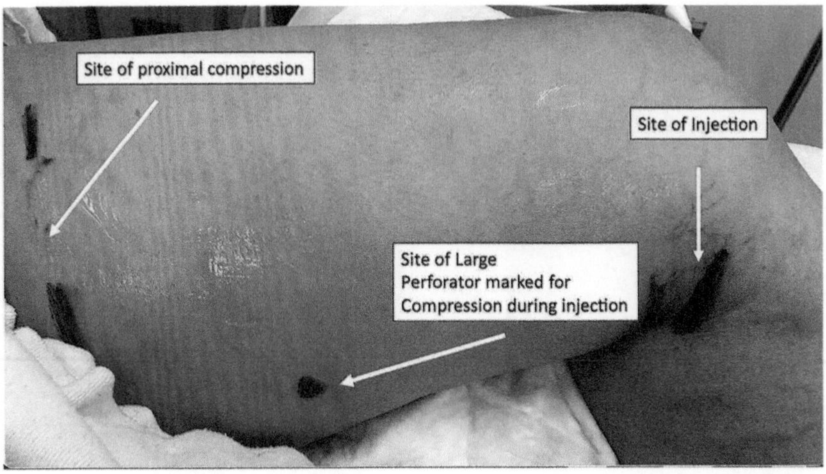

Figure 5.4 Intraoperative ultrasound vein mapping by the clinician localizes perforators in the target truncal vein prior to microfoam ablation and may minimize Varithena extension into the deep venous system.

5 minutes. Because increased foam volume has been associated with potentially increased passage into the deep venous system, we attempt to limit foam volume to as close to 5 mL as possible.[7,8] We also adhere to the Varithena Instructions for Use (IFU) of 15 mL maximal microfoam volume per session. During this time, we ask the patient to dorsiflex and plantar flex his/her ankle 20 times to increase flow through the deep venous system. Following 5 minutes of compression, ultrasound is used to ensure that vasospasm is present in the target vein and that no acute thrombus is noted in the femoral or popliteal veins (Figure 5.5). The treated limb is then compressed with abdominal (ABD) pads overlying the treated veins and long-stretch compression bandages. The patient is instructed to keep the compression bandage in place until the first post-procedure visit 48–72 hours later. They are then recommended to wear 20–30 mmHg compression stockings for 14 days. This is also recommended based on the Varithena IFU.

EVIDENCE SUPPORTING THE EFFICACY OF POLIDOCANOL MICROFOAM

Several level 1, randomized, blinded, controlled studies have demonstrated good clinical outcomes supporting the safety and efficacy of MFA.[9–11] King, et al. conducted the VANISH-1 study, a multicenter trial that randomized 279 patients to treatment with different concentrations of polidocanol MF (0.125%, 0.5%, 1%, 2%) or placebo.[9] Veins treated included the GSV, AASV, and associated superficial tributaries. Symptomatic improvement was the primary endpoint measured. Secondary endpoints included improved appearance of visible varicose veins from baseline to week 8. Objective quality-of-life evaluation demonstrated significant clinical relief in the MFA groups compared with the control group ($p < .0001$). The MFA cohort also demonstrated significantly improved appearance at all therapeutic dose concentrations. The most common adverse thrombotic event (ATE) was superficial thrombophlebitis which occurred in 10.5% of study patients. Twenty-seven patients experienced deep venous ATEs including 15 ablation related thrombus extensions (ARTE) and 12 peripheral deep venous thromboses (DVT). All resolved with oral anticoagulation, and no

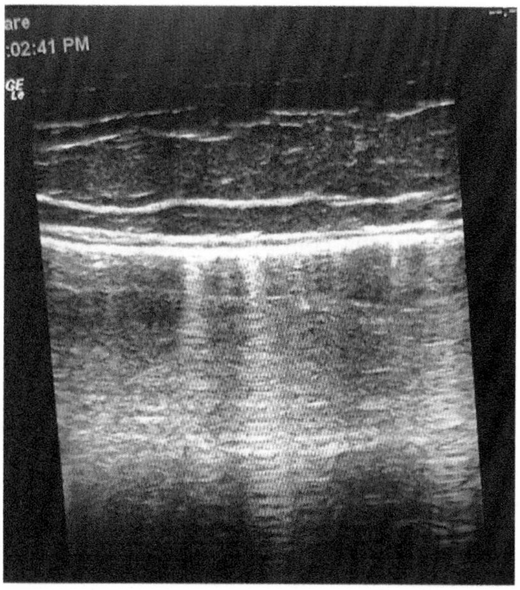

Figure 5.5 Varithena microfoam is highly echogenic on ultrasound. This figure demonstrates profound vasospasm following microfoam ablation of the GSV.

pulmonary emboli were noted. No neurologic complications or symptomatic embolic events were reported.

The VANISH-2 was a 5-year, randomized, multicenter, parallel group study. Patients (n = 232) were randomized to treatment with MF concentrations of 0.5%, 1%, and placebo.[9,10] Similar to VANISH-1, target veins included the GSV, AASV, and associated superficial tributaries. The mean vein diameter treated was 8.7 mm (range 3.1 mm–19.4 mm). The primary efficacy endpoint was patient-reported improvement in symptoms, as measured by the change from baseline to week 8 in the 7-day average electronic daily diary VVSymQ™ score. The co-secondary endpoints were the improvement in appearance of visible varicosities from baseline to week 8, as measured by patients and by an independent physician review panel.

There were significant improvements for both the 0.5% and 1.0% treatment groups compared with placebo. Overall, there was a 64% improvement in symptoms in the treatment groups compared with 22% in the placebo group ($p < 0.0001$). Statistically significant improvement in appearance was also noted in both treatment groups. Elimination of reflux and/or complete occlusion of the GSV was achieved in 83% and 86% of patients who received 0.5% and 1.0% polidocanol respectively. Adverse thrombotic events occurred in 10.4% of patients. Thrombus extension into the common femoral vein (CFV) occurred in nine patients (3.9%). None were occlusive. There were six proximal (2.6%) and seven distal (3%) DVTs. Two patients developed gastrocnemius thrombi. Half of the patients received anticoagulation, and the remainder were managed with non-steroidal anti-inflammatory medications and/or compression and observation.

Another study by Gibson and colleagues randomized 77 patients to treatment with 1% polidocanol MF (n = 39) or placebo (n = 38) during the blinded portion of the study.[8] Subsequently, 34 placebo-group patients were crossed over into treatment with 1% polidocanol microfoam. Like the VANISH trials, symptoms and appearance both improved significantly in the Varithena group. This study protocol initially allowed <30 mL of MF per treatment. However, because there was a trend suggesting higher occurrence of ATEs with higher volumes, the protocol was amended mid-study to a maximum of 15 mL per procedure (the current IFU recommended volume). Overall, the incidence of CFV ARTE was 4.1%, and the incidence of new DVT was 9.6%. All but one venous thrombus resolved without clinical significance. A summary of Level 1 evidence validating Varithena 1% polidocanol MF compared with placebo can be found in Table 5.1.

The literature supporting Varithena continues to reveal more specific indications, anatomic features, and techniques for microfoam use to optimize outcomes. We recently analyzed results following both MFA and radiofrequency ablation (RFA) in large-diameter truncal veins (> 8 mm). Results following treatment of 66 limbs with MFA and 66 with RFA during the same study period were analyzed.[12] Immediate closure rates were excellent in both groups (RFA–100%, MFA–95%) Overall, VCSS improved after treatment in both groups (RFA, from 9.5 to 7.8; $P < .001$) (MFA, from 11.3 to 9.0; $P < .001$). In the RFA and MFA groups, 83% and 79% of venous ulcers healed during the study period, respectively. Symptomatic superficial phlebitis occurred after RFA in 11% and 17% in MFA. The incidence of post-ablation ARTE was 3.0% in the RFA group and 6.1% in the MFA group, which was not statistically significant. All resolved with short-term oral anticoagulant therapy. No remote deep venous thromboses or pulmonary emboli occurred in either group.

Our group subsequently analyzed outcomes following primary closure of the GSV and AASV in the thigh.[13] A total of 200 consecutive thigh GSVs and ASVs were treated within the study period using either MFA (n = 100) or RFA (n = 100). Operative times were significantly shorter in the MFA group (42.4 ± 15.4 minutes in the RFA group and 33.8 ±16.9 minutes in the MFA group {$P < .001$}). The mean postoperative VCSS declined to 7.3 ± 2.1 in the RFA group and 7.8 ± 2.9 in the MFA group. Complete closure occurred in 100% of the limbs after RFA and 90% after MFA ($P = .005$). Overall, symptomatic relief was 90% following RFA and 89.5% following MFA. The complete ulcer healing rate for the entire cohort was 77.8%. Ablation related thrombus extension (RFA, 1%; vs MFA, 4%; $P = .37$) and remote DVT (RFA, 0%; vs MFA, 2%; $P = .5$) showed a trend toward being higher following MFA, but the difference did not reach statistical significance. All were asymptomatic and resolved with short-term anticoagulation therapy.

Deak demonstrated similar excellent outcomes following MFA compared with laser ablation (EVLA) of the saphenous veins.[14] In his large cohort, MFA was used for 550 procedures, and patients were followed for 43 ± 13 months; EVLA was used for 520 procedures and

Table 5.1 Summary of Randomized Trials Evaluating Polidocanol Microfoam

Study	*No. of Patients*	*Symptom Improvement (1% MF)*	*Elimination of Reflux and/or Closure (1% MF)*	*Mean Change in VCSS*	*Deep Venous Thrombosis*
King, et al. (VANISH-1)[9]	279	63%	80.4%	−3.70	2.5%
Todd, et al. (VANISH-2)[10]	232	77.8%	86%	−5.15	6.1%
Gibson, et al. (Varithena 013 Group)[8]	77	* HASTI Score Mean change from baseline 30.7 (Not reported as percentage)	90%	−3.4	9.6%

* HASTI: heaviness, achiness, swelling, throbbing, itching.

patients were followed for 57 ± 18 months. After complete treatment, the elimination of reflux was documented in 93.5% (514/550) and 92.8% (482/520) of the MFA and EVLA procedures, respectively. Ulcer healing rates were significantly improved following treatment with Varithena (MFA–69%; EVLA–5%).

Studies with increased duration of follow-up are currently required to determine whether the long-term closure rates and symptom relief following MFA compare favorably with thermal ablation and high ligation and stripping. Unlike those two modalities, there is no current randomized data comparing long-term results with Varithena to other closure methods.[15] This information is particularly important because strong evidence supports that long-term efficacy following PCF for truncal veins is inferior to thermal and surgical techniques.[16]

COMPLICATIONS FOLLOWING MICROFOAM ABLATION

The incidence of serious complications is rare (ie. pulmonary embolus, neurologic complications). Localized pain at the injection site is the most common patient complaint during early follow-up but resolves in a few weeks. Adverse thrombotic events (ie. superficial thrombophlebitis, ARTE, and DVT) continue to be reported and are potentially serious if left untreated.[17] A recent analysis of above knee GSVs treated with MFA at our institution found the incidence of ARTE to be 5.2% compared with 0.7% following RFA.[18] This difference was statistically significant. Based on our anecdotal experience and ATE rates in the recent literature, we continue to advocate the use of early (48–72-hour) post-procedure ultrasound to rule out ARTE and DVT following Varithena ablation of superficial truncal veins.

The most recent Clinical Practice Guidelines from the Society for Vascular Surgery (SVS), American Venous Forum (AVF), and American Vein and Lymphatic Society (AVLS) do not make specific recommendations for surveillance and treatment of superficial thrombophlebitis and ARTE following MFA (or other non-thermal treatments for truncal vein reflux) due to insufficient published evidence.[19] Superficial thrombophlebitis with subsequent hyperpigmentation can be a frustrating post-procedure event for patients. Incision and drainage with evacuation of thrombosed superficial veins can result in more rapid pain relief and can lead to quicker resolution of hyperpigmentation. We do not routinely anticoagulate patients for focal superficial thrombophlebitis. Patients with extensive and symptomatic superficial thrombophlebitis and ARTE (SVS EHIT II or greater) are treated with directly acting oral anticoagulants (DOACS) with reevaluation at 1-week intervals until the deep vein extension retracts or resolves. We have demonstrated excellent clinical outcomes utilizing this surveillance and selective anticoagulation protocol.[4]

CONCLUSIONS

Treatment of symptomatic, superficial, and incompetent truncal and tributary veins using commercially manufactured polidocanol microfoam results in successful early closure rates, excellent relief of symptoms, and effective ulcer healing rates. These early results compare favorably to thermal ablation in non-randomized, short-term comparisons. Further investigation is required to determine and characterize the optimal clinical indications and patient selection for MFA. Because the natural history of ARTE following MFA has not been fully elucidated, there are no formal clinical practice guidelines for surveillance and management of these post-procedure ATEs. Our clinical experience strongly suggests that early post-procedure ultrasound surveillance with selective anticoagulation following truncal vein MFA constitutes best practice and optimizes patient safety when this technique is utilized.

REFERENCES

1. Puggioni A, Kalra M, Carmo M, Mozes G, Gloviczki P. Endovenous laser therapy and radiofrequency ablation of the great saphenous vein: Analysis of early efficacy and complications. J Vasc Surg. 2005;42:488–93.
2. Food and Drug Administration. Highlights of Prescribing Information, n.d. www.accessdata.fda.gov/drugsatfda_docs/label/2013/205098s000lbl.pdf
3. Redondo P, Cabrera J. Microfoam sclerotherapy. Semin Cutan Med Surg. 2005;24:175–83.
4. Jimenez JC, Lawrence PF, Woo K, Chun TT, Farley SM, Rigberg DA, et al. Adjunctive techniques to minimize thrombotic complications following microfoam sclerotherapy of saphenous trunks and tributaries. J Vasc Surg Venous Lymphat Disord. 2021;9:904–9.
5. Regan JD, Gibson KD, Rush JE, Shortell CK, Hirsch SA, Wright DI. Clinical significance of cerebrovascular gas emboli during polidocanol endovenous ultra-low nitrogen microfoam ablation and correlation with magnetic resonance imaging in patients with right-to-left shunt. J Vasc Surg 2011;53:131–37.
6. Jimenez JC, Lawrence PF, Pavlyha M, Farley SM, Rigberg DA, DeRubertis BG, et al. Endovenous microfoam ablation of below knee superficial truncal veins is safe and effective in patients with prior saphenous treatment across a wide range of CEAP classes. J Vasc Surg Venous Lymphat Disord. 2022;10:390–94.
7. Yamaki T, Nozaki M, Sakurai H, Takeuchi M, Soejima K, Kono T. Multiple small-dose injections can reduce the passage of sclerosant foam into deep veins during foam sclerotherapy for varicose veins. Eur J Vasc Endovasc Surg. 2009;37:343–48.
8. Gibson K, Kabnick L; Varithena® 013 Investigator group. A multicenter, randomized, placebo-controlled study to evaluate the efficacy and safety of Varithena® (polidocanol endovenous microfoam 1%) for symptomatic, visible varicose veins with saphenofemoral junction incompetence. Phlebology. 2017;32:185–93.
9. King JT, O'Byrne M, Vasquez M, Wright D; VANISH-1 Investigator Group. Treatment of truncal incompetence and varicose veins with a single administration of a new polidocanol endovenous microfoam preparation improves symptoms and appearance. Eur J Vasc Endovasc Surg. 2015;50:784–93.
10. Todd KL, Wright DI; VANISH-2 Investigator Group. The VANISH-2 study: A randomized, blinded, multicenter study to evaluate the efficacy and safety of polidocanol endovenous microfoam 0.5% and 1.0% compared with placebo for the treatment of saphenofemoral junction incompetence. Phlebology. 2014;29:608–18.
11. Todd KL 3rd, Wright DI; VANISH-2 Investigator group. Durability of treatment effect with polidocanol endovenous microfoam on varicose vein symptoms and appearance (VANISH-2). J Vasc Surg Venous Lymphat Disord. 2015;3:258–64.e1.
12. Chin AL, Talutis SD, Lawrence PF, Jimenez JC. Early results following comparison of radiofrequency and microfoam ablation of large diameter truncal veins demonstrate high closure rates and symptomatic relief. J Vasc Surg Venous Lymphat Disord. 2023;11:716–22.
13. Talutis SD, Chin AL, Lawrence PF, Woo K, Jimenez JC. Comparison of outcomes following polidocanol microfoam and radiofrequency ablation of incompetent thigh great and accessory saphenous veins. J Vasc Surg Venous Lymphat Disord. 2023;11(5):916–20.
14. Deak ST. Treatment of superficial venous insufficiency in a large patient cohort with retrograde administration of ultrasound-guided polidocanol endovenous microfoam versus endovenous laser ablation. J Vasc Surg Venous Lymphat Disord. 2022;10:999–1006.e2.
15. Eggen CAM, Alozai T, Pronk P, Mooij MC, Gaastra MTW, Unlu C, et al. Ten-year follow up of a randomized controlled trial comparing saphenofemoral ligation and stripping of the great

saphenous vein with endovenous laser ablation (980 nm) using local tumescent anesthesia. J Vasc Surg Venous Lymphat Disord. 2022;10:646–53.

16. Brittenden J, Cooper D, Dimitrova M, Scotland G, Cotton SC, Elders A, et al. Five-year outcomes of a randomized trial of treatments for varicose veins. N Engl J Med. 2019;381:912–22.
17. Yang J, Chung S, Srivatsa S. Prospective randomized trial of antithrombotic strategies following great saphenous vein ablation using injectable polidocanol endovenous microfoam (Varithena). J Vasc Surg Venous Lymphat Disord. 2023;11:488–97.e4.
18. Chin AL, Talutis SD, Lawrence PF, Woo K, Rollo J, Jimenez JC. Factors associated with ablation related thrombus extension (ARTE) following GSV closure with endovenous microfoam ablation. [abstract]. In: Western Vascular Society 38th Annual Meeting; September 9–12, 2023 (Accepted for presentation).
19. Gloviczki P, Lawrence PF, Wasan SM, Meissner MH, Almeida J, Brown KR, et al. The 2023 Society for Vascular, American Venous Forum and American Vein and Lymphatic Society clinical practice guidelines for the management of varicose veins of the lower extremities. Part II. J Vasc Surg Venous Lymphat Disord. 2024;12:101670.

Chapter 6

Cyanoacrylate Treatment of Superficial Venous Insufficiency

Technique and Results

Amanda L. Chin and Johnathon C. Rollo

BACKGROUND

Cyanoacrylate is a liquid adhesive that was first approved by the US Food and Drug Administration (FDA) for endovascular application in 2000, when Trufill n-BCA Liquid Embolic System (Cordis, Miami Lakes, FL) obtained clearance for presurgical devascularizaton of cerebral arteriovenous malformations.[1] The monomeric form of cyanoacrylate consists of an ethylene molecule with a cyano group and an ester attached to one of the carbons. The specific hydrocarbon attached to the ester (the R position) contributes to the name of the cyanoacrylate. When exposed to an anion, such as those in blood, polymerization into a solid material is initiated with bonding of the ethylene units.[2] Instillation of cyanoacrylate within a vessel causes an inflammatory reaction in the wall followed by closure with coaptation.

Cyanoacrylate closure (CAC) of incompetent veins is a non-thermal, non-tumescent, and non-sclerosant endovenous ablation technique for the treatment of venous insufficiency. The concept was first developed by Dr. Rod Raabe, an interventional radiologist, at Inland Imaging in Spokane, WA. In 2011, the results from a pilot study on use of CAC of truncal veins in swine models were reported. Following adhesive delivery to swine superficial epigastric veins, chosen due to their similarities to human great saphenous veins, venous closure, segmental wall thickening, and fibrosis were observed on histologic examination at 60 days.[1] The first-in-human use of endovenous CAC in great saphenous veins was reported in 2013, demonstrating safety and efficacy.[3, 4] It was subsequently marketed as VenaSeal adhesive, a proprietary n-butyl-2-cyanoacrylate (n-BCA) based formulation that received FDA approval in 2015 for the treatment of symptomatic lower extremity varicose veins through endovascular embolization with coaptation. CAC offers advantages over other endovenous ablation techniques as it omits the need for tumescent anesthesia as well as post-procedure compression stockings.[3–6]

DEVICE

The VenaSeal closure system is a sterile, single patient kit that includes the delivery system and proprietary liquid adhesive. The adhesive, a proprietary n-butyl-2-cyanoacrylate (n-BCA) based formulation, is a clear liquid that is contained within a screw-capped vial, sterilized by exposure to dry heat. 5 mL total is provided within each kit. The delivery system is composed of the following components: dispenser gun, dispenser tips, catheter, introducer, dilator, 3 mL syringes, and 0.035" 180 cm straight floppy-tip guidewire. The dispenser gun consists of an integrated barrel and trigger, which delivers 0.10 mL of adhesive with each 3-second depression. The introducer is 7 Fr with an effective length of 80 cm. Along its length, there are circumferential markings spaced 10 mm apart to aid in calculated retraction of the delivery catheter during the procedure. The delivery catheter itself is 5 Fr with an effective length of

DOI: 10.1201/9781003316626-8

91 cm. Its high echogenicity enables the catheter tip to be easily visualized for precise adhesive administration. A laser marking at 3 cm from the tip indicates the optimal priming location for the adhesive at the start of the procedure, and another marking at 85 cm from the tip assists with catheter and introducer alignment.

INDICATIONS

Like other endovenous ablation techniques, the VenaSeal closure system is indicated for permanent closure of lower extremity superficial truncal veins, such as the great and small saphenous veins (GSV and SSV), in adults with symptomatic venous reflux as demonstrated by duplex ultrasound. While most studies discuss treatment of saphenous veins less than 2 cm in diameter, there have been reports of successful closure of incompetent veins up to 2.8 cm.[7]

CONTRAINDICATIONS

CAC with the VenaSeal adhesive is contraindicated in patients with previous hypersensitivity reactions to the VenaSeal adhesive or cyanoacrylates, acute superficial thrombophlebitis, thrombophlebitis migrans, and acute sepsis.

TECHNIQUE

The extremity is prepped and draped in standard sterile fashion. Ultrasound is first used to map out the course of the target truncal vein and locate its most distal point for intended access. Below the knee and/or above knee GSV is an acceptable target. The entire GSV can be treated in one application. Accurate and effective treatment of the small saphenous or anterior accessory GSV is also possible due to the lack of thermal action and viscosity of the glue embolic material. Local anesthetic is administered at the access site. Using standard micropuncture technique with a 5 Fr micropuncture access kit, the vein is accessed with a 21G needle under ultrasound guidance. An 0.018" microaccess wire is advanced into the vein followed by the microsheath/dilator. After removal of the microaccess wire and dilator, the 0.035" J-wire guidewire from the VenaSeal kit is advanced into the truncal vein via the microsheath. The microsheath is then exchanged with the 7 Fr blue introducer/dilator over the guidewire into the saphenofemoral junction (SFJ). Once fully advanced, the guidewire and dilator are removed, and the introducer is flushed with saline. Under ultrasound guidance, the introducer tip is then positioned 5 cm caudal to the SFJ.

The delivery catheter is then prepped per manufacturer instructions. Using the provided dispenser tip and 3 mL syringe, the VenaSeal adhesive is extracted from the vial and air bubbles removed. The dispenser tip is detached, and syringe is connected to the delivery catheter with a standard Luer lock. To insert the syringe into the dispenser gun, the release button is pushed and the plunger pulled back; the syringe can then be inserted and rotated firmly to secure. The delivery can now be primed by pulling the trigger of the dispenser gun until adhesive is advanced to the 3 cm laser marker from the tip; it is imperative that the adhesive is not advanced beyond this point to prevent premature exposure and polymerization of the glue upon insertion into the vein, as this will cause a glue plug in the delivery catheter. The catheter is then advanced into the introducer until the 85 cm laser marker on the catheter is aligned with the hub of the introducer. Once at this position, the introducer is pulled back 5 cm and the catheter advanced fully to spin-lock in place. This maneuver positions the delivery catheter tip at 5 cm from the SFJ, which should be verified on ultrasound prior to proceeding.

While applying constant compression with the ultrasound transducer in transverse position at 2–3 cm above the delivery catheter tip, the first 0.10 mL aliquot of adhesive is delivered into the vein by pulling and holding the dispenser trigger for 3 seconds. The catheter is immediately pulled back 1 cm, another 0.10 mL aliquot delivered, and again pulled back 3 cm. Manual compression is then applied to the treated venous segment in addition to compression with the transducer for a minimum of 3 minutes. The exact number of aliquots delivered at the initial treatment segment varies somewhat based on experience, but for larger veins (>1 cm) I recommend 3 aliquots delivered. Once complete, the delivery catheter tip is located with ultrasound. Compression is again applied just proximal to the tip, and the remaining length of incompetent vein may be treated with the following delivery sequence: administration of 0.10 mL adhesive by pulling trigger for 3 seconds, retraction of the catheter 3 cm, and compression for 30 seconds. It is important to cease delivery of adhesive 5 cm from the access site to avoid injection into the subcutaneous tissue. While holding the introducer stationary, the catheter is unlocked from the introducer and recaptured by retracting it through the introducer until the proximal laser mark is visible 1–5 cm outside of the introducer. The delivery catheter and introducer are then removed together, and compression held for hemostasis. A completion ultrasound duplex is performed at the conclusion of the procedure to confirm vein closure along the treated segment.

While post-procedure compression stockings are typically recommended following other endovenous ablation procedures, high closure rates of treated truncal veins have been demonstrated in the absence of the use of compression stockings (4–6). This offers a significant benefit of CAC given frequent patient dissatisfaction and limited compliance of compression stocking use. I recommend the patient is wrapped in compression ace wrap for 2 days post procedure to reduce inflammatory reaction.

CLINICAL OUTCOMES

Early Trials

Results from the first-in-human trial reported by Almeida et al.[3, 4] demonstrated closure of the great saphenous vein (GSV) in 92% of the patient cohort at 1 year, along with significant improvement of symptoms as measured by a reduction in Venous Clinical Severity Score (VCSS). In 2015, the initial results from the European Sapheon Closure System Observational Prospective (eSCOPE) Study were published by Proebstle et al.[8] This was a single-arm, prospective, multicenter study conducted at seven centers in four European countries evaluating outcomes of VenaSeal CAC for GSV reflux, which demonstrated a cumulative 12-month survival free from recanalization of 92.9% in a total of 70 treated veins. At the 3-year follow-up, closure rates remained high at 88.5%.[9]

Randomized Control Trial

The VenaSeal closure system (VeClose) pivotal study was a multicenter, prospective randomized control trial reported by Morrison et al. in which patients with venous reflux in the GSV were treated with either CAC utilizing the VenaSeal closure system or radiofrequency ablation (RFA) with the ClosureFast system (Medtronic, Minneapolis, MN).[10] A total of 222 patients were randomized, with 108 patients treated with CAC and 114 patients with RFA. All study participants were symptomatic with documented reflux of the GSV >0.5 seconds, GSV diameter measuring 3–12 mm while standing, and CEAP classification C2-C4b. 3-month closure rates were 99% for CAC and 96% for RFA with all primary end point analyses supporting the study's non-inferiority hypothesis. Pain during the procedure and immediately post-procedure were similar between groups, however ecchymosis at day 3 was *absent* in significantly more patients treated with CAC than RFA (48% vs. 68%, $p < 0.01$). VCSS improved by approximately 3.5 from baseline in both groups, with no statistical differences. No patients developed deep venous thrombosis or pulmonary embolism.

Follow-up results of the VeClose trial at 36 months[11] and 5 years[12] were also reported, again demonstrating non-inferiority of CAC compared with RFA. At 5 years, Kaplan-Meier estimates for freedom from recanalization in the randomized CAC and RFA groups were 91.4% and 85.2%, respectively. Both groups also demonstrated sustained improvements in EuroQol-Five Dimension and quality of life measures.

Post-Market Trial

Gibson et al. reported the results of the first post-market, prospective trial in the United States of CAC for incompetent non-GSV truncal veins in the Lake Washington Vascular VenaSeal Post-Market Evaluation (WAVES) Study.[5] It was a single-center, multi-investigator, single-arm prospective study investigating the use of CAC in a cohort of subjects with symptomatic venous reflux disease in the GSV, small saphenous vein (SSV), and/or accessory saphenous vein (ASV). Inclusion criteria included CEAP class C2–5, target vein diameters 4–20 mm, and a refluxing segment >0.5 seconds of at least 10 mm in length. Notably, unlike the prior VeClose randomized trial that utilized post-procedure compression stockings for comparison of CAC and RFA, the WAVES study did not.

A total of 70 truncal veins were treated in 50 patients. All treated veins (48 GSV, 14 ASV, and 8 SSV) had complete closure as demonstrated by ultrasound duplex at 1 month. At 36 months, GSV and SSV closures remained 100%, and ASV closure was 92.9%.[6] The one patient with recanalization of the ASV had successful closure of the primary target vein, the GSV, at 36 months. Venous quality of life indices utilized including the revised VCSS, Aberdeen Varicose Vein Questionnaire, and the EQ Visual Analogue Scale all demonstrated statistically significant improvement between baseline and both 1- and 3-month follow-up ($p < 0.001$). Forty-nine patients (98%) indicated that they were either "completely" or "somewhat" satisfied with the procedure. The most common adverse event was phlebitis, which occurred in 10 patients (20%), all of which resolved by 1 month except in one patient.

Treatment in CEAP Class 6

Prior studies described excluded patients with advanced venous disease and active venous ulcers. However, O'Banion et al. reported a multi-institutional retrospective review of all patients with CEAP class 6 who underwent VenaSeal CAC versus ClosureFast RFA from 2015 to 2020.[13] A total of 119 patients were included in this study, with 68 patients treated with RFA and 51 patients with CAC. CAC showed a superior time to wound healing (43 days) compared to RFA (104 days) in patients with active venous ulcers at time of treatment ($p = 0.001$). On multivariate analysis, treatment modality was the only significant predictor of time to wound healing.

An adjunct study performed by the authors with the same study population demonstrated a less frequent need to treat perforator veins following VenaSeal CAC compared to ClosureFast RFA in patients with CEAP class 6 venous ulcers.[14] They hypothesized that the increased treatment length below the knee afforded by CAC compared to RFA affected refluxing perforators and thus the need for subsequent perforator treatment in patients with active venous ulcers. More broadly, these findings may suggest that any non-thermal treatment modality that does not confer the risk of nerve injury can eliminate a longer length of saphenous vein, particularly the crucial below knee segment, thus inherently decreasing the need for subsequent procedures and shortening time to ulcer healing.

Adverse Events and Complications

Hypersensitivity Reactions

Hypersensitivity reactions (HSR) are a unique risk following treatment with CAC.[15–19] While studies have had varying definitions of HSR, it is generally recognized as the development of a diffuse erythematous rash overlying the treated vein frequently associated with itching, occurring within the first few weeks after CAC. HSR is noted to be distinct from post-procedure phlebitis, which is a known adverse event following endothermal ablation of incompetent saphenous veins presenting as localized pain, tenderness, or swelling over the treated vein without significant erythema.

Gibson et al. performed a combined retrospective/prospective review of CAC at a single institution over 5 years to evaluate the frequency and severity of HSR.[15] In this study, 379 limbs were treated with CAC in 286 patients, with an incidence of 18 HSRs (6% patients, 5.8% treated limbs). These were further subdivided into mild presentations (4.3%) requiring either no treatment or over-the-counter medications, moderate (1.3%) treated with a 6-day tapered course of oral steroids, or severe (0.3%) if reaction prolonged >30 days or required vein excision. The one patient with severe HSR developed a rash on the torso in addition to the overlying treated area, initially resolving with oral steroids but returning on several occasions, months to a year later. The patient ultimately underwent excision of the treated vein with histology revealing a giant cell foreign body reaction within the specimen and chronic inflammation. The symptoms resolved fully after vein excision.

There have been numerous other studies describing HSR following CAC with a wide range of frequency reported. Sermsathanasawadi et al. showed an incidence of HSR in 15.8% of patients following CAC in a study performed in Thailand.[18] Park et al. reported an incidence as high as 25.4% in Korean patients.[16] Differences in reported incidence among studies may be secondary to differing definitions of HSR or cofounding factors such as racial differences.

Careful patient selection for CAC is important in prevention of HSR. Avoidance in patients with known allergies to adhesives and glues including artificial nails, eyelashes, or bandages as well as patients with history of skin conditions such as atopic dermatitis or psoriasis is recommended.[15] Recapture of the delivery catheter within the blue introducer sheath may avoid inadvertent spillage of adhesive into the subcutaneous tissues and dermis and also help to prevent a rarer complication such as granuloma or abscess formation at the access site.[20]

Endovenous Glue-Induced Thrombosis

Similar to endothermal heat-induced thrombosis (EHIT), endovenous glue-induced thrombosis (EGIT) is a complication of CAC in which there is thrombus extension into the deep vein after the procedure. Initial trials of VenaSeal reported a wide range of incidence of EGIT from 0% to 21.1% (3, 8, 10), treated with either observation on serial duplex ultrasound or short course of anticoagulation. Retrospective reviews have also been performed which suggest possible risk factors for EGIT. Pillutla et al. demonstrated a 13% rate of EGIT following CAC in 76 GSV. Within those patients who developed EGIT, older age was found to be a significant risk factor ($p = 0.03$). Furthermore, Cho et al. performed a retrospective analysis of CAC in 191 patients, demonstrating EGIT in 5.8%.[21] Interestingly, preoperative saphenous vein diameter of <5 mm was the only associated risk factor for development of EGIT ($p = 0.04$). This is contrary to current literature on EHIT following RFA, which suggests a significantly higher rate with larger saphenous vein diameters, particularly >8 mm.[22] Presently, there are no consensus guidelines that exist for anticoagulation treatment of EGIT after CAC.

CONCLUSIONS

CAC is a safe and effective endovenous therapy for treatment of saphenous vein reflux that promotes closure with coaptation. Unlike other endovenous techniques, it does not require the use of tumescent anesthesia or post-procedure compression stockings to result in high rates of long-term target vein occlusion. Due to the non-thermal closure, it is safe and effective for below knee GSV, SSV, and AAGSV. However, it is important to adhere to instructions for use to and avoid in patients with allergies to adhesives and certain dermatologic or autoimmune conditions as to prevent the distinct complication of hypersensitivity reaction following treatment.

REFERENCES

1. Almeida JI, Min RJ, Raabe R, McLean DJ, Madsen M. Cyanoacrylate adhesive for the closure of truncal veins: 60-day swine model results. Vascular and Endovascular Surgery. 2011 Oct 1;45(7):631–35.
2. Pollak JS, White RI. The use of cyanoacrylate adhesives in peripheral embolization. Journal of Vascular and Interventional Radiology. 2001 Aug 1;12(8):907–13.
3. Almeida JI, Javier JJ, Mackay E, Bautista C, Proebstle TM. First human use of cyanoacrylate adhesive for treatment of saphenous vein incompetence. Journal of Vascular Surgery: Venous and Lymphatic Disorders. 2013 Apr 1;1(2):174–80.
4. Almeida JI, Javier JJ, Mackay EG, Bautista C, Cher DJ, Proebstle TM. Thirty-sixth-month follow-up of first-in-human use of cyanoacrylate adhesive for treatment of saphenous vein incompetence. Journal of Vascular Surgery: Venous and Lymphatic Disorders. 2017 Sep;5(5):658–66.
5. Gibson K, Ferris B. Cyanoacrylate closure of incompetent great, small and accessory saphenous veins without the use of post-procedure compression: Initial outcomes of a post-market evaluation of the VenaSeal system (the WAVES Study). Vascular. 2017 Apr 1;25(2):149–56.
6. Gibson K, Minjarez R, Gunderson K, Ferris B. Need for adjunctive procedures following cyanoacrylate closure of incompetent great, small and accessory saphenous veins without the use of postprocedure compression: Three-month data from a postmarket evaluation of the VenaSeal system (the WAVES Study). Phlebology. 2019 May 1;34(4):231–37.
7. Park I. Successful use of VenaSeal system for the treatment of large great saphenous vein of 2.84-cm diameter. Annals of Surgical Treatment and Research. 2018 Apr;94(4):219–21.
8. Proebstle TM, Alm J, Dimitri S, Rasmussen L, Whiteley M, Lawson J, et al. The European multicenter cohort study on cyanoacrylate embolization of refluxing great saphenous veins. Journal of Vascular Surgery: Venous and Lymphatic Disorders. 2015 Jan 1;3(1):2–7.

9. Proebstle T, Alm J, Dimitri S, Rasmussen L, Whiteley M, Lawson J, et al. Three-year follow-up results of the prospective European multicenter cohort study on cyanoacrylate embolization for treatment of refluxing great saphenous veins. Journal of Vascular Surgery: Venous and Lymphatic Disorders. 2021 Mar 1;9(2):329–34.
10. Morrison N, Gibson K, McEnroe S, Goldman M, King T, Weiss R, et al. Randomized trial comparing cyanoacrylate embolization and radiofrequency ablation for incompetent great saphenous veins (VeClose). Journal of Vascular Surgery. 2015 Apr 1;61(4):985–94.
11. Morrison N, Kolluri R, Vasquez M, Madsen M, Jones A, Gibson K. Comparison of cyanoacrylate closure and radiofrequency ablation for the treatment of incompetent great saphenous veins: 36-month outcomes of the VeClose randomized controlled trial. Phlebology. 2019 Jul;34(6):380–90.
12. Morrison N, Gibson K, Vasquez M, Weiss R, Jones A. Five-year extension study of patients from a randomized clinical trial (VeClose) comparing cyanoacrylate closure versus radiofrequency ablation for the treatment of incompetent great saphenous veins. Journal of Vascular Surgery: Venous and Lymphatic Disorders. 2020 Nov;8(6):978–89.
13. O'Banion LA, Reynolds KB, Kochubey M, Cutler B, Tefera EA, Dirks R, et al. A comparison of cyanoacrylate glue and radiofrequency ablation techniques in the treatment of superficial venous reflux in CEAP 6 patients. Journal of Vascular Surgery: Venous and Lymphatic Disorders. 2021 Sep 1;9(5):1215–21.
14. Kiguchi MM, Reynolds KB, Cutler B, Tefera E, Kochubey M, Dirks R, et al. The need for perforator treatment after VenaSeal and ClosureFast endovenous saphenous vein closure in CEAP 6 patients. Journal of Vascular Surgery: Venous and Lymphatic Disorders. 2021 Nov 1;9(6):1510–16.
15. Gibson K, Minjarez R, Rinehardt E, Ferris B. Frequency and severity of hypersensitivity reactions in patients after VenaSeal™ cyanoacrylate treatment of superficial venous insufficiency. Phlebology. 2020 Jun 1;35(5):337–44.
16. Park I, Jeong MH, Park CJ, Park WI, Park DW, Joh JH. Clinical features and management of "phlebitis-like abnormal reaction" after cyanoacrylate closure for the treatment of incompetent saphenous veins. Annals of Vascular Surgery. 2019 Feb 1;55:239–45.
17. Tang TY, Tiwari A. The VenaSeal™ Abnormal red skin reaction: Looks like but is not phlebitis! European Journal of Vascular and Endovascular Surgery. 2018 Jun 1;55(6):841.
18. Sermsathanasawadi N, Hanaroonsomboon P, Pruekprasert K, Prapassaro T, Puangpunngam N, Hongku K, et al. Hypersensitivity reaction after cyanoacrylate closure of incompetent saphenous veins in patients with chronic venous disease: A retrospective study. Journal of Vascular Surgery: Venous and Lymphatic Disorders. 2021 Jul;9(4):910–15.
19. Jones AD, Boyle EM, Woltjer R, Jundt JP, Williams AN. Persistent type IV hypersensitivity after cyanoacrylate closure of the great saphenous vein. Journal of Vascular Surgery Cases, Innovations and Techniques. 2019 Aug 7;5(3):372–74.
20. Sermsathanasawadi N, Pruekprasert K, Chinsakchai K, Wongwanit C, Ruangsetakit C. Cyanoacrylate granuloma after cyanoacrylate closure of incompetent saphenous veins. Dermatol Surgery. 2021 Oct;47(10):1372–75.
21. Cho S, Gibson K, Lee SH, Kim SY, Joh JH. Incidence, classification, and risk factors of endovenous glue-induced thrombosis after cyanoacrylate closure of the incompetent saphenous vein. Journal of Vascular Surgery: Venous and Lymphatic Disorders. 2020 Nov 1;8(6):991–98.
22. Lawrence PF, Chandra A, Wu M, Rigberg D, DeRubertis B, Gelabert H, et al. Classification of proximal endovenous closure levels and treatment algorithm. Journal of Vascular Surgery. 2010 Aug 1;52(2):388–93.

Chapter 7

Mechanochemical Ablation of the Saphenous Veins

Benjamin J. DiPardo and Jesus G. Ulloa

BACKGROUND

The standard of care for superficial venous insufficiency has shifted from open high ligation and stripping to minimally invasive endovenous ablation procedures, resulting in less postoperative pain, improved cosmesis, earlier return to normal activity, and decreased cost.[1–6] Numerous endovenous ablation techniques have been developed, including endovenous laser ablation (EVLA), radiofrequency ablation (RFA), endovenous foam sclerotherapy or cyanoacrylate closure, and mechanochemical ablation (MOCA). MOCA was developed in 2005 by Dr. Tal at Yale University and subsequently marketed as the ClariVein device (Merit Medical, West Jordan, UT). ClariVein received approval from the US Food and Drug Administration (FDA) in 2008 and entered clinical use in the United States and Europe in 2010.[7] It employs a catheter with a rotating wire at the tip to cause vasospasm and endothelial damage, with concurrent instillation of liquid sclerosant.[8] The resulting wire tip vasospasm serves to increase contact between the endothelium and sclerosant. Unlike thermal ablation techniques, the ClariVein device is disposable and does not require purchase and maintenance of an energy source. Additionally, MOCA does not risk thermal injury to surrounding structures, and therefore unlike thermal endovenous ablation techniques, MOCA does not require the use of tumescent anesthesia.

DEVICE

There are two single-use components to the ClariVein device: the catheter and the motor drive unit (MDU). The catheter has an outer diameter of 0.035" and therefore can be introduced through a 4Fr micropuncture sheath. The catheter contains a rotating wire and infusion lumen, which connects to a 5 mL syringe via a Luer lock for flushing and instillation of sclerosant. The catheter is available in 45 cm and 65 cm lengths, which includes 2 cm of angled exposed wire at the distal aspect. The diameter of rotation of the wire tip is 6.5 mm. The wire can be sheathed and unsheathed from the catheter. After positioning the catheter appropriately in the vein, the catheter is connected to the MDU and cannot be removed. The MDU contains a 9V battery and motor which can be set to speeds between 2000 and 3500 rpm and is activated by depressing a finger trigger.

INDICATIONS

Indications for MOCA to treat great saphenous vein (GSV) or small saphenous vein (SSV) reflux are similar to those for other methods of endovenous ablation discussed elsewhere. Veins up to 20 mm diameter have been treated with MOCA. Although the diameter of excursion of the wire tip is 6.5 mm, endothelial damage of larger veins can be effectively accomplished with ultrasound-guided compression. The length of vein treatable in one session is

DOI: 10.1201/9781003316626-9

limited by sclerosant dosage. Bilateral long-segment GSV ablation is therefore not possible, but bilateral short segment ablations may be done concurrently.

TECHNIQUE

The extremity is prepped and draped in the usual sterile fashion, and ultrasound is used to map out the course of the incompetent truncal vein. If the entire GSV is to be treated, two access sites may be necessary given the maximum catheter length of 65 cm. Local anesthesia is administered at the access site, and the vein is accessed under ultrasound guidance using the micropuncture technique with a micropuncture access kit. The patient is placed into a reverse Trendelenburg position to permit distension of the incompetent truncal vein. The 21G needle is introduced into the vein allowing passage of the 0.018" micropuncture wire, which is visualized in the vein using ultrasound. The needle is then exchanged for a 4 or 5 Fr micropuncture sheath. The ClariVein device is prepared according to manufacturer instructions and the catheter is flushed with saline. Sclerosant is prepared. Use of sodium tetradecyl sulfate (STS) and polidocanol (Pol.) are described. We use STS diluted to a concentration of 1.5% for the GSV and 1% for the SSV. The total volume of sclerosant is calculated based on the treatment length and vein diameter (Table 7.1). The catheter is then advanced through the target vein under ultrasound guidance. For treatment of the GSV, the catheter is advanced to place the tip

Table 7.1 Typical Volume of STS (left) and Polidocanol (right) Instilled (in mL), Determined by the Vein Length and Diameter

	STS								*Polidocanol*							
	Length (cm)								*Length (cm)*							
Diameter (mm)	*15*	*20*	*25*	*30*	*35*	*40*	*45*	*50*	*15*	*20*	*25*	*30*	*35*	*40*	*45*	*50*
3	1	2	2	2	3	3	3	4	1	2	2	2	3	3	3	4
4	2	2	3	3	4	4	5	5	2	2	3	3	4	4	5	5
5	2	3	3	4	5	6	6	7	2	3	3	4	5	6	6	7
6	3	3	4	5	6	7	8	9	3	3	4	5	6	7	8	8
7	3	4	5	6	7	8	9	10	3	4	5	6	7	8	8	8
8	4	5	6	7	8	9	10	10	4	5	6		8	8	8	8
9	4	5	7	8	9	10	10	10	4	5	7	7	8	8	8	8
10	4	6	7	9	10	10	10	10	4	6	7	8	8	8	8	8
11	5	7	8	10	10	10	10	10	5	7	8	8	8	8	8	8
12	5	7	9	10	10	10	10	10	5	7	8	8	8	8	8	8
13	6	8	10	10	10	10	10	10	6	8	8	8	8	8	8	8
14	6	8	10	10	10	10	10	10	6	8	8	8	8	8	8	8
15	7	9	10	10	10	10	10	10	7	8	8	8	8	8	8	8
16	7	10	10	10	10	10	10	10	7	8	8	8	8	8	8	8
17	8	10	10	10	10	10	10	10	8	8	8	8	8	8	8	8
18	8	10	10	10	10	10	10	10	8	8	8	8	8	8	8	8
19	9	10	10	10	10	10	10	10	8	8	8	8	8	8	8	8
20	9	10	10	10	10	10	10	10	8	8	8	8	8	8	8	8

Note: STS concentrations of 1.5% and 1% are used for the GSV and SSV, respectively. Volumes above represent 2% polidocanol for the GSV and SSV.

2 cm distal to the saphenofemoral junction (SFJ). It may also be placed immediately distal to the inferior epigastric vein if this is more proximal. For SSV ablation, the wire tip is placed just distal to the fascial curve. Care must be taken to confirm visualization of the distal aspect of the catheter on ultrasound using a longitudinal view in order to avoid inadvertent treatment too centrally and consequent risk of DVT. After the device is appropriately positioned the catheter is connected to the MDU. The patient is now positioned in a Trendelenburg position to flatten the incompetent truncal vein against the wire tip. The wire is then unsheathed, confirming no change in position on ultrasound. The vein is then treated by turning on the motor of the device. The device is slowly pulled back 5 mm over 3 seconds to induce vasospasm at the proximal aspect of the ablation zone. We also routinely compress the SFJ with the ultrasound probe to further prevent central embolization of sclerosant. The vein is then treated with a pullback rate of 6–7 s/cm with slow continuous instillation of sclerosant. As the device reaches the sheath, the sheath is withdrawn over the catheter to allow treatment of the distal aspect of the vein. The wire tip is re-sheathed and the device is removed. Pressure is held for hemostasis. A completion duplex ultrasound is performed before leaving the procedure suite in order to confirm technical success.

Histological Effects

A caprine animal model demonstrated complete saphenous vein occlusion after MOCA but not after mechanical irritation or STS instillation alone. Veins treated with MOCA showed complete fibrotic obliteration of the lumen and fibrotic changes to the media.[9]

Sclerosant

MOCA may be performed with STS or polidocanol, and there is no consensus on the ideal sclerosant agent or concentration. Lam et al. performed a randomized controlled trial comparing MOCA performed with polidocanol concentrations of 3%, 2%, and 1% microfoam. The 1% microfoam formulation resulted in a closure rate of 30% at 6 weeks[10] and was therefore abandoned. At 6 months follow-up, technical success was 69.8% in the 2% polidocanol group compared to 78.0% in the 3% polidocanol group ($p = 0.027$). However, Venous Clinical Severity Score (VCSS) and Aberdeen Varicose Vein Questionnaire (AVVQ) scores were similarly improved after MOCA between the two groups, and thus the clinical significance of this difference is unclear.[11]

Phlebectomy

Studies have shown lower reintervention rates with concomitant phlebectomy but possible overtreatment of patients who would not go on to need phlebectomy after truncal vein ablation.[12, 13] As with other methods of endovenous ablation, concomitant phlebectomy is frequently performed with MOCA and is described both before and after the ablation procedure. When phlebectomy is indicated we routinely perform it after completion of the MOCA procedure. In the case of MOCA, concomitant phlebectomy carries a theoretical risk of sclerosant extravasation from avulsed vein segments with tissue necrosis; however this complication has not been reported in the literature nor has it been observed in our practice.

Post-Procedure

A dressing is placed over the access site, and the leg is compressed with an elastic bandage. Early ambulation and calf flexion are encouraged to clear the deep veins of sclerosant. We routinely obtain follow-up duplex ultrasound within 1 week after the procedure to assess closure level and possible need for anticoagulation.[14]

OUTCOMES

Anatomic and Clinical Success

Since the initial report by van Eekeren in 2011,[15] numerous prospective and retrospective observational studies have described MOCA for treatment of both GSV and SSV reflux,[10, 16–25] summarized in Table 7.2. Initial technical success is reported as >98%. At 6 months, durable anatomical success is described in 87–97% of patients treated with MOCA. At 1 year follow-up, vein closure remains durable in 77–95%. Witte et al. reported 3-year follow-up of a prospective series of patients treated with MOCA. In this series, persistent vein closure was maintained in 87% of patients at 3 years.[26] The clinical success rate at 3 years was 83%, with statistically significant deterioration between 1 and 3 years as measured by the Venous Clinical Severity Score (VCSS) or Aberdeen Varicose Vein Questionnaire (AVVQ). However, not all recanalizations were clinically significant, and of the 15 patients with ultrasound-documented GSV recanalization, only four had undergone reintervention at 3 years.

Procedural Pain and Complications

Several observational and randomized studies have shown statistically significant decreased pain during MOCA compared to other methods of endovenous ablation, although absolute differences in pain scores are relatively small.[18, 23, 27, 29]

Serious complications after MOCA are rare. Superficial thrombophlebitis, hematoma, ecchymosis, and skin hyperpigmentation are the most commonly reported complications. A systematic review of 1521 MOCA procedures described a DVT rate of 0.2%, PE rate of 0.1%, and paresthesia rate of <0.1%.[33] With close post-procedure ultrasound follow-up within 1 week, we reported a 13.5% rate of thrombus extending central to the SFJ (comparable to endothermal heat induced thrombosis [EHIT] level greater than 2) and routinely treat these patients with a course of anticoagulation.[32] Specifically, among 92.7% of patients with successful ablation, 86.5% showed EHIT 1 level closure, 3.4% level 2 closure, 8.9% level 3 closure, and 1% level 4 closure. Other series describe initial duplex surveillance at 1 to 2 months and report venous thromboembolism (VTE) rates of less than 2%. Inadvertent arterial instillation of sclerotherapy through an unrecognized arteriovenous fistula has been described which resulted in amputation.[34]

Randomized Controlled Trials (RCTs)

Four RCTs have been completed comparing MOCA to thermal endovenous ablation procedures. Lane et al.[23] and Bootun et al.[22] performed an RCT comparing MOCA to RFA in a total of 170 patients with GSV or SSV reflux. Of those randomized, 82 patients underwent MOCA, and 82 patients underwent RFA, with 74% undergoing concomitant phlebectomy. The primary outcomes were maximum and average procedural pain which were significantly

Table 7.2 Studies Evaluating MOCA

Author	*Year*	*Ref*	*Design*	*Treatments*	*Sample Size*[c]	*Vein*	*Sclerosant*	*MOCA Closure Rate, n (%)*	*MOCA Clinical Outcomes*	*MOCA Complications (%)*	*Comparisons*
van Eekeren	2011	(15)	Prospective	MOCA	30	GSV	1.5% Pol.	Initial 30/30 (100) 6 weeks: 26/30 (87)	VCSS initial: 3 VCSS 6 weeks: 1*	Ecchymosis (30) Superficial phlebitis (13)	
Elias	2012	(16)	Prospective	MOCA	30	GSV	1.5% STS	Initial 30/30 (100) 6 months: 29/30 (97)	VCSS initial 4.5	Ecchymosis (10)	
van Eekeren	2013	(27)	Prospective, observational comparative	MOCA or RFA	34 MOCA 34 RFA	GSV	1.5%/2% Pol.	n/a	AVVQ initial: 7.1 AVVQ 6 weeks: 5.0*	Hematoma (6) Induration (12) Hyperpigmentaiton (9)	Less postoperative pain in first two weeks after MOCA compared to RFA, with earlier return to activity and work
Boersma	2013	(17)	Prospective	MOCA	50	SSV	1.5%/2% Pol.	Initial 50/50 (100) 6 weeks: 50/50 (100) 1 year 44/47 (94)	VCSS initial 3 VCSS 6 weeks 1*	Ecchymosis (12) Induration (12) Superficial phlebitis (14)	
van Eekeren[a] Witte	2014 2017	(25) (26)	Prospective	MOCA	106	GSV	1.5%/2% Pol.	Initial 105/106 (99) 6 months: 96/103 (93) 1 year: (92) 3 years: (87)	VCSS initial 4 VCSS 1 year: 1* VCSS 3 years: 1*	Hematoma (9) Thrombophlebitis (3) Hyperpigmentation (5)	

(Continued)

Table 7.2 Studies Evaluating MOCA *(Continued)*

Author	*Year*	*Ref*	*Design*	*Treatments*	*Sample Size*[c]	*Vein*	*Sclerosant*	*MOCA Closure Rate, n (%)*	*MOCA Clinical Outcomes*	*MOCA Complications (%)*	*Comparisons*
Vun	2015	(18)	Retrospective	MOCA	57 MOCA 50 RFA 40 EVLT	MOCA: 51 GSV 6 SSV	1.5% STS	4–6 weeks: 52/57 (91)	n/a	n/a	Shorter procedure, less postoperative pain with MOCA compared to EVLT and RFA
Deijen	2016	(21)	Retrospective	MOCA	570	GSV 438 SSV 132	1.5%/2% Pol.	6–12 weeks: 457/506 (90)	n/a	Phlebitis (2) DVT (0.4) PE (0.4) Sural nerve injury (0.2)	
Bishawi Kim	2014 2017	(19) (20)	Prospective	MOCA	126	GSV	1.5% STS or 1.5% Pol.	Initial 125/125 (100) 3 months: 98/100 (98) 6 months 84/89 (94) 1 year: 75/79 (95) 2 years 60/65 (92)	VCSS initial: 9.5 VCSS 6 months: 3*	Hematoma (1) Ecchymosis (9) Phlebitis (10)	
Bootun Lane	2016 2017	(22) (23)	RCT	MOCA vs RFA	83 MOCA 82 RFA	MOCA: 77 GSV 6 SSV	2% STS	1 month: 64/69 (93) 6 months: 54/62 (87)	VCSS initial: 6 VCSS 1 month: 2 VCSS 6 months: 2 AVVQ initial: 19.5 AVVQ 1 month: 12.1 AVVQ 6 months: 11.8	Phlebitis (4) DVT (1)	Less procedural pain with MOCA, similar occlusion rates, VCSS, AVVQ, quality of life at 1 and 6 months follow-up

Lam[b]	2016	(10)	RCT	MOCA	76	GSV	2% Pol.: 25 3% Pol.: 28 1% Pol. microfoam: 23	6 weeks 7/23 (30)	VCSS initial 6.7 (1% microfoam) VCSS 6 weeks: 3.4	n/a	
Lam	2022	(11)	RCT	MOCA	375	GSV	2% POLI: 189 3% POLI: 186	6 weeks: 2%: 168/189 (89) 3%: 156/186 (84)	VCSS initial: 5.4 vs 5.4 (2% vs 3%) VCSS 6 weeks: 4.2 vs 4.2 VCSS 6 months:: 4.1 vs 4.2	PE: (0.5) DVT: (0.5)	
Tang	2017	(28)	Prospective	MOCA	393	GSV 333 SSV 60	2% STS	Initial 393/393 (100) 8 weeks: 382/393 (97)	n/a	Phlebitis (4)	
Holewijn	2019	(29)	RCT	MOCA vs RFA	105 MOCA 104 RFA	GSV	1.5%/3% Pol.	4 weeks: 98/102 (96) 1 year: 66/81 (81) 2 years: 55/76 (72)	VCSS initial 4.9 VCSS 4 weeks 1.8 VCSS 1 year 1.8 VCSS 2 years 1.0 AVVQ initial 14.3 AVVQ 1 month 8.9 AVVQ 1 year 7.5 AVVQ 2 years 5.0	Hyperpigmentation (7) Phlebitis (12) Induration (17) Hematoma (14)	Compared to RFA, MOCA associated with less postoperative pain, faster improvement in VCSS, higher rates of hyperpigmentation

(Continued)

Table 7.2 Studies Evaluating MOCA *(Continued)*

Author	*Year*	*Ref*	*Design*	*Treatments*	*Sample Size*[c]	*Vein*	*Sclerosant*	*MOCA Closure Rate, n (%)*	*MOCA Clinical Outcomes*	*MOCA Complications (%)*	*Comparisons*
Vähääho	2019	(30)	RCT	MOCA vs RFA vs EVLA	65 MOCA 34 EVLA 33 RFA	GSV	1.5% STS	1 month: 65/65 (100) 1 year: 45/55 (82)	AVVQ initial 15.8 AVVQ 1 year 6.2 *		Pigmentation (11)
Mohamed	2021	(31)	RCT	MOCA vs EVLA	75 MOCA 75 EVLA	MOCA: 61 GSV 6 ASV 8 SSV	1.5% STS	1 year: 53/69 (77)	AVVQ initial 13.4 AVVQ 1 year 2.0 * VCSS initial 6.5 VCSS 1 year 0 *	DVT (1)	No significant differences in procedural pain, recovery time. Higher technical success at one year, but comparable VCSS and AVVQ improvements
Chen	2022	(32)	Retrospective	MOCA	104	GSV	1.5% STS	<1 week: 89/96 (93)	n/a	EHIT class >2 (14)	

Notes:
Abbreviations: randomized controlled trial (RCT); mechanochemical ablation (MOCA); endovenous laser ablation (EVLA); radiofrequency ablation (RFA); greater saphenous vein (GSV); accessory saphenous vein (ASV); short saphenous vein (SSV); sodium tetradecyl sulfate (STS); polidocanol (Pol.); Venous Clinical Severity Score (VCSS); Aberdeen Varicose Vein Questionnaire (AVVQ); endothermal heat induced thrombosis (EHIT); deep venous thrombosis (DVT); pulmonary embolism (PE).
[a]Two studies describing same patient population
[b]Given low technical success in the 1% polidochanol microfoam arm, the study design dropped this arm and went on to enroll additional patients in the 2% and 3% polidochaenol arms, published as Lam et al. 2022
*p<0.05

lower in the MOCA group compared to RFA. Secondary outcomes of disease-specific and general quality of life were not different between MOCA and RFA. Disease severity measured by VCSS was improved after treatment and similar between MOCA and RFA. Technical success rates were similar at 1 month (MOCA 93%, RFA 92%, p = 0.40) and at 6 months (MOCA 87%, RFA 93%, p = 0.48).

Vähääho et al.(30) randomized 125 patients to MOCA, EVLA, or RFA. Of the planned 160 patients, 132 patients with GSV reflux were randomized: 65 to MOCA, 34 to EVLA, and 34 to RFA. The primary outcome was technical success, with 45/55 (82%) of patients after MOCA showing GSV ablation at 1 year, compared to 100% in the EVLA and RFA groups (p = 0.002). However, disease-specific quality of life (AVVQ) was significantly improved from baseline and similar between groups at 1 year. There was a trend toward higher rates of nerve injury in EVLA (9%) and RFA (7%) compared to MOCA (0%), which did not reach significance (p = 0.090). Perioperative pain scores were similar between groups.

Holewijn et al. recently published the 2-year follow-up results of the MARADONA trial, a multicenter prospective randomized controlled trial comparing MOCA to RFA for GSV incompetence.(29) The trial randomized 209 patients with primary GSV insufficiency to MOCA(105) or RFA.(104) The study design planned for randomization of 460 patients, but enrollment ended early due to funding issues. Initial technical success was >99% in both groups. In the first 14 days after the procedure pain scores were slightly lower with MOCA over RFA (0.2 vs 0.5, p = 0.010). Anatomic closure rates at 30 days were higher after RFA (97.2% vs 100%, p = 0.045) with four cases of complete or partial recanalization after MOCA. This difference persisted at 1 and 2-year follow-up (1 year 83.5% vs 94.2%, p = 0.025; 2 year 80.0% vs 88.3%, p = 0.066) due to partial recanalization in the MOCA patients. Complication rates were similar with the exception of higher incidence of hyperpigmentation at 30 days after MOCA than RFA (6.7% vs 1.9%, p = 0.038). There were similar rates of induration and edema. Aberdeen Varicose Vein Questionnaire (AVVQ) scores were similar between MOCA and RFA at 4 weeks, 1 year, and 2 year follow ups, with comparable decrease from baseline in both groups. Venous Clinical Severity Score (VCSS) improved faster in the MOCA group and were lower at 4 weeks after MOCA compared to RFA (1.8 vs 2.6 p = 0.001). VCSS scores were similar between groups at 1 and 2 years.

The LAMA trial, published in 2021, randomized 150 patients evenly to MOCA and EVLA.(31) Procedural pain was similar between groups. Technical success at 1 year was higher after EVLA compared to MOCA (persistent GSV occlusion in 91% vs 77%, p = 0.020). Disease-specific quality of life, however, was significantly decreased from baseline in both groups, with no differences between AVVQ at 1 year between MOCA and EVLA.

CONCLUSIONS

MOCA is an effective endovenous therapy for saphenous reflux, with high technical success rates comparable to other endovenous therapies. An advantage of MOCA is that it does not use thermal energy for vein ablation, and therefore it avoids the risk of thermal injury, does not require tumescent anesthesia, and is a single-use device which does not require an external energy source. Studies show similar or decreased procedural pain with MOCA compared to thermal endovenous ablation. Long-term durability of vein closure may be lower after MOCA, but the clinical significance of this is unclear and requires further investigation.

REFERENCES

1. Whing J, Nandhra S, Nesbitt C, Stansby G. Interventions for great saphenous vein incompetence. Cochrane Database Syst Rev. 2021;8(8):CD005624.
2. Brittenden J, Cotton SC, Elders A, Ramsay CR, Norrie J, Burr J, et al. A randomized trial comparing treatments for varicose veins. N Engl J Med. 2014;371(13):1218–27.
3. Siribumrungwong B, Noorit P, Wilasrusmee C, Attia J, Thakkinstian A. A systematic review and meta-analysis of randomised controlled trials comparing endovenous ablation and surgical intervention in patients with varicose vein. Eur J Vasc Endovasc Surg. 2012;44(2):214–23.
4. van den Bos R, Arends L, Kockaert M, Neumann M, Nijsten T. Endovenous therapies of lower extremity varicosities: A meta-analysis. J Vasc Surg. 2009;49(1):230–39.
5. Gloviczki P, Comerota AJ, Dalsing MC, Eklof BG, Gillespie DL, Gloviczki ML, et al. The care of patients with varicose veins and associated chronic venous diseases: Clinical practice guidelines of the Society for Vascular Surgery and the American Venous Forum. J Vasc Surg. 2011;53(5 Suppl):2S–48S.
6. Rautio T, Ohinmaa A, Perala J, Ohtonen P, Heikkinen T, Wiik H, et al. Endovenous obliteration versus conventional stripping operation in the treatment of primary varicose veins: A randomized controlled trial with comparison of the costs. J Vasc Surg. 2002;35(5):958–65.
7. Mueller RL, Raines JK. ClariVein mechanochemical ablation: Background and procedural details. Vasc Endovascular Surg. 2013;47(3):195–206.
8. Boersma D, van Haelst ST, van Eekeren RR, Vink A, Reijnen MM, de Vries JP, et al. Macroscopic and histologic analysis of vessel wall reaction after mechanochemical endovenous ablation using the ClariVein oc device in an animal model. Eur J Vasc Endovasc Surg. 2017;53(2):290–98.
9. Tal MG, Dos Santos SJ, Marano JP, Whiteley MS. Histologic findings after mechanochemical ablation in a caprine model with use of ClariVein. J Vasc Surg Venous Lymphat Disord. 2015;3(1):81–85.
10. Lam YL, Toonder IM, Wittens CH. Clarivein(R) mechano-chemical ablation an interim analysis of a randomized controlled trial dose-finding study. Phlebology. 2016;31(3):170–76.
11. Lam YL, Alozai T, Schreve MA, de Smet A, Vahl AC, Nagtzaam I, et al. A multicenter, randomized, dose-finding study of mechanochemical ablation using ClariVein and liquid polidocanol for great saphenous vein incompetence. J Vasc Surg Venous Lymphat Disord. 2022;10(4):856–64.e2.
12. Aherne TM, Ryan EJ, Boland MR, McKevitt K, Hassanin A, Tubassam M, et al. Concomitant vs. staged treatment of varicose tributaries as an adjunct to endovenous ablation: A systematic review and meta-analysis. Eur J Vasc Endovasc Surg. 2020;60(3):430–42.
13. Welch HJ. Endovenous ablation of the great saphenous vein may avert phlebectomy for branch varicose veins. J Vasc Surg. 2006;44(3):601–5.
14. Lawrence PF, Chandra A, Wu M, Rigberg D, DeRubertis B, Gelabert H, et al. Classification of proximal endovenous closure levels and treatment algorithm. J Vasc Surg. 2010;52(2):388–93.
15. van Eekeren RR, Boersma D, Elias S, Holewijn S, Werson DA, de Vries JP, et al. Endovenous mechanochemical ablation of great saphenous vein incompetence using the ClariVein device: A safety study. J Endovasc Ther. 2011;18(3):328–34.
16. Elias S, Raines JK. Mechanochemical tumescentless endovenous ablation: Final results of the initial clinical trial. Phlebology. 2012;27(2):67–72.
17. Boersma D, van Eekeren RR, Werson DA, van der Waal RI, Reijnen MM, de Vries JP. Mechanochemical endovenous ablation of small saphenous vein insufficiency using the ClariVein((R)) device: One-year results of a prospective series. Eur J Vasc Endovasc Surg. 2013;45(3):299–303.
18. Vun SV, Rashid ST, Blest NC, Spark JI. Lower pain and faster treatment with mechanicochemical endovenous ablation using ClariVein(R). Phlebology. 2015;30(10):688–92.
19. Bishawi M, Bernstein R, Boter M, Draughn D, Gould CF, Hamilton C, et al. Mechanochemical ablation in patients with chronic venous disease: A prospective multicenter report. Phlebology. 2014;29(6):397–400.

20. Kim PS, Bishawi M, Draughn D, Boter M, Gould C, Koziarski J, et al. Mechanochemical ablation for symptomatic great saphenous vein reflux: A two-year follow-up. Phlebology. 2017;32(1):43–48.
21. Deijen CL, Schreve MA, Bosma J, de Nie AJ, Leijdekkers VJ, van den Akker PJ, et al. Clarivein mechanochemical ablation of the great and small saphenous vein: Early treatment outcomes of two hospitals. Phlebology. 2016;31(3):192–97.
22. Bootun R, Lane TR, Dharmarajah B, Lim CS, Najem M, Renton S, et al. Intra-procedural pain score in a randomised controlled trial comparing mechanochemical ablation to radiofrequency ablation: The Multicentre Venefit versus ClariVein(R) for varicose veins trial. Phlebology. 2016;31(1):61–65.
23. Lane T, Bootun R, Dharmarajah B, Lim CS, Najem M, Renton S, et al. A multi-centre randomised controlled trial comparing radiofrequency and mechanical occlusion chemically assisted ablation of varicose veins – final results of the venefit versus Clarivein for varicose veins trial. Phlebology. 2017;32(2):89–98.
24. Tang TY, Kam JW, Gaunt ME. ClariVein(R) – Early results from a large single-centre series of mechanochemical endovenous ablation for varicose veins. Phlebology. 2017;32(1):6–12.
25. van Eekeren RR, Boersma D, Holewijn S, Werson DA, de Vries JP, Reijnen MM. Mechanochemical endovenous ablation for the treatment of great saphenous vein insufficiency. J Vasc Surg Venous Lymphat Disord. 2014;2(3):282–88.
26. Witte ME, Holewijn S, van Eekeren RR, de Vries JP, Zeebregts CJ, Reijnen MM. Midterm outcome of mechanochemical endovenous ablation for the treatment of great saphenous vein insufficiency. J Endovasc Ther. 2017;24(1):149–55.
27. van Eekeren RR, Boersma D, Konijn V, de Vries JP, Reijnen MM. Postoperative pain and early quality of life after radiofrequency ablation and mechanochemical endovenous ablation of incompetent great saphenous veins. J Vasc Surg. 2013;57(2):445–50.
28. Tang TY. Commentary: ClariVein: MOCA's Midterm report – still the flavor of the month or a sustainable trend? J Endovasc Ther. 2017;24(1):156–58.
29. Holewijn S, van Eekeren R, Vahl A, de Vries J, Reijnen M; MARADONA Study Group. Two-year results of a multicenter randomized controlled trial comparing Mechanochemical endovenous Ablation to RADiOfrequeNcy ablation in the treatment of primary great saphenous vein incompetence (MARADONA trial). J Vasc Surg Venous Lymphat Disord. 2019;7(3):364–74.
30. Vähäaho S, Mahmoud O, Halmesmaki K, Alback A, Noronen K, Vikatmaa P, et al. Randomized clinical trial of mechanochemical and endovenous thermal ablation of great saphenous varicose veins. Br J Surg. 2019;106(5):548–54.
31. Mohamed AH, Leung C, Wallace T, Smith G, Carradice D, Chetter I. A randomized controlled trial of endovenous laser ablation versus mechanochemical ablation with clarivein in the management of superficial venous incompetence (LAMA Trial). Ann Surg. 2021;273(6):e188–95.
32. Chen AJ, Ulloa JG, Torrez T, Yeh SL, de Virgilio CM, Gelabert HA, et al. Mechanochemical endovenous ablation of the saphenous vein: A look at contemporary outcomes. Ann Vasc Surg. 2022;82:7–12.
33. Witte ME, Zeebregts CJ, de Borst GJ, Reijnen M, Boersma D. Mechanochemical endovenous ablation of saphenous veins using the ClariVein: A systematic review. Phlebology. 2017;32(10):649–57.
34. Grommes J, Franzen EL, Binnebosel M, Toonder IM, Wittens C, Jacobs M, et al. Inadvertent arterial injection using catheter-assisted sclerotherapy resulting in amputation. Dermatol Surg. 2011;37(4):536–38.

Chapter 8

High Ligation and Stripping of the Saphenous Veins

Samuel Eric Wilson, Samuel P. Arnot, and Juan Carlos Jimenez

INTRODUCTION

Ligation of the great saphenous vein (GSV) was first described by Ambroise Pare in the 16th century and further advocated by Friedrich Trendelenburg in 1890.[1] Jerry Moore further modified this technique and described flush ligation and division of the GSV at the saphenofemoral junction (SFJ) for treatment of venous reflux to the lower leg.[2] Internal stripping of the GSV was first described by Keller in 1905, and these principles still apply to selected patients undergoing venous surgery in the contemporary era.[3]

At the outset, one should acknowledge that most procedures for correction of reflux in the truncal veins are accomplished today by endovenous techniques. Medicare provider data analyzed for practice trends by Crawford et al in 2019 showed up to 60% growth in venous ablation procedures.[4] Vascular and general surgeons performed 43% of these procedures with cardiologists and multiple other specialties accounting for the remainder. Nevertheless, certain indications remain for open surgical treatment.

Comparative studies show only slight difference in outcomes between surgical and endovascular methods, although the latter is preferred because it is less invasive and usually does not require overnight hospitalization.[5,6] This chapter will review the clinical and anatomical situations which are more suitable for open surgery, describe the technique for high ligation and stripping (HL/S) of the saphenous veins, and detail potential complications.

INDICATIONS FOR SAPHENOUS VEIN LIGATION AND STRIPPING

The 2023 guidelines of the Society for Vascular Surgery, American Venous Forum, and American Vein and Lymphatic Society (in Section 2.3.1),

> For patients with symptomatic varicose veins and axial vein reflux in the great or small saphenous vein, we recommend treatment with ligation and stripping of the saphenous vein if technology or expertise in endovenous ablation is not available or if the venous anatomy precludes endovenous treatment.[7]

The level of recommendation is Grade 1 (strong) and the quality of evidence is considered B (moderate). These most recent guidelines also support the use of HL/S for the anterior and posterior accessory saphenous veins for similar indications (Table 8.1). Lack of equipment is increasingly uncommon since the technology is relatively simple and widely available. Yet certain patient specific factors favor the use of truncal vein HL/S over less invasive techniques.

Anatomical abnormalities favoring HL/S over endovenous treatment include aneurysmal dilatation of the GSV. This may take the form of dilation at the saphenofemoral junction (SFJ) preventing successful endovenous ablation. In addition to the increased risk of

 DOI: 10.1201/9781003316626-10

Table 8.1 Current Clinical Practice Guidelines (2023) Applicable to High Ligation and Stripping of the Saphenous Veins[7]

Guideline 2.2.
2.2.1. For patients with symptomatic varicose veins and axial reflux in the great saphenous vein who are candidates for intervention, we recommend treatment with endovenous ablation over high ligation and stripping of the great saphenous vein because of less postprocedure pain and morbidity and an earlier return to regular activity. Level of recommendation: grade 1 (strong), quality of evidence: B (moderate)
2.2.2. For patients with symptomatic varicose veins and axial reflux in the SSV who are candidates for intervention, we recommend treatment with endovenous ablation over ligation and stripping of the small saphenous vein because of less postprocedure pain and morbidity and an earlier return to regular activity. Level of recommendation: grade 1 (strong), quality of evidence: C (low to very low)
2.2.3. For patients with symptomatic varicose veins and axial reflux in the AAGSV or PAGSV who are candidates for intervention, we suggest treatment with endovenous ablation, with additional phlebectomy, if needed, over ligation and stripping of the accessory great saphenous vein because of less early pain and morbidity and an earlier return to regular activity. Level of recommendation: grade 2 (weak), quality of evidence: C (low to very low)
Guideline 2.3.
2.3.1. For patients with symptomatic varicose veins and axial reflux in the great saphenous or small saphenous veins, we recommend treatment with ligation and stripping of the saphenous vein if the technology or expertise in endovenous ablation is not available or the venous anatomy precludes endovenous treatment. Level of recommendation: grade 1 (strong), quality of evidence: B (moderate)
2.3.2. For patients with symptomatic varicose veins and axial reflux in the anterior accessory great saphenous vein or posterior accessory great saphenous vein, we suggest treatment with ligation and stripping of the accessory great saphenous vein, with additional phlebectomy, if needed, if the technology or expertise in endovenous ablation is not available or the venous anatomy precludes endovenous treatment. Level of recommendation: grade 2 (weak), quality of evidence: C (low to very low)

non-closure and early recanalization following thermal ablation, large saphenous vein diameters have also been found to be a risk factor for ablation related thrombus extension (ARTE) into the deep venous system.[8,9] Although no absolute maximal truncal vein diameter has been established in the literature as a contraindication to thermal ablation, we use an approximate diameter of 15 mm as an indication to ligate and strip the GSV in the thigh.

In thin patients, the saphenous veins may be close to the skin surface in which case thermal endoluminal ablation may result in skin injury, such as a burn. Thus, HL/S (along with phlebectomies) may also be preferred. A tortuous saphenous vein prevents passage of endovenous wires and catheters required for thermal ablation. Tortuous saphenous veins may be excised through stripping of an isolated non-tortuous segment and multiple stab phlebectomies. A short main trunk just caudal to the SFJ and/or saphenopopliteal (SPJ) junctions also frequently precludes endovenous ablation.

The saphenous nerve is particularly vulnerable to thermal injury and will cause troublesome numbness over the medial aspect of the knee and lower leg. Similarly, injury to the sural nerve during ablation of the SSV will cause pain and numbness in the posterior calf, heel, and ankle. In these instances, open surgical technique affords oversewing of the saphenous vein flush to the SFJ and/or SPJ. The truncal vein is divided close to the common femoral vein (CFV) and oversewn leaving minimal residual cuff. This minimizes the risk of thrombus propagation into the CFV and possible embolism.

TECHNIQUE FOR LIGATION AND STRIPPING OF SAPHENOUS VEINS

The potential benefits and risks of endovenous ablation versus HL/S should be agreed upon by patient and surgeon during the preoperative visit. Since HL/S is performed less frequently today, it is wise to check with the operating room staff that the equipment including vein stripper and various attachments are available on the day of operation (Figure 8.1). If phlebectomies are planned at the same operative setting, the veins to be removed should be marked in the standing position with a surgical marker so that there will be no disappointment with appearance postoperatively if some unrecognized unsightly veins remain. A general anesthetic is preferred for HL/S, and we prefer to avoid regional, spinal anesthesia since this may induce vasodilatation. Intraoperative ultrasound is preferred to map the target vein and associated anatomic landmarks. The SFJ, which usually lies just medial to the superficial femoral artery and a few centimeters below the inguinal ligament, is identified through a small transverse incision facilitated with ultrasound (Figure 8.2). It is important to ligate and divide the superficial tributary veins entering the proximal GSV at the fossa ovalis. Although often inconsistent, the tributaries usually include the circumflex iliac vein, superficial epigastric vein, pudendal vein, and the anterior and posterior accessory veins. Leaving one or more of these veins intact can lead to recurrence of varicosities. In patients who have a duplicated saphenous veins, care should be taken to identify the main, refluxing GSV prior to the introduction of the internal venous stripper.

After exposing the GSV distally just below the knee, the internal venous stripper is introduced into the vein lumen by advancing from distal to proximal for smoother crossing of valves. If the tip of the stripper meets resistance prior to reaching the SFJ, segmental stripping of the vein can be performed (Figure 8.3). After intraluminal passage to the proximal thigh, the stripper is exposed through a small venotomy, just caudal to the SFJ. We attach the cone (or mushroom tip) to the distal end and the vein is securely ligated with the suture around the

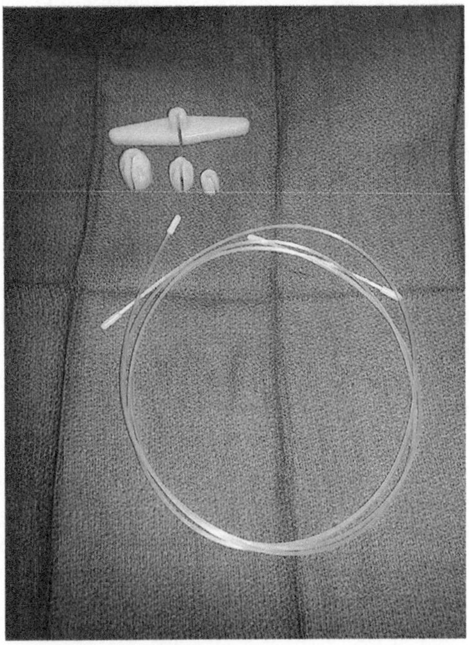

Figure 8.1 Commercially available vein stripper for high ligation and stripping of the saphenous veins. It may be comprised of either metal or plastic based on manufacturer.

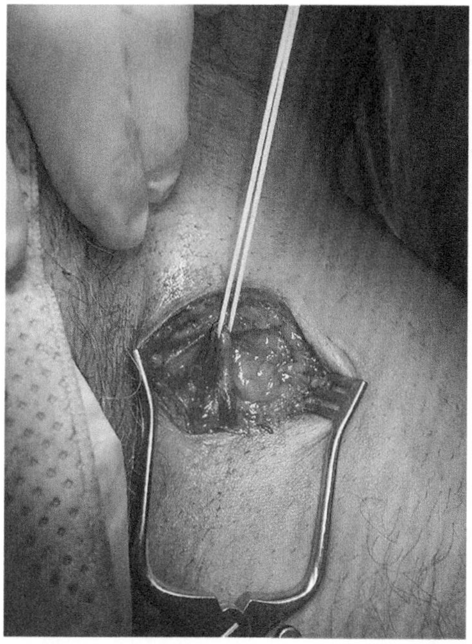

Figure 8.2 Surgical exposure of the great saphenous vein at the saphenofemoral junction. We recommend utilization of ultrasound to minimize the length and optimize location of the skin incision.

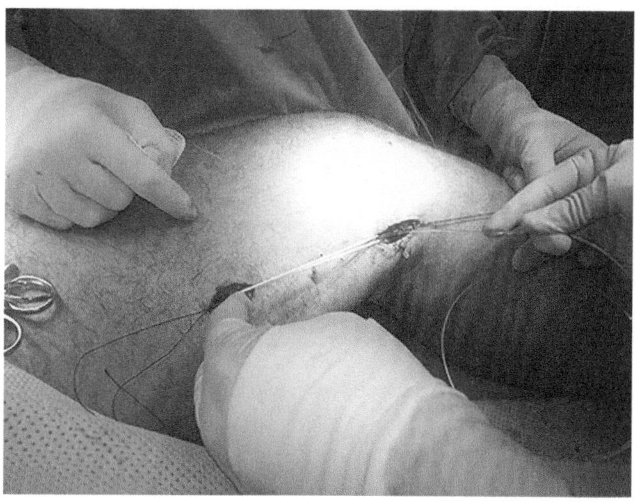

Figure 8.3 Endoluminal passage of the vein stripper toward the saphenofemoral junction. In this particular case, we performed segmental stripping of the great saphenous vein due to resistance during placement of the device.

stripper (Figure 8.4). At this time, we use a spinal needle to inject tumescent solution to the perivenous tissues within the saphenous fascia surrounding the target vein. This solution consists of 1% lidocaine, sodium bicarbonate, and normal saline. Administration of tumescent solution decreases bleeding from the saphenous vein tunnel following the stripping process and decreases pain in the immediate postoperative period.

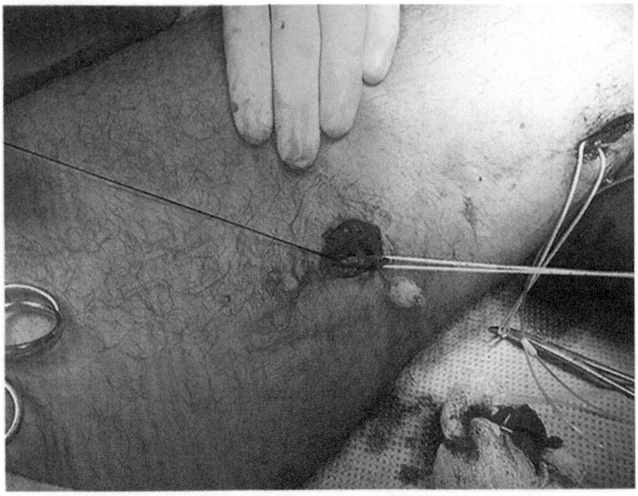

Figure 8.4 Placement of the conical tip on the distal end of the vein stripper. This device is sutured firmly to the saphenous vein prior to inversion stripping.

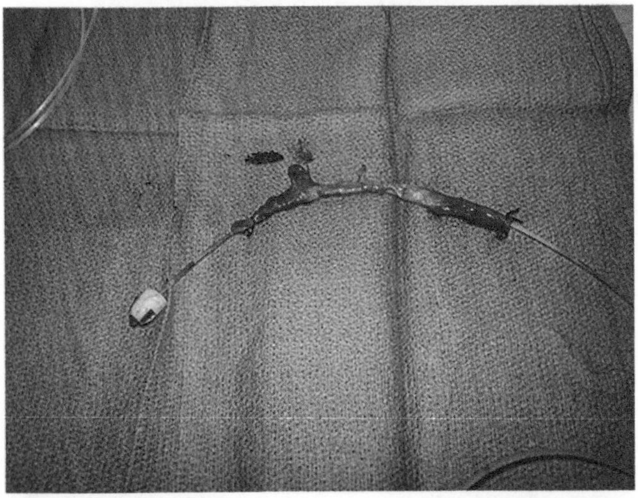

Figure 8.5 The great saphenous vein with associated vein stripper following removal.

A T shaped handle is present at the proximal end which is used to pull the venous stripper. An assistant uses towels to compress the venous bed, and with steady traction the vein is removed (Figure 8.5). Pressure is held on the elevated leg for 10 minutes, which helps avoid hematoma and minimize swelling postoperatively. Previously identified and marked accessory veins can be removed by avulsion with stab phlebectomies. Sterile gauze and compression bandages are firmly wrapped around the leg beginning at the foot.

For the SSV, the vein is ligated flush to the SPJ and divided. We prefer to limit stripping of the SSV to the segment immediately caudal to the SPJ because of the proximity of the sural nerve to the SSV in the lower calf. In general, the venous anatomy of the SSV is less predictable and more variable than that of the GSV. Preoperative and intraoperative duplex ultrasound guidance allows clear anatomical delineation of the SPJ and associated venous branches and should be used routinely.

RESULTS FOLLOWING SAPHENOUS VEIN LIGATION AND STRIPPING

Good clinical evidence continues to demonstrate that saphenous HL/S is a safe, effective, and durable technique for the treatment of symptomatic reflux and varicose veins.[10] Over the past decade, several randomized trials have compared this conventional surgical technique with endovenous methods for truncal vein closure with favorable and comparable outcomes.

Brittenden and colleagues performed a randomized controlled trial in the United Kingdom that compared quality of life and cost-effectiveness in 595 patients following HL/S, laser ablation, and foam sclerotherapy.[11] At 5 years, disease-specific quality of life was improved (and similar) following laser ablation and surgery compared with foam sclerotherapy. Laser ablation was found to be the most cost-effective option amongst the different treatments.

Another randomized study compared clinical outcomes at 10 years following HL/S with laser ablation.[12] The trial cohort consisted of 130 limbs (68 limbs treated with HL/S and 62 limbs with EVLA). The 10-year estimated freedom from groin recurrence was higher in the HL/S group compared with laser. The same trend was noted for clinically evident recurrence. There were no significant differences between quality of life and relief of venous symptoms between the two groups. Long-term cosmetic outcomes also favored the HL/S group.

Joh and colleagues compared short-term outcomes following saphenous HL/S and cyanoacrylate closure (CAC).[13] The primary outcome studied was complete closure of the target vein at 3 months. The study included 126 randomized subjects (63 with CAC and 63 with HL/S). At 3 months, all patients demonstrated complete vein closure in both groups. Postoperative pain was significantly lower in the CAC group. Venous Clinical Severity Scores (VCSS) and quality of life improved equally in both groups.

Clinical outcomes following HL/S for the SSV are also good when compared to non-thermal techniques. Nandhra and colleagues performed a randomized clinical trial comparing HL/S and laser ablation of the SSV.[14] Although elimination of axial reflux was superior following laser ablation, there were no significant differences in clinical recurrence, sensory disturbance, or quality of life at 2 years between the two groups.

COMPLICATIONS OF HIGH LIGATION AND STRIPPING OF THE SAPHENOUS VEINS

The most immediate negative sequela of HL/S is postoperative pain. The current literature and our anecdotal clinical experience suggest that HL/S requires more anesthesia and is more painful compared with thermal ablation and CAC.[15] Clinical recurrence of varicose veins may occur following both surgical and endovenous saphenous vein closure.[16]

Postoperative seroma or lymphocele may develop at the groin wound if a lymph node has been injured or divided.[17] When recognized, complete excision of the node will prevent leakage of serum and minimize postoperative collections.

In past years the stripper was often passed as far as the ankle level to allow removal of the entire vein, however this approach may injure the saphenous nerve, which is closely adjacent to the GSV in the lower leg.[18] Many surgeons limit stripping from just below the knee to the

SFJ. Injuries to the saphenous and sural nerves nerve may occur following HL/S of the GSV and SSV, respectively. The literature suggests that the incidence of nerve injury in this setting is low and rarely results in long-term impairment or decreased quality of life.[18]

As impossible as it may seem, there are patients who have had the superficial femoral artery mistaken for a thick wall saphenous vein resulting in arterial injury.[19] The expected severe consequences have ensued.

CONCLUSIONS

High ligation and stripping of the saphenous veins have a lesser role in therapy than endovenous ablation in the contemporary era. Today they are indicated primarily for those who have a contraindication to percutaneous methods primarily because the morbidity is less, general anesthesia is not required, and recovery is faster. Specific indications, however, remain for surgical HL/S, and both short and long-term clinical outcomes are favorable when compared with less invasive techniques for patients with symptomatic varicose veins. Vascular surgeons and venous specialists should be familiar with its anatomical indications and technique.

REFERENCES

1. van den Bremer J, Moll FL. Historical overview of varicose vein surgery. Ann Vasc Surg. 2010;24:426–32.
2. Royle J, Somjen GM. Varicose veins: Hippocrates to jerry moore. ANZ J Surg. 2007;77:1120–27.
3. Cheatle T. The long saphenous vein: To strip or not to strip? Semin Vasc Surg 2005;18:10–14.
4. Crawford JM, Gasparis A, Almeida J, et al. A review of United States endovenous ablation practice trends from the Medicare data utilization and payment database. J Vasc Surg Venous Lymphatic Disorders. 2019;7:471–79.
5. Garcia-Madrid C, Manrique OP, Gomez-Blasco F, et al. Update on endovenous radio-frequency closure ablation of varicose veins. Ann Vasc Surg. 2012;26:281–91.
6. Bountouroglu DG, Azzam M, Kakkos SK, et al. Ultrasound-guided foam sclerotherapy combined with sapheno-femoral ligation compared to surgical treatment of varicose veins: Early results of a randomized controlled trial. Eur J Vasc Endovasc Surg. 2006;31:93–100
7. Gloviczki P, Lawrence PF, Wasan SM, Meissner MH, Almeida J, Brown KR, et al. The 2022 Society for Vascular Surgery, American Venous Forum, and American Vein and Lymphatic Society clinical practice guidelines for the management of varicose veins of the lower extremities. Part I. Duplex scanning and treatment of superficial truncal reflux: Endorsed by the Society for Vascular Medicine and the International Union of Phlebology. J Vasc Surg Venous Lymphat Disord. 2023;11:231–36.e6.
8. Kemaloglu C. Saphenous vein diameter is a single risk factor for early recanalization after endothermal ablation of incompetent great saphenous vein. Vascular. 2019;27:537–41.
9. Lawrence PF, Chandra A, Wu M, Rigberg D, Derubertis B, Gelabert H, et al. Classification of proximal endovenous closure levels and treatment algorithm. J Vasc Surg. 2010;52:388–93.
10. Shahzad N, Elsherif M, Abaidat I, Brar R. A systematic review and meta-analysis of randomized controlled trials comparing thermal versus non-thermal endovenous ablation in superficial venous incompetence. Eur J Vasc Endovasc Surg. 2023;66:687–95.
11. Brittenden J, Cooper D, Dimitrova M, Scotland G, Cotton SC, Elders A, et al. Five-year outcomes of a randomized trial of treatments for varicose veins. N Engl J Med. 2019;381:912–22.
12. Eggen CA, Alozai T, Pronk P, Mooij MC, Gaastra MTW, Unlu C, et al. Ten-year follow up of a randomized controlled trial comparing saphenofemoral ligation and stripping of the great

saphenous vein with endovenous laser ablation (980 nm) using local tumescent anesthesia. J Vasc Surg Venous Lymphat Disord. 2022;10:646–53.e1.

13. Joh JH, Lee T, Byun SJ, Cho S, Park HS, Yun WS, et al. A multicenter randomized controlled trial of cyanoacrylate closure and surgical stripping for incompetent great saphenous veins. J Vasc Surg Venous Lymphat Disord. 2022;10:353–59.
14. Nandhra S, El-Sheikha J, Carradice D, Wallace T, Souroullas P, Samuel N, et al. A randomized clinical trial of endovenous laser ablation versus conventional surgery for small saphenous varicose veins. J Vasc Surg. 2015;61:741–46.
15. Kanber EM, Cetin HK. Comparison of radiofrequency ablation and saphenous vein stripping for the treatment of recurrent lower extremity venous insufficiency. Vasc Endovasc SUrg. 2023;57:726–731.
16. Nesbitt C, Bedenis R, Bhattacharya V, Stansby G. Endovenous ablation (radiofrequency and laser) and foam sclerotherapy versus open surgery for great saphenous vein varices. Cochrane Database Syst Rev. 2014;(7):CD005624.
17. Dessalvi S, Villa G, Campisi CC, Boccardo F. Decreasing and preventing lymphatic-injury-related complications in patients undergoing venous surgery: A new diagnostic and therapeutic protocol. Lymphology. 2018;51:57–65.
18. Morrison C, Dalsing MC. Signs and symptoms of saphenous nerve injury after greater saphenous vein stripping: Prevalence, severity, and relevance for modern practice. J Vasc Surg. 2003;38:886–90.
19. Marcucci G, Accrocca F, Antonelli R, Siani A. The management of arterial and venous injuries during saphenous vein surgery. Interact Cardiovasc Thorac Surg. 2008;7:432–33.

Chapter 9

Ambulatory (Stab) Phlebectomy

William Duong and David Rigberg

THE ORIGIN OF PHLEBECTOMY

Varicose veins are a common condition managed by the vascular provider, affecting 23% of adults in the United States, with an estimated 22 million women and 11 million men between the ages of 40 and 80 years old.[1] From Latin, "*varicosus*" means "dilated veins;" varicose veins are enlarged superficial veins that exist on the spectrum of chronic venous disease, alongside subdermal spider veins, telangiectasis, and reticular veins. By definition, varicose veins are dilated, tortuous, subcutaneous veins measuring greater than or equal to 3 mm in diameter.[2] Running in the superficial space above the saphenous fascia, these are tributaries of and ultimately drain into the greater saphenous vein.[3]

The treatment of a venous varix by phlebotomy was first conceptualized by Hippocrates in 400 BC,[4] by performing multiple punctures in the vein. However, it was Aulus Cornelius Celsus (25 BC–45 AD) who was first to perform a phlebectomy to treat a varicose vein in ancient Rome around 0 CE.[5] Without the assistance of anesthesia, patients experienced great pain from the procedure, and the technique eventually fell out of favor.[6] The idea was rediscovered in 1956 by Dr. Robert Muller, a Swedish surgeon, who developed and refined his own method, now referred to as Muller's phlebectomy, or ambulatory/stab phlebectomy.[5]

INDICATIONS

Ambulatory phlebectomy is directed toward the treatment of primary or secondary truncal and accessory varicose veins. These are often large and symptomatic, as they can cause sensations of extremity heaviness, discomfort, or even pain.[3] Areas that may be appropriate for the procedure of phlebectomy include the accessory saphenous veins of the thigh, pudendal veins of the groin, reticular varicose veins of the popliteal fossa, as well as the lateral portion of the thigh and leg, and the veins of the ankle and dorsum of the foot.[7] Although not commonly practiced, phlebectomy could be carried out for dilated veins in the upper extremity or even dilated venous networks within the face.[7] Within the Society for Vascular Surgery and American Venous Forum clinical practice guidelines, there is strong recommendation with moderate quality of evidence for, "[recommending] ambulatory phlebectomy for treatment of varicose veins, performed with saphenous vein ablation, either during the same procedure or at a later stage. If general anesthesia is required for phlebectomy, we suggest concomitant saphenous ablation."[8]

CONTRAINDICATIONS

Although often a minor outpatient procedure, ambulatory phlebectomy should be avoided in select patients, particularly in patients with high risk for bleeding or with legs where wound healing would be prohibitive, including those with significant swelling and edema. Conversely, patients with hypercoagulable states should be approached cautiously with careful attention

DOI: 10.1201/9781003316626-11

given to their medical management. Contraindications include extremities with active infection or inflammation, such as cellulitis or dermatitis. Finally, as stab phlebectomy is most often pursued in an elective fashion, patients who are generally poor surgical candidates or have ongoing illness with active threat to life should not undergo this procedure.[4]

PREPARATION FOR PROCEDURE

Preoperative marking of the patient is an important step to the ambulatory phlebectomy procedure. With the patient standing, the varicosities are marked with indelible ink as they are often more visible in this position (Figure 9.1). Palpation can be helpful. This is best done with ambient lighting that falls tangentially over the varicosities being examined.[6] A vein transilluminator can be utilized. The patient is, as well, useful in identifying the symptomatic veins that require attention.

MULLER'S TECHNIQUE

Once the patient has been marked, they are brought into the office procedure room or operating room and positioned as needed. Although general anesthesia, monitored anesthesia care, or regional anesthesia are all acceptable options for anesthesia, local anesthesia is usually sufficient, with 0.5% or 1% lidocaine with or without epinephrine. It is important to note the amount of local anesthetic given, as for 1% lidocaine with epinephrine, the maximum recommended dosage is 7 mg/kg.

Hair removal is optional, as hair rarely interferes with the procedure. The operating leg is then elevated to minimize the venous bleeding and ecchymosis associated with the procedure. With the veins marked, and following infiltration of local anesthetic, a 1–3 mm incision is made with an 11-scalpel adjacent to each varicosity. An 18 gauge needle can also be used to make the incision.[9] We recommend beginning proximally and moving distally. When done in

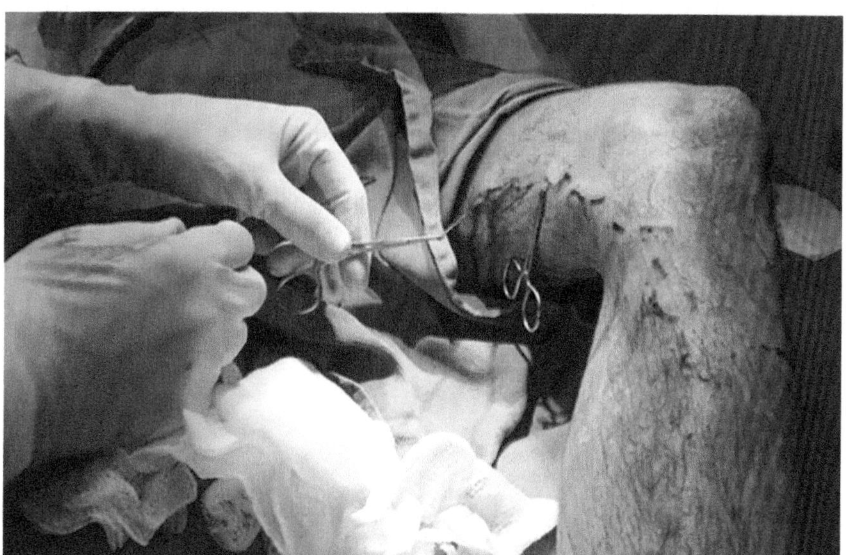

Figure 9.1 Patient has been pre-operatively marked and is undergoing stab phlebectomy.

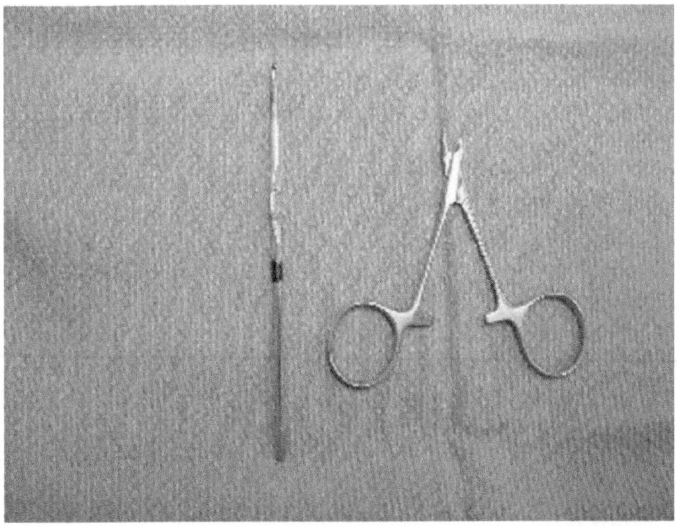

Figure 9.2 A crochet hook (left) and a Halsted mosquito hemostat (right) is pictured.

the lower extremity, a longitudinal incision is often preferred; however transverse incisions in the groin, knee, and ankle may be more cosmetic as they align with the lines of Langer.[9]

A hook instrument is then used to capture the varicosity, such as the Oesch-style hook or a crochet hook (Figure 9.2). Once captured, the vein will appear pearly white[6] (Figure 9.3). Although smaller subdermal varicosities can simply be avulsed, longer and larger varicosities should be grasped with pointed clamp, such as a Halsted mosquito hemostat. Once the vein is doubly clamped, it is sharply divided between the two clamps. Each end is slowly and gently pulled from the adhering subcutaneous fat and slowly rolled onto the clamp in the direction of the vein (Figure 9.3). Successive clamps can be applied to improve traction. Effort should be directed toward preventing premature avulsion of the vein; if this occurs, a separate incision can be made proximally or distally to recapture the vein and maximize length of vein removed.[9] It is important to remove as much of the varicosity as possible as this will reduce the potential inflammation that arises from the thrombosis of a retained segment.[4] This should be repeated as many times as necessary, commonly requiring in excess of 20 or more phlebectomies.[9] Following each phlebectomy, pressure can be held over the site to ensure hemostasis.

Closure of the skin can be completed with steri-strip bandages, or the incisions can simply be left open. Rarely, a single interrupted subcuticular stitch with absorbable suture such as 4–0 Monocryl is sufficient. A 2×2 or 4×4 gauze can be used to cover the incision. The extremity is then dressed with a compression dressing, either with an elastic bandage or a fitted compression hose with 20 to 30 mmHg of compression. The compression should continue for at least 48 hours before removal and followed by 6 weeks of compression during the day. Follow-up is arranged for the patient in 1 to 2 weeks with imaging as needed.

COMPLICATIONS

Although rare and often benign, the surgeon should be aware of potential complications from the procedure; divided into cutaneous, vascular, and neurological.[10] Commonly, skin complications, such as dimpling or pigmentation can occur, however blistering or infection, while rare, can also

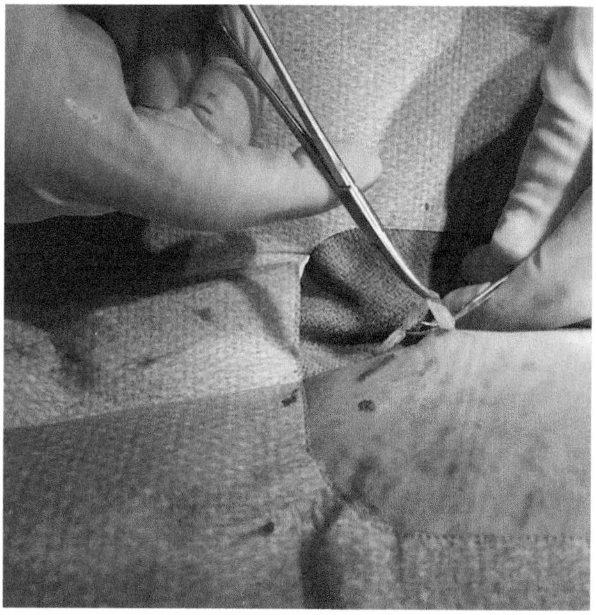

Figure 9.3 A vein (pearly white) is pictured and gently grasped and pulled from the subcutaneous tissue.

occur. Bleeding can also occur resulting in ecchymosis or hematoma formation. Additionally, the improper application of the compressive elastic bandage can lead to pain and soft tissue injury if placed too tight. The local anesthetic may lead to an allergic reaction especially when given in large quantities such as with concomitant saphenous ablation. Local thrombophlebitis can occur from thrombosis of remnant varix. Very rarely, nerve injury to the saphenous, sural, or branches of the peroneal can occur, although the majority of nerve injuries are often sensory.[11]

TRANSILLUMINATED POWERED PHLEBECTOMY

Transilluminated powered phlebectomy (TIPP) was developed in 1996 as the TriVex system utilizing three technologies to complete the dissection.[12] Often using the same incision as the ablation of the greater saphenous vein, an endoscopic device is first used to transilluminate the subcutaneous varicosities and deliver tumescent anesthesia.[12] A separate device, an endoscopic powered tissue dissector, is then delivered through an opposing incision, which contains a rotating blade which destroys and aspirates the varicose veins.[12] Initial studies were promising, as early results demonstrated efficacy and required a decreased number of incisions and shorter operative time.[13] However, further studies including a meta-analysis by Luebke et al found that despite the decreased number of incisions and operative time, there was an increased incidence of calf hematoma and higher pain scores with the TIPP compared to the conventional stab phlebectomy technique.[14,15] In actuality, the relative benefits and drawbacks of the TIPP have not been consistently demonstrated in future studies. A randomized control trial by Aremu et al, comparing 100 limbs with conventional stab phlebectomy to 88 limbs with TIPP found that TIPP had significantly less incisions (5 vs. 29), but there was no difference in operative time. In their study there was no difference in pain score, bruising, numbness, or overall satisfaction.[16] A separate randomized control trial from Chetter et al had similar findings regarding operative time and number of incisions but found that bruising and pain were significantly higher in the TIPP groin, with a greater negative impact on quality of life and recovery time.[17] Given the mixed data, need for additional equipment, and learning curve, this has led to the recommendation that TIPP should be reserved in select cases, for example, in patients with a large number of varicosities, reoperations, or patients with obesity.[18]

STAGING OF PHLEBECTOMY

Although ambulatory phlebectomy is often completed in conjunction with ablation of axial reflux, it does not necessarily need to be completed within the same operation. Treatment of axial reflux within the greater saphenous vein initially may decrease the pressure within the tributary veins and cause them to shrink, making them more appropriate for sclerotherapy and obviating the need for stab phlebectomy.[9] Thus, staging of the two procedures allows the practitioner to potentially decrease the extent of the procedure and potentially avoid additional ones.[19] On the other hand, combining the procedures leads to fewer office visits and less anesthetic at the cost of increased procedure time with potentially increased recovery time.

The literature is conflicted on the benefit of one approach over the other. Monahan studied 45 patients and 222 varicose veins in the treatment of greater saphenous vein insufficiency with radiofrequency ablation without treating the varicose veins directly. He found that 88.7% of varicose veins decreased in size, with 28.4% of veins spontaneously resolved. Of the veins that resolved, 41.9% were above the knee and 25.6% were below the knee.[20] This was supported by a retrospective study by Welch, who reviewed 184 endovenous ablation procedures, and of the 155 patients who had total occlusion or partial patency of the greater saphenous vein, only 25.2% went on to receive subsequent stab phlebectomy for persistent symptomatic varicosities.[21] Similarly, Schanzer et al studied 86 lower extremities with endovenous ablation alone and found that only 41.8% of extremities required a second stage procedure, with complete resolution of varicosities in 41.8% extremities.[22] On the other hand, other studies, such as Harlander-Locke et al, have found concomitant phlebectomy to be safe and effective for patients, particularly those with refluxing tributary veins >3 mm.[23]

Carradice et al was the first to complete a randomized control trial comparing stab phlebectomy in the concomitant or staged format. They randomized 50 patients to endovenous laser therapy alone or endovenous laser therapy with concomitant ambulatory phlebectomy.[24] While there was an increase in average procedure time, there was no difference in post-procedural pain. Furthermore, median Venous Clinical Severity Score at 3 months (0 vs. 2) was lower for the concomitant procedure as well as lower Aberdeen Varicose Vein Questionnaire scores at 6 weeks (7.9 vs. 13.5) and 3 months (2 vs. 9.6).[24] There were no differences in these scores at 1 year.

The AVULS study, Ambulatory Varicosity Avulsion Later or Synchronized, is the largest randomized control trial to date and is by Lane et al.[25] With 101 recruited patients, they compared quality of life and clinical outcomes between staged and concomitant phlebectomies. 36% of the delayed group required further treatment compared with only 2% of the simultaneous group. Although both groups had a decrease in the Aberdeen Varicose Vein Questionnaire, the simultaneous group had a greater decrease by 5.48 at 6 weeks, although no difference was seen at 6 or 12 months. Quality of life (using EuroQol 5 level) was also improved in the simultaneous group at 6 weeks (0.866 vs. 0.773), but this difference disappeared at future follow-ups. Interestingly, of the patients who had been recruited for the trial and refused participation, 95% cited wanting a single sitting treatment as their reason.[25]

Saphenous ablation has also been performed with a concomitant TIPP, as studied by Obi et al.[26] As expected, there was a greater improvement in Venous Clinical Severity Score with the ablation plus phlebectomy group compared to the ablation alone (3.8 vs. 3.2). Notably, the powered phlebectomy group did have a higher incidence of hematoma (7.8% vs. 1.2%) and superficial thrombosis (6.4% vs. 2.8%).[26]

One concerning finding was a potentially increased rate of endovenous heat-induced thrombosis in patients undergoing concomitant procedures. In Hicks et al's retrospective study of 299 patients undergoing radiofrequency ablation with and without stab phlebectomy, endovenous heat-induced thrombosis occurred more often in concomitant procedures (14% vs. 6%), with an odds ratio of 3.46 on multivariate analysis.[27] Hicks hypothesized the increased pain from phlebectomy may have led to decreased activity level and thus increased risk of thrombosis. Worsened venous disease requiring the additional phlebectomy may also be contributive.[27]

A meta-analysis of 15 studies comparing concomitant versus staged treatment of varicose veins by Aherne et al was completed in 2020. Overall disease severity, measured by Venous Clinical Severity Score, and quality of life, measured by the Aberdeen Varicose Vein Questionnaire, both favored the concomitant group when measured at 3 months and between 3 and 12 months.[28] There was no difference in rates of deep venous thrombosis or complication rate inclusive of endovenous heat-induced thrombosis.

Ultimately, the decision to undergo a staged versus concomitant procedure is left to the practitioner. In the specific setting of general anesthesia, it may be favorable to complete them at the same time to reduce the dosage of anesthesia. However, with the advent of tumescence, local anesthesia, and when completed in an office or at an outpatient surgery center, a patient-centered discussion of risk, benefit, convenience, and patient preference may be prudent to optimize patient care.

CONCLUSIONS

The treatment of varicose veins has evolved over time to the refined technique of ambulatory stab phlebectomy by Dr. Muller. It has become the gold standard for the treatment of this subset of chronic venous disease. Although there can be variability in anesthetic choice, procedural method, or even staging of the procedure, thorough discussion with the patient can ensure optimal outcomes.

REFERENCES

1. Piazza G. Varicose veins. *Circulation*. 2014;130(7):582–587. doi:10.1161/CIRCULATIONAHA.113.008331
2. Hamdan A. Management of varicose veins and venous insufficiency. *JAMA*. 2012;308(24):2612–2621. doi:10.1001/jama.2012.111352
3. Moore's Vascular and Endovascular Surgery (9th ed.). Accessed February 20, 2023. www.elsevier.com/books/moores-vascular-and-endovascular-surgery/moore/978-0-323-48011-6
4. Kabnick LS, Ombrellino M. Ambulatory phlebectomy. *Semin Interv Radiol.* 2005;22(3):218–224. doi:10.1055/s-2005-921955
5. Ramelet AA, Weiss RA. Principles and technique of ambulatory phlebectomy. In: *Advanced Techniques in Dermatologic Surgery*. CRC Press, 2006.

6. Andrews RH, Dixon RG. Ambulatory phlebectomy and sclerotherapy as tools for the treatment of varicose veins and telangiectasias. *Semin Interv Radiol.* 2021;38(2):160–166. doi:10.1055/s-0041-1727151
7. Ramelet AA. Phlebectomy – cosmetic indications. *J Cosmet Dermatol.* 2002;1(1):13–19. doi:10.1046/j.1473-2130.2001.00004.x
8. Gloviczki P, Comerota AJ, Dalsing MC, et al. The care of patients with varicose veins and associated chronic venous diseases: Clinical practice guidelines of the Society for Vascular Surgery and the American Venous Forum. *J Vasc Surg.* 2011;53(5, Supplement):2S–48S. doi:10.1016/j.jvs.2011.01.079
9. Iafrati MD. Varicose Veins: Surgical Treatment. Rutherford's Vascualr Surgery and Endovascular Therapy 10th Edition, Chapter 154,2031-2048.e2.
10. Ramelet AA. Phlebectomy. Technique, indications and complications. *Int Angiol J Int Union Angiol.* 2002;21(2 Suppl 1):46–51.
11. Olivencia JA. Complications of ambulatory phlebectomy. Review of 1000 consecutive cases. *Dermatol Surg Off Publ Am Soc Dermatol Surg Al.* 1997;23(1):51–54.
12. Arumugasamy M, McGreal G, O'Connor A, Kelly C, Bouchier-Hayes D, Leahy A. The technique of transilluminated powered phlebectomy – a novel, minimally invasive system for varicose vein surgery. *Eur J Vasc Endovasc Surg.* 2002;23(2):180–182. doi:10.1053/ejvs.2001.1553
13. Spitz GA, Braxton JM, Bergan JJ. Outpatient varicose vein surgery with transilluminated powered phlebectomy. *Vasc Surg.* 2000;34(6):547–555. doi:10.1177/153857440003400608
14. Luebke T, Brunkwall J. Meta-analysis of transilluminated powered phlebectomy for superficial varicosities. *J Cardiovasc Surg (Torino).* 2008;49(6):757–764.
15. Scavée V, Lesceu O, Theys S, Jamart J, Louagie Y, Schoevaerdts JC. Hook phlebectomy versus transilluminated powered phlebectomy for varicose vein surgery: Early results. *Eur J Vasc Endovasc Surg Off J Eur Soc Vasc Surg.* 2003;25(5):473–475. doi:10.1053/ejvs.2002.1908
16. Aremu MA, Mahendran B, Butcher W, et al. Prospective randomized controlled trial: Conventional versus powered phlebectomy. *J Vasc Surg.* 2004;39(1):88–94. doi:10.1016/j.jvs.2003.09.044
17. Chetter IC, Mylankal KJ, Hughes H, Fitridge R. Randomized clinical trial comparing multiple stab incision phlebectomy and transilluminated powered phlebectomy for varicose veins. *Br J Surg.* 2006;93(2):169–174. doi:10.1002/bjs.5261
18. Kantarovsky A, Vinogradski D, Mankowitsch E, Ashkenazi I. Pain is a limiting factor in patients suitable for transilluminated powered phlebectomy. *Rambam Maimonides Med J.* 2019;10(4):e0023. doi:10.5041/RMMJ.10377
19. Hager ES, Ozvath KJ, Dillavou ED. Evidence summary of combined saphenous ablation and treatment of varicosities versus staged phlebectomy. *J Vasc Surg Venous Lymphat Disord.* 2017;5(1):134–137. doi:10.1016/j.jvsv.2016.07.009
20. Monahan DL. Can phlebectomy be deferred in the treatment of varicose veins? *J Vasc Surg.* 2005;42(6):1145–1149. doi:10.1016/j.jvs.2005.08.034
21. Welch HJ. Endovenous ablation of the great saphenous vein may avert phlebectomy for branch varicose veins. *J Vasc Surg.* 2006;44(3):601–605. doi:10.1016/j.jvs.2006.06.003
22. Schanzer H. Endovenous ablation plus microphlebectomy/sclerotherapy for the treatment of varicose veins: Single or two-stage procedure? *Vasc Endovascular Surg.* 2010;44(7):545–549. doi:10.1177/1538574410375126
23. Harlander-Locke M, Jimenez JC, Lawrence PF, Derubertis BG, Rigberg DA, Gelabert HA. Endovenous ablation with concomitant phlebectomy is a safe and effective method of treatment for symptomatic patients with axial reflux and large incompetent tributaries. *J Vasc Surg.* 2013;58(1):166–172. doi:10.1016/j.jvs.2012.12.054
24. Carradice D, Mekako AI, Hatfield J, Chetter IC. Randomized clinical trial of concomitant or sequential phlebectomy after endovenous laser therapy for varicose veins. *Br J Surg.* 2009;96(4). doi:10.1002/bjs.6556
25. Lane TRA, Kelleher D, Shepherd AC, Franklin IJ, Davies AH. Ambulatory varicosity avulsion later or synchronized (AVULS): A randomized clinical trial. *Ann Surg.* 2015;261(4):654–661. doi:10.1097/SLA.0000000000000790

26. Obi AT, Reames BN, Rook TJ, et al. Outcomes associated with ablation compared to combined ablation and transilluminated powered phlebectomy in the treatment of venous varicosities. *Phlebology*. 2016;31(9):618–624. doi:10.1177/0268355515604257
27. Hicks CW, DiBrito SR, Magruder JT, Weaver ML, Barenski C, Heller JA. Radiofrequency ablation with concomitant stab phlebectomy increases risk of endovenous heat-induced thrombosis. *J Vasc Surg Venous Lymphat Disord*. 2017;5(2):200–209. doi:10.1016/j.jvsv.2016.10.081
28. Aherne TM, Ryan ÉJ, Boland MR, et al. Concomitant vs. staged treatment of varicose tributaries as an adjunct to endovenous ablation: A systematic review and meta-analysis. *Eur J Vasc Endovasc Surg Off J Eur Soc Vasc Surg*. 2020;60(3):430–442. doi:10.1016/j.ejvs.2020.05.028

Chapter 10

The Management of Incompetent Perforating Veins

Mary A. Binko, Misaki M. Kiguchi, Peter F. Lawrence, and Eric S. Hager

INTRODUCTION

Incompetent perforating veins (IPVs) are usually associated with advanced stages of chronic venous insufficiency (CVI) including ulcerations, although they may also occur in patients with CEAP C2 with varicose veins.[1] Most large refluxing IPVs are associated with more severe clinically significant venous disease with higher rates of ulcer recurrence.[2] The refluxing perforator veins located beneath venous ulcers contribute to local ambulatory venous hypertension, causing impaired wound healing secondary to fibrin cuffing and impaired oxygen delivery. The ablation of IPVs has become an important treatment for patients with advanced CVI who fail standard compression therapy, ablation of superficial venous axial reflux, and/or deep venous stenting.

The treatment of IPVs has evolved dramatically from invasive, open surgery to minimally invasive modern techniques. Dr. Linton originally described open ligation of perforating veins through incisions in already lipodermatosclerotic and ulcerated skin, often leading to delayed wound healing and infection.[3,4] The development of subfascial endoscopic perforator surgery (SEPS) revived interest in the treatment of IPVs, as this endoscopic technique involved placement of ports in unaffected skin remote to the lipodermatosclerotic skin for access to the subfascial space and allowed dividing of IPVs. By eliminating incisions in affected skin, SEPS improved the healing of venous ulcers with fewer wound complications as well as shorter recovery times.[4–6] However, the mid-term results from the North American Subfascial Endoscopic Perforator Surgery registry required general or regional anesthesia and reported ulcer recurrence rates of 16% and 28% at 1 and 2 years respectively, similar to the recurrence rates for open ligation.[7,8] The failure of perforator closure following SEPS was shown to be a risk factor for ulcer recurrence.[9] The development of minimally invasive venous devices and techniques ushered in the percutaneous ablation of incompetent perforator veins. Currently, the three most common percutaneous modalities are ultrasound-guided foam sclerotherapy (UGFS), radiofrequency ablation (RFA), and endovenous laser ablation (EVLA). There have recently been reports of ultrasound-guided glue ablation of the perforator vein at the level of the fascia.[10,11] The success of IPV ablation closure using percutaneous modalities is predictive of venous ulcer healing as well as reduced ulcer recurrence.[12–15]

ANATOMY AND PATHOPHYSIOLOGY OF PERFORATING VEINS

Relevant anatomy to management of IPVs is detailed in this section. Normal perforators allow venous flow from the superficial to the deep system across the fascia. The bicuspid venous valves maintain unidirectional flow by preventing flow reversal during muscle contraction. However, there is a subset of perforators without valves in normal limbs, allowing

 DOI: 10.1201/9781003316626-12

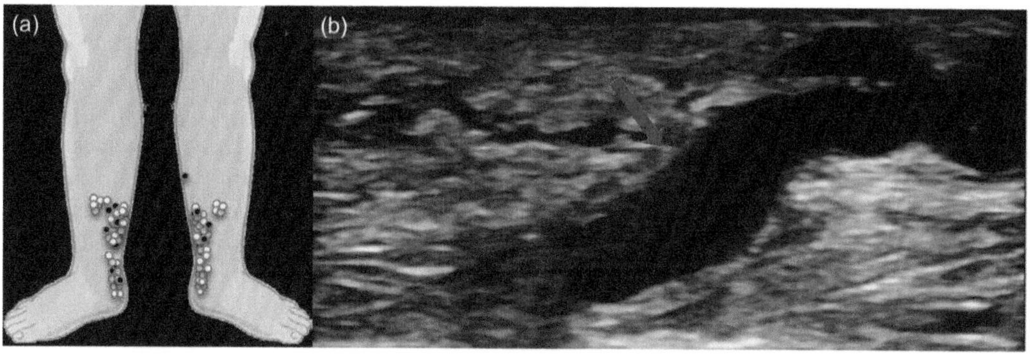

Figure 10.1 (a) Schematic depicting the most common location and distribution of venous ulcers. (b) Duplex ultrasound showing a pathologic perforating vein above a venous ulcer targeted for ablation.

for bidirectional flow between the venous systems.[16] Pathologic perforators allow venous flow from the deep to superficial system, causing ambulatory venous hypertension.

Early cadaveric dissections found an abundance of large perforating veins in the medial calf and ankle, where venous ulcers most commonly form (Figure 10.1a).[3] Following the introduction of SEPS, further anatomic study focused on characterizing the perforators in the medial leg between the medial malleolus and the tibial tuberosity.[17] The posterior tibial perforators, also historically known as Cockett perforators, connect the posterior accessory great saphenous vein to the posterior tibial veins. Cockett perforators are classified as I, II, and III based on the distance from the sole of the foot or the medial malleolus (currently we measure IPV by the distance from the sole of the foot). Cockett II and III perforators are most commonly targeted for ablation and found 7–9 cm and 10–12 cm from the medial malleolus, respectively.[17] Delis confirmed on ultrasound the most common location for IPVs was the middle and lower third of the medial calf.[18] In the proximal half of the leg, the paratibial perforators connect the great saphenous vein (GSV) to the posterior tibial veins. Boyd's perforator, also located in the proximal leg near the tibial tuberosity, connects the GSV to the popliteal vein.[17]

On duplex ultrasound, there is an increase in both the number and diameter of IPVs in patients with venous ulcers.[2,19] Stuart et al.[19] found patients with venous ulcers had one to four IPVs in the medial calf. These dilated and low resistance pathologic perforators allow for larger volumes of blood flow from the deep to superficial system at rates as high as 60 mL per minute during muscle contraction.[19,20] The venous pressures are elevated in the supramalleolar area due to pathologic perforators, akin to 'leaking bellows'.[21] The local venous hypertension leads to fibrin cuff formation, white-cell mediated inflammation, and impaired oxygen and nutrient delivery.[22] This creates a milieu that is susceptible to ulceration and poor healing. Therefore, the IPVs usually selected for ablation are those adjacent to the area of lipodermatosclerosis and venous ulceration (Figure 10.1b).[12]

TREATMENT INDICATIONS

Given the minimally invasive nature of percutaneous ablation techniques, most patients with advanced CVI and IPVs are eligible for treatment. The main contraindications to treatment include DVT within the last 3 months. Based on grade 2B evidence, the practice guidelines from the Society for Vascular Surgery and the American Venous Forum currently recommend treatment of pathologic IPVs with reflux ≥ 500 ms and diameter ≥ 3.5 mm in patients with CEAP C5 and C6 disease.[23,24] In addition, patients with C4b disease who are at risk for developing venous ulcers, indicated by skin changes such as progressive lipodermatosclerosis or peri-malleolar pain, can also be considered for treatment.[24] However, there is still less evidence to support the treatment of IPVs in the early stages of CVI, including C2 and C3 disease.[23,25,26] Updated guidelines from the Society for Vascular Surgery, American Venous Forum, and American Vein and Lymphatic Society continue to oppose the initial treatment of pathologic perforators concurrently with ablation of superficial axial reflux in patients with C2 disease.[26] No further recommendations regarding C3 disease have been established.

As perforator vein reflux most commonly occurs with superficial axial venous reflux, the treatment of IPVs can be concurrent or subsequent to the treatment of superficial axial venous reflux.[24] However, the treatment of IPVs is usually staged, as ablation of superficial axial reflux alone can correct pathologic perforator vein reflux and contributes to the successful healing of ulceration.[27,28] Therefore, patients with incompetent perforators after ablation of axial veins (saphenous and small saphenous) who have persistent symptoms and a persistently dilated and refluxing perforator are appropriate candidates for perforator ablation (Figure 10.2). A recent study of all three procedural options for the treatment of venous ulcers, truncal vein ablation, perforator vein ablation, and iliac vein stenting demonstrated that each contributes independently to ulcer healing.[29] Since truncal vein ablation (great saphenous, small saphenous, or anterior accessory saphenous) is relatively simple and

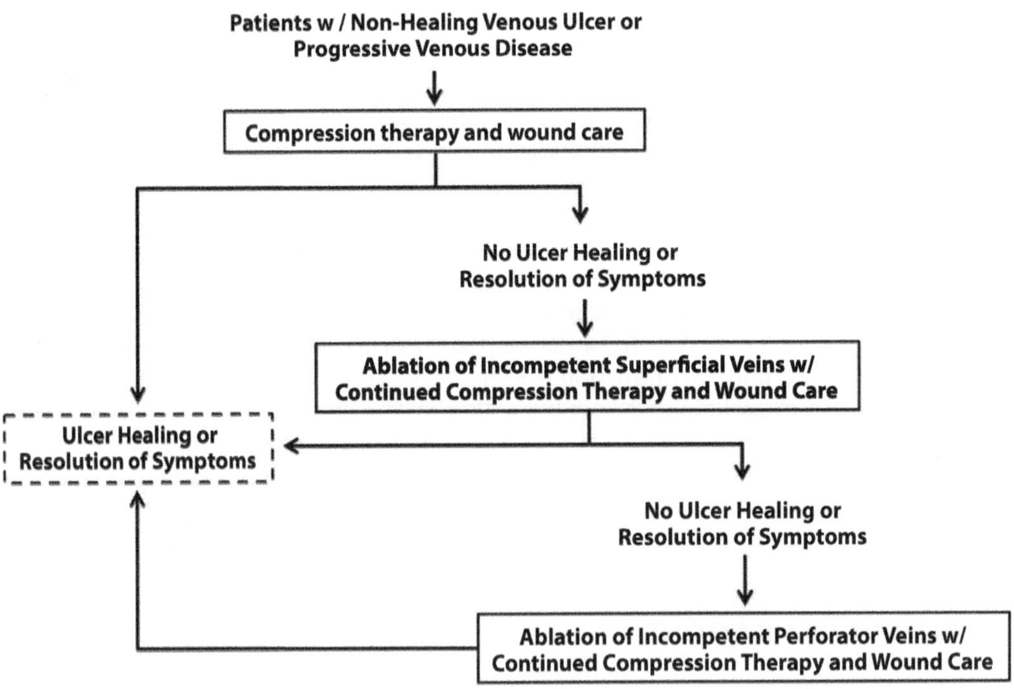

Figure 10.2 Treatment algorithm for management of non-healing venous ulcers and indication for ablation of IPVs.

efficient procedure, most venous specialists start with that procedure, although some begin with iliac vein stenting, if there is clinically significant iliac vein pathology.[29]

PREOPERATIVE EVALUATION

The preoperative evaluation requires comprehensive imaging with duplex ultrasound by a certified technologist. The exam should be performed with the patient standing or in reverse Trendelenburg position to characterize and delineate the superficial, deep, and perforating veins, and to evaluate for reflux and occlusive pathology.

The saphenous vein should be imaged in transverse and longitudinal views to systematically identify perforators passing through the fascia. To determine if a perforator is pathologic, color Doppler should be used while eliciting reflux.[30] There are several methods for eliciting reproducible reflux, including manually squeezing the calf or automatically inflating pneumatic cuffs.[30]

PERCUTANEOUS ABLATION TECHNIQUES

Ultrasound-Guided Foam Sclerotherapy

Under ultrasound guidance, the perforator vein is imaged in both transverse and longitudinal views as it allows for triangulation of the IPV for access planning. A 23-gauge needle is inserted into a varicose vein connected to the IPV. Confirmation of intraluminal access is demonstrated by back-bleeding. Although not approved for specific use by the FDA, either proprietary 1% polidocanol foam (Varithena, Boston Scientific Corporation, Marlborough, MA) or physician compounded foam (PCF) can be used. The foam sclerosant is introduced into the IPV through the 23-gauge needle. While injecting, compression of the deep vein by the ultrasound transducer can be an effective way of limiting the amount of foam that enters the deep system. A maximum of 10 cc of foam is used per session to limit the amount of gas introduced. The patient is also asked to repeatedly dorsiflex the ankle to augment flow through the deep system. The deep veins should also be imaged after injection to confirm the absence of foam.

Radiofrequency Ablation

Radiofrequency ablation has gained popularity for the treatment of IPVs. There are two techniques for perforator ablation that are frequently used and are often determined by IPV anatomy, physician expertise, and available equipment. The radiofrequency stylet catheter (ClosureFast, Medtronic, Minneapolis, MN) can be used in a direct puncture technique or with a Seldinger technique over a glide wire. In long straight IPVs, direct access can be achieved by interrogating the IPV with an ultrasound and anesthetizing the skin with lidocaine near the junction of the superficial vein and IPV (Figure 10.3a and 10.3b). A direct puncture can then be performed and the catheter advanced.

With short or tortuous IPVs, direct puncture can be challenging, and therefore, the Seldinger technique is preferred. Puncture of the vein can be achieved with a standard micropuncture kit and a glidewire advanced through the IPV into the deep system. This allows the RFA catheter to be introduced safely to the target area. The perforator vein is imaged in the longitudinal view, and the catheter is advanced within the perforator vein to 2 to 3 mm from the deep

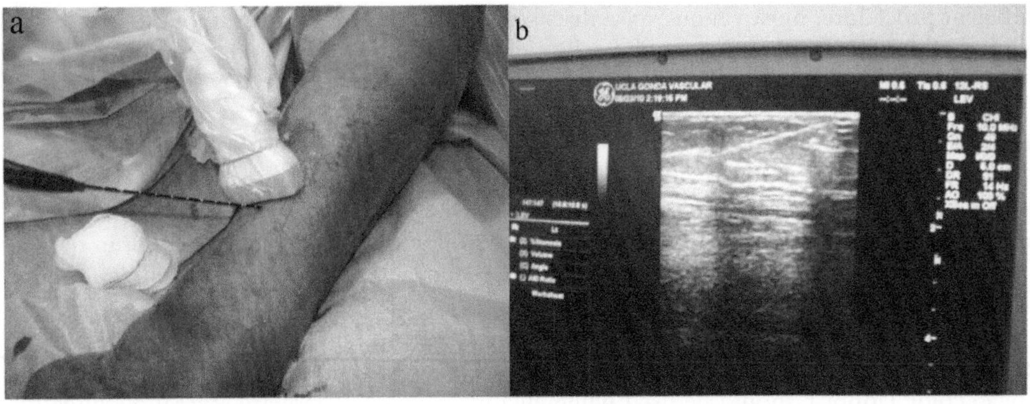

Figure 10.3 (a) Under ultrasound guidance, the RFA catheter is advanced within the perforator until 2–3 mm from the deep vein. (b) Duplex ultrasound showing the RFA catheter within the lumen of the perforating vein.

vein. Once the final catheter position is confirmed, tumescent anesthesia of 1% lidocaine is infiltrated surrounding the perforator vein. The vein is treated in four quadrants (0, 90, 180, 270 degrees) for 30–90 seconds at a temperature of 85°C with an impedance of less than 400 Ohms. The catheter is removed in 3 to 5 mm increments with repeated treatment of the four quadrants. A retrospective case-control study found no difference between a protocol time of 6-minutes at 85°C, 4 minutes at 90°C, and 3-minutes at 95°C.[31] The transducer is used to apply external pressure during the procedure to improve contact of the catheter with the vein wall. Once the catheter is removed, ultrasound imaging is repeated to confirm the absence of DVT as well as the closure of the perforating vein.

Endovenous Laser Ablation

Under ultrasound guidance, the 400-µm laser microfiber (Angiodynamics, Latham, NY) is inserted through a 21-gauge needle. The perforating vein is imaged in the longitudinal view, and the fiber is advanced within the perforator, up to 2 to 3 mm from the deep vein. Once the final position of the fiber tip is confirmed, tumescent anesthesia of 1% lidocaine is infiltrated surrounding the perforating vein. The fiber is connected to the 1470-nm diode laser (AngioDynamics, Latham, NY). The generator is set at a power of 5–10 W in continuous pullback mode. Higher energy levels are needed for perforator ablation compared to superficial axial ablation.[32] Instead of a bare fiber, a slim radial fiber (ELVeS-Radial slim kit, Biolitec Biomedical Technology GmbH, Jena, Germany) was also relatively recently used for perforator ablation.[15,32] The radial fiber emits 360 degrees of laser energy through a small diameter tip. Following the procedure, ultrasound imaging is repeated to confirm the absence of DVT as well as the closure of the perforating vein.

Postoperative Care

Following treatment of perforating veins, patients are advised to continue with daily compression therapy and wound care. Patients can resume all activities. A post-procedure ultrasound is typically performed within 72 hours to 2 weeks to assess the closure of the treated perforator as well as the absence of DVT.

CLINICAL OUTCOMES OF PERFORATING VEIN ABLATION

The treatment of IPVs developed as an adjunct for venous ulcers since compression therapy alone often failed to heal non-healing ulcers and prevent recurrent ulcers. The Effect of Surgery and Compression on Healing and Recurrence (ESCHAR) trial demonstrated surgical treatment of superficial axial reflux reduced ulcer recurrence at 4 years compared to compression alone (Figure 10.4).[33] Although only superficial axial reflux was corrected, this trial shifted treatment paradigms toward intervention for patients who cannot heal venous ulcers using compression alone. The treatment of IPVs has also been shown to improve ulcer healing and reduce ulcer recurrence, historically through SEPS and currently through percutaneous ablation of perforators (Table 10.1). Alden et al.[34] compared compression alone with multiple concurrent interventions, including RFA of superficial veins and UGFS of perforating veins, for the treatment of 95 venous ulcers. In comparison to compression alone, ulcer healing time was shorter in the intervention group (7.9 versus 22 weeks, $p < 0.001$) and recurrence was reduced at 1 year (22.9% versus 48.9%, $p = 0.004$).[34] In another study, patients undergoing RFA of perforating veins showed improved ulcer healing, increasing at a rate of 0.9 cm^2/month with compression alone to healing at a rate of 2.9 cm^2/month following IPV ablation ($p < 0.05$) (Figure 10.5).[35]

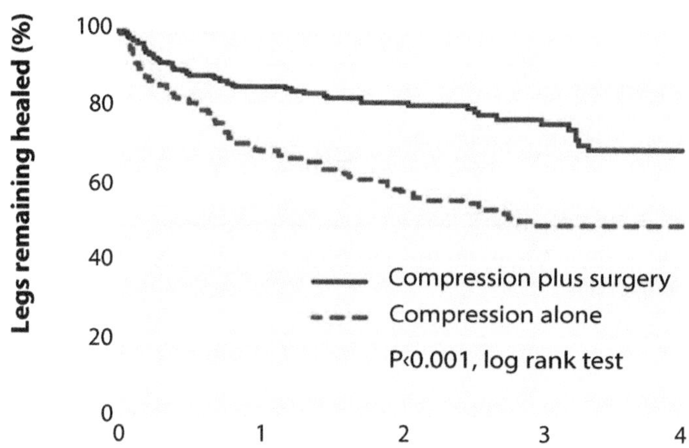

Numbers at risk					
Compression plus surgery	216	166	124	68	27
Compression alone	226	139	98	45	10

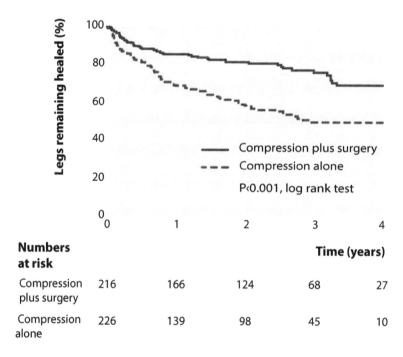

Gohel M S et al. BMJ 2007;335:83

Figure 10.4 Ulcer recurrence for patients who underwent compression alone compared to compression plus surgery, including superficial venous surgery or calf perforator surgery. At 4 years, ulcer recurrence was significantly reduced in the compression plus surgery group compared to compression alone. (From Gohel et al.[33])

Table 10.1 Clinical Results of Percutaneous Ablation Techniques

Author, Year	*Treatment Modality*	*No of Ulcers*	*Ulcer Healing %*	*Ulcer Recurrence %*	*Mean or Median Follow-Up (months)*
Masuda et al.,[36] 2006	UGFS	37+	68	32	
Alden et al.,[34] 2013	UGFS	48	65	23	12
Kiguchi et al.,[14] 2014	UGFS	73	59		34
Marsh et al.,[37] 2010	RFA	3	100		14
Lawrence et al.,[12] 2011	RFA	75	90*	4	13
Harlander-Locke et al.,[13] 2012	RFA	21++		5	25
Harlander-Locke et al.,[35] 2012	RFA	110	76	7	12
Hissink et al.,[38] 2010	EVLA	5	80		3
Dumantepe et al.,[39] 2012	EVLA	5	80		
Seren et al.,[15] 2017	EVLA	40	95*	6	20

+ Number of Limbs with Ulcers.
++ Number of Limbs with CEAP 5 Disease.
* Healing with closure of at least one perforator.

Table 10.2 Guidelines of the Society for Vascular Surgery and American Venous Forum on the Treatment of Perforating Veins[23]

No.	*Guideline*	*GRADE of Recommendation (1, strong; 2, weak)*	*Level of Evidence (A, high quality; B, moderate quality; C, low or very low quality)*
13.1	We recommend against selective treatment of incompetent perforating veins in patients with simple varicose veins (CEAP class C_2).	1	B
13.2	We suggest treatment of "pathologic" perforating veins that includes those with an outward flow duration of ≥ 500 ms, with a diameter of ≥ 3.5 mm, located beneath a healed or open venous ulcer (CEAP class C_5-C_6).	2	B
13.3	For treatment of "pathologic" perforating veins, we suggest subfascial endoscopic perforating vein surgery, ultrasonographically guided sclerotherapy, or thermal ablations.	2	C

(Continued)

Table 10.2 (Continued)

No.	*Guideline*	*GRADE of Recommendation (1, strong; 2, weak)*	*Level of Evidence (A, high quality; B, moderate quality; C, low or very low quality)*
Guidelines 6.5–6.8 of the Society for Vascular Surgery and American Venous Forum on the Treatment of Perforating Veins for Management of Venous Leg Ulcers[24]			
6.5	Combined Superficial and Perforator Venous Reflux With or Without Deep Venous Reflux and Active Venous Leg Ulcer In a patient with a venous leg ulcer (C6) and incompetent superficial veins that have reflux to the ulcer bed in addition to pathologic perforating veins (outward flow of >500 ms duration, with a diameter of >3.5 mm) located beneath or associated with the ulcer bed, we suggest ablation of both the incompetent superficial veins and perforator veins in addition to standard compressive therapy to aid in ulcer healing and to prevent recurrence.	2	C
6.6	Combined Superficial and Perforator Venous Reflux With or Without Deep Venous Disease and Skin Changes at Risk for Venous Leg Ulcer (C4b) or Healed Venous Ulcer (C5) In a patient with skin changes at risk for venous leg ulcer (C4b) or healed venous ulcer (C5) and incompetent superficial veins that have reflux to the ulcer bed in addition to pathologic perforating veins (outward flow of >500 ms duration, with a diameter of >3.5 mm) located beneath or associated with the healed ulcer bed, we suggest ablation of the incompetent superficial veins to prevent the development or recurrence of a venous leg ulcer. Treatment of the incompetent perforating veins can be performed simultaneously with correction of axial reflux or can be staged with re-evaluation of perforator veins for persistent incompetence after correction of axial reflux.	2	C
6.7	Pathologic Perforator Venous Reflux in the Absence of Superficial Venous Disease, With or Without Deep Venous Reflux, and a Healed or Active Venous Ulcer In a patient with isolated pathologic perforator veins (outward flow of >500 ms duration, with a diameter of >3.5 mm) located beneath or associated with the healed (C5) or active ulcer (C6) bed, regardless of the status of the deep veins, we suggest ablation of the "pathologic" perforating veins in addition to standard compression therapy to aid in venous ulcer healing and to prevent recurrence.	2	C
6.8	Treatment Alternatives for Pathologic Perforator Veins For those patients who would benefit from pathologic perforator vein ablation, we recommend treatment by percutaneous techniques that include ultrasound-guided sclerotherapy or endovenous thermal ablation (radiofrequency or laser) over open venous perforator surgery to eliminate the need for incisions in areas of compromised skin.	1	C

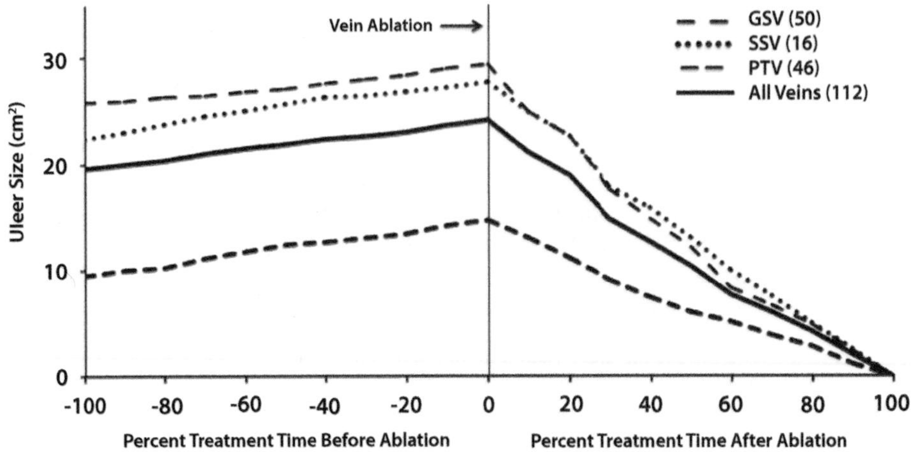

Figure 10.5 The effect of ablation of incompetent superficial and perforating veins on the healing rate of venous ulcers that healed completely. Ulcer size increased with compression alone prior to the ablation of incompetent veins and decreased following vein ablation. The number of incompetent veins treated is indicated in parentheses. GSV, great saphenous vein; SSV, small saphenous vein; PTV posterior tibial perforator vein. (From Harlander-Locke et al.[35])

The ablation of IPVs has been controversial as perforator reflux rarely occurs alone, but rather in combination with superficial or deep reflux.[1,2] Many studies simultaneously treat both superficial and perforator reflux making it difficult to discriminate between the role of perforator ablation alone in ulcer healing and recurrence. Lawrence et al.[12] treated IPVs in patients with recalcitrant venous ulcers despite ablation of superficial axial reflux. At a mean of 4.5-months, 90% of ulcers healed following the ablation of at least one perforator with RFA.[12] Harlander-Locke et al.[13] studied ulcer recurrence in patients with C5 disease presenting with signs of imminent ulceration despite treatment with compression therapy for at least 3 months followed by superficial axial ablation, if indicated, for at least 3 months before IPV ablation was performed. Following RFA ablation of IPV, ulcer recurrence rates were 0% at 6 months and 4.8% at 12 and 18 months.[13] Seren et al.[15] examined the treatment of IPVs in patients with recalcitrant venous ulcers, where 28 of 36 patients were treated with IPV ablation alone and 8 of 36 were treated with concomitant superficial axial ablation. At a mean of 11.5 months, 95% of ulcers healed following the ablation of at least one perforator with EVLA. The ulcer recurrence rates were 0% at 6 months, 2.7% at 12 months, and 5.5% at 18 months.[15] Furthermore, two studies examined ulcer healing in patients undergoing isolated treatment of IPVs with UGFS.[14,36] Masuda and colleagues reported a healing rate of 67.6% with an average healing time of 35.6 days following IPV treatment with UGFS.[36] The ulcer recurrence rate was 32.4% in this study and was associated with recurrent perforators.[36] Kiguchi et al.[14] demonstrated higher rates of IPV thrombosis in patients with healed rather than non-healed ulcers following UGFS (69% versus 38%, $p < 0.001$). The only positive predictor of ulcer healing in this study was successful thrombosis of IPVs.[14] In a multi-institution retrospective review, Reitz and colleagues analyzed ulcer healing and recurrence for 232 patients who underwent percutaneous ablation of perforators by UGFS, EVLA, or RFA during their index procedure despite 6 weeks of compression therapy.[40] At a median follow-up of 13-months, ulcer healing occurred in 57% and recurred in 25% of venous ulcers.[40] All the patients had combined IPV and superficial or deep venous insufficiency, and 10 patients (4%)

underwent only IPV treatment at their index procedure. These studies strongly suggest that percutaneous ablation of perforator veins independently improves ulcer healing.

Although there are no randomized control trials examining percutaneous ablation of perforators, two trials were conducted using SEPS with countering results. A multicenter randomized controlled trial was performed comparing surgical intervention, including SEPS, to compression alone in 170 patients with venous ulcers.[41] At a mean follow-up of 29-months in the surgical cohort and 26-months in the control cohort, there was no difference in the ulcer-free legs (72% versus 53%, $p = 0.11$).[41] In a 10-year follow-up of this cohort, 41% of the legs were evaluated in 73 of 170 patients.[42] At a mean follow-up of 97-months, the percent of ulcer-free legs was significantly higher in the surgical group compared to the control group (59% versus 40%, $p = 0.007$).[42] Van Gent et al.[42] identified the number of IPVs as a risk factor for those who are not ulcer-free. The Swedish SEPS Study Group performed a randomized controlled trial to compare saphenous surgery with and without SEPS in 75 patients with healed or active venous ulcers.[43] There was no difference in the ulcer healing rate or ulcer recurrence rate at the 12-month follow-up. Further validation of the independent role of perforator ablation using percutaneous modalities requires comparison in randomized controlled trials.

PROCEDURAL SUCCESS OF PERFORATING VEIN ABLATION

There is no consensus on the superior modality for the ablation of IPVs. The technical success, measured by the rate of closure, varies broadly across percutaneous techniques.[44] UGFS is commonly used as a modality that is technically simple, relatively inexpensive, and fast. However, there may be a greater risk that the sclerosing agent will enter the deep venous system and cause calf vein DVT. In addition to ablating the perforator, the varicosities connected to the perforating vein can be simultaneously treated. Masuda et al.[36] showed an initial closure rate of 98% after undergoing ablation of IPVs with 5% liquid sodium morrhuate and reported no instances of DVT. In this study, three-quarters of patients were diagnosed with C4 and C6 disease and showed improvement of venous clinical severity scores following treatment.[36] In a study of patients with C6 disease, the closure rate was 54% using polidocanol or sodium tetradecyl sulfate and had a low rate of DVT at 3%.[14]

The rigid catheter used for RFA makes the modality technically challenging, with a significant learning curve. At a high-volume institution, the perforator closure rate improved from 56% to 79% over a 4-year period.[12] If cannulation is successful, there are high rates of procedural success. Hingorani et al.[45] demonstrated an initial closure rate of 88% for patients undergoing ablation of 93 IPVs using RFA. In his study, only pulsatile venous flow predicted treatment failure. This bidirectional cardiac phasicity may represent patients with congestive heart failure, valvular regurgitation, and other systemic contributions to increased venous hypertension, contributing to the failure of IPV closure. Of the 38 patients, four (11%) had pulsatile flow with a 20% closure rate.[45] Marsh et al.[37] treated 124 IPVs and demonstrated a closure rate of 82% at a median follow-up of 14 months. Twelve percent of limbs in this study suffered neuropraxia.[37] In a recent study, Wang and colleagues reported an initial closure rate of 100% for 165 IPVs.[46] At 1-year follow-up, the closure rate was 98% with an associated improvement of the Venous Clinical Severity Score (5.77 ± 1.88 versus 2.70 ± 1.39, $p < 0.05$).

In comparison to RFA, EVLA is more user friendly, due to the flexible laser fiber but with similar complications due to the thermal mechanism of both modalities. There are two wavelengths, 810-nm and 1470-nm, which are most commonly used for EVLA. Hissink et al.[38] treated 58 IPVs using an 810-nm laser diode and showed a closure rate of 78% at a 3-month follow-up. In a large cohort of 534 IPVs, treated using an 808-nm laser diode, Corcos and colleagues demonstrated a closure rate of 72.2% at a mean follow-up of 27.5 months.[47] Zerweck et al.[32] treated 69 IPVs using a 1470-nm laser diode with a 95.6% closure rate at 1 month. In a study with longer follow-up, Dumantepe and colleagues treated 23 IPVs using a 1470-nm laser diode and showed a closure rate of 86.9% at 1-year follow-up.[39] There was an associated improvement in the Venous Clinical Severity Score by the third month of follow-up (15.1 ± 3.2 versus 4.2 ± 1.3, $p < 0.001$).[39] As there are high closure rates with both wavelengths, there is no consensus on the best protocol for the treatment of IPVs. However, one study compared the effects of two laser wavelengths on the treatment of 67 IPVs and found closure rates were better with 1,320 nm at 10 W compared to 940 nm at 30 W.[48]

Although there are no randomized control trials comparing treatment modalities, two published comparative analyses are available.[40,49] In a retrospective single-institution analysis of 112 patients, 296 perforator ablations were performed by UGFS (141, 48%), RFA (93, 31%), and EVLA (62, 21%).[49] At the 2-week follow-up, closure rates were lower for UGFS compared to RFA (57% versus 73%; $p = 0.05$). However, there was no statistical difference between UGFS compared to EVLA (57% versus 61%; $p = 0.09$). The patients who failed closure by UGFS showed significantly higher closure rates when IPVs were subsequently treated with EVLA (85%, $p = 0.03$) and RFA (89%, $p = 0.003$). The main factor that predicted failure across all modalities was BMI > 50 kg/m^2.[49] A retrospective multi-institution analysis compared the rate of venous ulcer healing in 232 patients following IPV ablation during the index procedure.[40] Of 232 patients with recalcitrant venous ulcers, 14 (6%) underwent UGFS, 127 (55%) RFA, and 91 (39%) EVLA. At 1 year, there was no significant difference in the rate of ulcer healing or frequency of repeat procedures across treatment modalities. However, there was a non-significant trend toward RFA having the highest rate of ulcer healing.[40]

All treatment modalities are reported to be safe with minimal risk of complications. The most common risks include local pain, ecchymosis, paresthesia, neuropraxia, phlebitis, skin necrosis, and DVT. Compared to thermal ablation techniques, there is a higher risk of DVT with UGFS as the sclerosant could be introduced into the deep veins. However, this risk is minimized by using ultrasound-guided compression of the deep vein connection, in addition to instructing the patient to repeatedly flex the ankle to prevent the sclerosant from adhering to the deep veins. The thermal modalities have a higher risk of paresthesia and neuropraxia than UGFS. One group reported neuropraxia in 12% of limbs following ablation of IPV with RFA.[37]

CONCLUSIONS

Dilated and high-refluxing pathologic perforators, abundant in the medial calf and ankle, contribute to local ambulatory venous hypertension, ultimately causing progressive lipodermatosclerosis and ulcer formation. Therefore, pathologic perforators should be treated in patients with C5 and C6 disease.[23] In 2022, joint guidelines from the Society for Vascular Surgery, American Venous Forum, and American Vein and Lymphatic Society continue to oppose the treatment of incompetent perforators concurrently with ablation of superficial axial reflux in patients with C2 disease.[26] However, incompetent perforator veins should be treated after incompetent truncal veins are treated in patients with persistent or recurrent symptoms and often before proximal iliac vein obstruction is treated.

There is no consensus on the best treatment modality for percutaneous ablation of incompetent perforators, as all techniques have been shown to be technically successful with a low risk of complications. However, long-term studies indicate that there may be lower closure rates using UGFS, even though this modality is less technically challenging than EVLA and RFA. The risk factors for ablation failure include pulsatile venous flow and BMI > 50 kg/m^2. All percutaneous treatment modalities, when successful, have also been shown to improve ulcer healing and reduce ulcer recurrence. As perforator reflux rarely occurs in isolation, future studies need to further validate the independent contribution of perforator ablation in ulcer healing and recurrence.

REFERENCES

1. Delis KT. Perforator vein incompetence in chronic venous disease: A multivariate regression analysis model. J Vasc Surg. 2004;40(4):626–33.
2. Labropoulos N, Mansour MA, Kang SS, Gloviczki P, Baker WH. New insights into perforator vein incompetence. Eur J Vasc Endovasc Surg. 1999;18(3):228–34.
3. Linton RR. The communicating veins of the lower leg and the operative technic for their ligation. Ann Surg. 1938;107(4):582–93.
4. Pierik EG, van Urk H, Hop WC, Wittens CH. Endoscopic versus open subfascial division of incompetent perforating veins in the treatment of venous leg ulceration: A randomized trial. J Vasc Surg. 1997;26(6):1049–54.
5. Stuart WP, Adam DJ, Bradbury AW, Ruckley CV. Subfascial endoscopic perforator surgery is associated with significantly less morbidity and shorter hospital stay than open operation (Linton's procedure). Br J Surg. 1997;84(10):1364–65.
6. Lee DW, Chan AC, Lam YH, Wong SK, Fung TM, Mui LM, et al. Early clinical outcomes after subfascial endoscopic perforator surgery (SEPS) and saphenous vein surgery in chronic venous insufficiency. Surg Endosc. 2001;15(7):737–40.
7. Gloviczki P, Bergan JJ, Rhodes JM, Canton LG, Harmsen S, Ilstrup DM. Mid-term results of endoscopic perforator vein interruption for chronic venous insufficiency: Lessons learned from the North American subfascial endoscopic perforator surgery registry. The North American Study Group. J Vasc Surg. 1999;29(3):489–502.
8. Sybrandy JE, van Gent WB, Pierik EG, Wittens CH. Endoscopic versus open subfascial division of incompetent perforating veins in the treatment of venous leg ulceration: Long-term follow-up. J Vasc Surg. 2001;33(5):1028–32.
9. Tenbrook JA, Iafrati MD, O'Donnell TF, Wolf MP, Hoffman SN, Pauker SG, et al. Systematic review of outcomes after surgical management of venous disease incorporating subfascial endoscopic perforator surgery. J Vasc Surg. 2004;39(3):583–89.
10. Toonder IM, Lam YL, Lawson J, Wittens CH. Cyanoacrylate adhesive perforator embolization (CAPE) of incompetent perforating veins of the leg, a feasibility study. Phlebology. 2014;29(1 Suppl):49–54.
11. Mordhorst A, Yang GK, Chen JC, Lee S, Gagnon J. Ultrasound-guided cyanoacrylate injection for the treatment of incompetent perforator veins. Phlebology. 2021;36(9):752–60.
12. Lawrence PF, Alktaifi A, Rigberg D, DeRubertis B, Gelabert H, Jimenez JC. Endovenous ablation of incompetent perforating veins is effective treatment for recalcitrant venous ulcers. J Vasc Surg. 2011;54(3):737–42.
13. Harlander-Locke M, Lawrence P, Jimenez JC, Rigberg D, DeRubertis B, Gelabert H. Combined treatment with compression therapy and ablation of incompetent superficial and perforating veins reduces ulcer recurrence in patients with CEAP 5 venous disease. J Vasc Surg. 2012;55(2):446–50.
14. Kiguchi MM, Hager ES, Winger DG, Hirsch SA, Chaer RA, Dillavou ED. Factors that influence perforator thrombosis and predict healing with perforator sclerotherapy for venous ulceration without axial reflux. J Vasc Surg. 2014;59(5):1368–76.

15. Seren M, Dumantepe M, Fazliogullari O, Kucukaksu S. Combined treatment with endovenous laser ablation and compression therapy of incompetent perforating veins for treatment of recalcitrant venous ulcers. Phlebology. 2017;32(5):307–15.
16. Sarin S, Scurr JH, Smith PD. Medial calf perforators in venous disease: The significance of outward flow. J Vasc Surg. 1992;16(1):40–46.
17. Mozes G, Gloviczki P, Menawat SS, Fisher DR, Carmichael SW, Kadar A. Surgical anatomy for endoscopic subfascial division of perforating veins. J Vasc Surg. 1996;24(5):800–8.
18. Delis KT. Leg perforator vein incompetence: Functional anatomy. Radiology. 2005;235(1):327–34.
19. Stuart WP, Adam DJ, Allan PL, Ruckley CV, Bradbury AW. The relationship between the number, competence, and diameter of medial calf perforating veins and the clinical status in healthy subjects and patients with lower-limb venous disease. J Vasc Surg. 2000;32(1):138–43.
20. Bjordal RI. Circulation patterns in incompetent perforating veins of the calf in venous dysfunction. Perforating Veins. Munich: Urban & Schwarzenberg; 1981.
21. Negus D, Friedgood A. The effective management of venous ulceration. Br J Surg. 1983;70(10):623–27.
22. Weingarten MS. State-of-the-art treatment of chronic venous disease. Clin Infect Dis. 2001; 32(6):949–54.
23. Gloviczki P, Comerota AJ, Dalsing MC, Eklof BG, Gillespie DL, Gloviczki ML, et al. The care of patients with varicose veins and associated chronic venous diseases: Clinical practice guidelines of the Society for Vascular Surgery and the American Venous Forum. J Vasc Surg. 2011;53(5 Suppl):2S–48S.
24. O'Donnell TF, Passman MA, Marston WA, Ennis WJ, Dalsing M, Kistner RL, et al. Management of venous leg ulcers: Clinical practice guidelines of the Society for Vascular Surgery® and the American Venous Forum. J Vasc Surg. 2014;60(2 Suppl):3S–59S.
25. Farah MH, Nayfeh T, Urtecho M, Hasan B, Amin M, Sen I, et al. A systematic review supporting the Society for Vascular Surgery, the American Venous Forum, and the American Vein and Lymphatic Society guidelines on the management of varicose veins. J Vasc Surg Venous Lymphat Disord. 2022;10(5):1155–71.
26. Gloviczki P, Lawrence PF, Wasan SM, Meissner MH, Almeida J, Brown KR, et al. The 2022 Society for Vascular Surgery, American Venous Forum, and American Vein and Lymphatic Society clinical practice guidelines for the management of varicose veins of the lower extremities. Part I. Duplex scanning and treatment of superficial truncal reflux: Endorsed by the Society for Vascular Medicine and the International Union of Phlebology. J Vasc Surg Venous Lymphat Disord. 2022;11(2):231–61.
27. Stuart WP, Adam DJ, Allan PL, Ruckley CV, Bradbury AW. Saphenous surgery does not correct perforator incompetence in the presence of deep venous reflux. J Vasc Surg. 1998;28(5):834–38.
28. Stuart WP, Lee AJ, Allan PL, Ruckley CV, Bradbury AW. Most incompetent calf perforating veins are found in association with superficial venous reflux. J Vasc Surg. 2001;34(5):774–78.
29. Lawrence PF, Hager ES, Harlander-Locke MP, Pace N, Jayaraj A, Yohann A, et al. Treatment of superficial and perforator reflux and deep venous stenosis improves healing of chronic venous leg ulcers. J Vasc Surg Venous Lymphat Disord. 2020;8(4):601–9.
30. Allan PL. Role of ultrasound in the assessment of chronic venous insufficiency. Ultrasound Q. 2001;17(1):3–10.
31. Aurshina A, Hingorani A, Blumberg S, Alsheekh A, Marks N, Iadagarova E, et al. Shortened protocol for radiofrequency ablation of perforator veins. J Vasc Surg Venous Lymphat Disord. 2017;5(6):824–28.
32. Zerweck C, von Hodenberg E, Knittel M, Zeller T, Schwarz T. Endovenous laser ablation of varicose perforating veins with the 1470-nm diode laser using the radial fibre slim. Phlebology. 2014;29(1):30–36.
33. Gohel MS, Barwell JR, Taylor M, Chant T, Foy C, Earnshaw JJ, et al. Long term results of compression therapy alone versus compression plus surgery in chronic venous ulceration (ESCHAR): Randomised controlled trial. BMJ. 2007;335(7610):83.

34. Alden PB, Lips EM, Zimmerman KP, Garberich RF, Rizvi AZ, Tretinyak AS, et al. Chronic venous ulcer: Minimally invasive treatment of superficial axial and perforator vein reflux speeds healing and reduces recurrence. Ann Vasc Surg. 2013;27(1):75–83.
35. Harlander-Locke M, Lawrence PF, Alktaifi A, Jimenez JC, Rigberg D, DeRubertis B. The impact of ablation of incompetent superficial and perforator veins on ulcer healing rates. J Vasc Surg. 2012;55(2):458–64.
36. Masuda EM, Kessler DM, Lurie F, Puggioni A, Kistner RL, Eklof B. The effect of ultrasound-guided sclerotherapy of incompetent perforator veins on venous clinical severity and disability scores. J Vasc Surg. 2006;43(3):551–56; discussion 6–7.
37. Marsh P, Price BA, Holdstock JM, Whiteley MS. One-year outcomes of radiofrequency ablation of incompetent perforator veins using the radiofrequency stylet device. Phlebology. 2010;25(2):79–84.
38. Hissink RJ, Bruins RM, Erkens R, Castellanos Nuijts ML, van den Berg M. Innovative treatments in chronic venous insufficiency: Endovenous laser ablation of perforating veins: A prospective short-term analysis of 58 cases. Eur J Vasc Endovasc Surg. 2010;40(3):403–6.
39. Dumantepe M, Tarhan A, Yurdakul I, Ozler A. Endovenous laser ablation of incompetent perforating veins with 1470 nm, 400 μm radial fiber. Photomed Laser Surg. 2012;30(11):672–7.
40. Reitz KM, Salem K, Mohapatra A, Liang NL, Avgerinos ED, Singh MJ, et al. Complete venous ulceration healing after perforator ablation does not depend on treatment modality. Ann Vasc Surg. 2021;70:109–15.
41. van Gent WB, Hop WC, van Praag MC, Mackaay AJ, de Boer EM, Wittens CH. Conservative versus surgical treatment of venous leg ulcers: A prospective, randomized, multicenter trial. J Vasc Surg. 2006;44(3):563–71.
42. van Gent WB, Catarinella FS, Lam YL, Nieman FH, Toonder IM, van der Ham AC, et al. Conservative versus surgical treatment of venous leg ulcers: 10-year follow up of a randomized, multicenter trial. Phlebology. 2015;30(1 Suppl):35–41.
43. Nelzén O, Fransson I, Swedish SEPS Study Group. Early results from a randomized trial of saphenous surgery with or without subfascial endoscopic perforator surgery in patients with a venous ulcer. Br J Surg. 2011;98(4):495–500.
44. Dillavou ED, Harlander-Locke M, Labropoulos N, Elias S, Ozsvath KJ. Current state of the treatment of perforating veins. J Vasc Surg Venous Lymphat Disord. 2016;4(1):131–35.
45. Hingorani AP, Ascher E, Marks N, Shiferson A, Patel N, Gopal K, et al. Predictive factors of success following radio-frequency stylet (RFS) ablation of incompetent perforating veins (IPV). J Vasc Surg. 2009;50(4):844–88.
46. Wang CM, Zhao SL, Feng QC, Gai S, Li X. One-year outcomes of radiofrequency ablation of incompetent perforator veins using the radiofrequency stylet device: Cohort study from East Asia. Phlebology. 2021;36(4):268–74.
47. Corcos L, Pontello D, Anna DDE, Dini S, Spina T, Barucchello V, et al. Endovenous 808-nm diode laser occlusion of perforating veins and varicose collaterals: A prospective study of 482 limbs. Dermatol Surg. 2011;37(10):1486–98.
48. Proebstle TM, Herdemann S. Early results and feasibility of incompetent perforator vein ablation by endovenous laser treatment. Dermatol Surg. 2007;33(2):162–68.
49. Hager ES, Washington C, Steinmetz A, Wu T, Singh M, Dillavou E. Factors that influence perforator vein closure rates using radiofrequency ablation, Laser ablation, or foam sclerotherapy. J Vasc Surg Venous Lymphat Disord. 2016;4(1):51–56.

Chapter 11

Thrombotic Complications Following Treatment of Peripheral Varicose Veins

Johnathon C. Rollo and Juan Carlos Jimenez

INTRODUCTION

Patients treated for lower extremity varicose veins are at risk for adverse thrombotic events (ATEs) despite a profound evolution in treatment methods over the past two decades.[1] The main principle of treatment involves correction of venous reflux (or reversal of venous flow) in diseased superficial truncal, tributary, and perforator veins. The primary method of reflux correction is controlled occlusion (and possibly removal) of the incompetent superficial vein. Whether this is performed with thermal energy (radiofrequency and laser ablation), non-thermal methods (polidocanol microfoam, cyanoacrylate, mechanochemical ablation), or surgical methods (high ligation and stripping, stab phlebectomy), deep venous extension of this controlled "thrombosis" or occlusion is rare but reported in the peer reviewed literature. Fortunately, this is a relatively infrequent complication that has a low incidence of serious clinical consequences to patients if diagnosed and treated properly.

CLASSIFICATION OF ADVERSE THROMBOTIC EVENTS FOLLOWING VARICOSE VEIN TREATMENTS

Extension of thrombus from the target superficial truncal vein into the adjacent deep vein following endovenous thermal ablation (RFA, EVLA) has traditionally been referred to as endovenous heat induced thrombus (EHIT). A newer term, ablation related thrombus extension (ARTE), was coined by the most recent clinical practice guidelines by the Society for Vascular Surgery (SVS), the American Venous Forum (AVF), and the American Vein and Lymphatic Society (AVLS).[2] The term ARTE is more general and refers to extension of thrombus into the adjacent deep vein following both thermal and non-thermal closure.

In 2021, a standardized classified system for EHIT was published by the AVF and SVS.[3] This combines elements from two prior distinct classification systems (Lawrence and Kabnick)[4,5] and is a four-tiered classification based on the anatomic location of adjacent deep venous thrombus extension following thermal ablation (Figure 11.1). The following terms were also formally defined in this paper. Non-EHIT DVT refers to a DVT occurring in a venous segment not contiguous with the thermally ablated vein. Post-ablation superficial venous thrombosis refers to the presence of thrombus in a superficial vein other than the treated vein. This vein may or may not be contiguous with the ablated vein.

DOI: 10.1201/9781003316626-13

Classification and Treatment of Endothermal Heat Induced Thrombosis

Recommendations from the American Venous Forum (AVF) and the Society for Vascular Surgery (SVS)

AVF EHIT CLASS	DEFINITION	TREATMENT RECOMMENDATION	STRENGTH OF RECOMMENDATION* AND LEVEL OF EVIDENCE**
I	Thrombus without propagation into deep vein a. **Peripheral to superficial epigastric vein** b. **Central to superficial eprgastric vein, up to** and including the deep vein junction	No treatment or surveillance.	2C
II	Thrombus propagation into the adjacent deep vein, but comprising <50% of the deep vein lumen	No treatment, weekly surveillance until thrombus resolution. In high risk patients consider antiplatelet therapy vs. anticoagulation. Discontinue treatment following thrombus retraction or resolution	2C
III	Thrombus propagation into the adjacent deep vein but comprising >50% of the deep vein lumen	Therapeutic anticoagulation, weekly surveillance. Discontinue treatment following thrombus retraction or resolution	1B
IV	Occlusive deep vein thrombosis contiguous **with the treated superficial vein**	Treatment should be individualized, taking into account risks and **benefits to patient. Reference may be made to CHEST guidelines** for treatment of DVT.	1A

*1=Strong, 2=Weak. ** A-High, B=Moderate, C= Low to very low

Figure 11.1 Classification and Treatment of Endovenous Heat Indused Thrombosis by the American Venous Forum and the Society for Vascular Surgery.

INCIDENCE OF ADVERSE THROMBOTIC EVENTS FOLLOWING VARICOSE VEIN TREATMENTS

Incidence of Deep Venous Thrombosis following Varicose Vein Surgery

Prior to the introduction of percutaneous endovenous methods for treatment of saphenous venous insufficiency, high ligation, and stripping (HL/S) with ambulatory phlebectomy were the most common techniques utilized. This involves surgical exposure of the great and/or accessory saphenous veins (GSV, AASV) at the saphenofemoral junction (SFJ) and a more distal incision (most commonly at the knee). For HL/S of the small saphenous vein (SSV), the incision is made overlying the saphenopopliteal junction and the more distal incision is made in the lower calf or leg. The GSV, AASV, or SSV is then ligated flush to its junction to the deep vein and divided. An endovenous stripper is introduced retrograde in the venous lumen and exposed through a venotomy near the junction. Inversion stripping of the vein is then performed.

Despite less frequent use of routine postoperative ultrasound during this era, the incidence of deep venous thrombosis (DVT) was reported to be approximately 5%.[6,7] A study by van Rij and colleagues reported an incidence of 5.3% (20 out of 377 limbs).[6] Only eight were symptomatic, and 90% were calf vein DVTs. No propagation of thrombus occurred in the study, and 50% of the thrombotic events resolved without complication. Puttaswamy and colleagues demonstrated a similar incidence of 4.8%.[7] More recently, Wolkowski et al reported an incidence of 3.5% (5 out of 377 limbs) following saphenous vein stripping and phlebectomy.[8] Similar to van Rij's study, all postoperative DVTs were in the distal leg. No pulmonary emboli were reported in any of these studies.

Incidence of Adverse Thrombotic Events following Endovenous Thermal Ablation (Radiofrequency and Laser)

Immediately following the advent of thermal ablation, early reports documented DVT rates as high as 16% following RFA of the GSV.[9] Twenty years later, with the continued improvement of technology and techniques, strong evidence has validated the safety of thermal ablation for saphenous vein insufficiency and the estimated incidence of ARTE and DVT associated with this treatment is between 1.3%–1.7%.[10–12] As a result, the most recent SVS clinical guidelines recommend against routine ultrasound surveillance following RFA or EVLA of truncal veins[2] (Table 11.1).

Incidence of Adverse Thrombotic Events following Endovenous Non-Thermal Ablation

Commercially Manufactured Polidocanol Microfoam and Physician Compounded Foam Sclerotherapy

Newer, non-thermal endovenous occlusion techniques have emerged for treatment of symptomatic truncal vein reflux over the past decade. One modality approved by the United States Food and Drug Administration (FDA) in 2013 is commercially manufactured polidocanol microfoam (Varithena®, Boston Scientific, Marlborough, MA, USA). Following direct venous injection, this compound adheres to the lipid cell membrane of the endothelial lining resulting in interruption of the osmotic barrier and damage to the endothelium with resultant vasospasm.[13] The endothelial disruption leads to acute thrombosis and occlusion of the venous

Table 11.1 Summary of Society for Vascular Surgery, American Venous Forum, and American Vein and Lymphatic Society Guidelines Pertaining to Post-Procedural Ultrasound Screening for Adverse Thrombotic Events

11.1. Post-Procedure Duplex Ultrasound
11.1.1. In asymptomatic, average-risk patients undergoing thermal ablation of the saphenous vein, we recommend against routine early post-procedural duplex ultrasound scanning (DUS) for ablation-related thrombus extension (ARTE) or deep vein thrombosis (DVT).
GUIDELINE. Grade of recommendation 1 (strong), Quality of Evidence B (moderate)
11.1.2. In asymptomatic, average-risk patients undergoing non-thermal ablation of the saphenous vein, early post-procedural DUS may be performed following procedures that have been reported to have increased risk of ablation-related thrombus extension (ARTE).
CONSENSUS STATEMENT
11.1.3. In asymptomatic, high-risk patients undergoing thermal or non-thermal saphenous ablation, early DUS to exclude ablation-related thrombus extension (ARTE) or DVT should be performed. Observation alone increases the risk of thrombotic complications.
CONSENSUS STATEMENT
11.1.4. In symptomatic patients who have undergone either thermal or non-thermal ablation, we recommend early DUS to exclude ablation-related thrombus extension (ARTE) or DVT.
GUIDELINE. Grade of recommendation 1 (strong), Quality of Evidence A (high)

Source: Adapted from Gloviczki P, Lawrence PF, Wasan SM, Meissner MH, Almeida J, Brown KR. The 2023 Society for Vascular Surgery, American Venous Forum, and American Vein and Lymphatic Society Clinical Practice Guidelines for the Management of Varicose Veins of the Lower Extremities. Part II, J Vasc Surg Venous Lymphat Disord. 2023. In Press (Elsevier).[2]

lumen. Chronic thrombosis of the vein results in filling of the venous lumen with fibrous connective tissue.

The incidence of ARTE and DVT following microfoam ablation (MFA) of truncal veins varies widely in the current literature. In the initial randomized trials leading to FDA approval of Varithena, the incidence of DVT following this treatment was reported between 2.5%–9.6%.[14–16] In a large (n = 250) single-center study by Deak, the incidence of DVT and ARTE was 0.8% and 0.4% respectively.[17] The differences in reported ATEs following MFA compared with catheter-directed thermal ablation may be due to increased variability in MFA techniques between procedures and operators (ie. amount of microfoam used, target veins, etc.).

In a study from our institution following early experience with MFA, we treated 157 limbs (truncal and tributary veins) over a 2-year period using adjunctive techniques not specifically outlined in the prior phase III clinical trials for Varithena[18] (Table 11.2). The overall incidence of ATEs in this study was 2.5% (ARTE–1.25% and DVT–1.25%). Three patients required short-term anticoagulation, and one asymptomatic patient resolved without treatment. In a follow-up comparison of above knee GSVs treated with both MFA (n = 127) and RFA (n = 150), the incidence of ARTE was higher in the Varithena group (MFA–6.3% vs. RFA–1.3%, p = 0.045).[19]

Physician compounded foam sclerotherapy (PCF) mixed using the Tessari method has been performed for many years prior to the advent of Varithena. The reported rate of venous thromboembolism is also highly variable (<1%–8.8%).[20,21] Differences in technique,

Table 11.2 Adjunctive Techniques Utilized during Microfoam Ablation

1. Preoperative duplex ultrasound examination performed by our *vascular ultrasound* laboratory and also performed by the proceduralist at the time of operation. Large perforator veins were localized and mapped before injection of microfoam.
2. Limb elevation to greater than 45°.
3. Injection of 10 mL of sterile saline before microfoam infusion to displace blood from the vein. In theory, the purpose is to limit the volume of foam administered and maximize microfoam contact with luminal surface.
4. Attempted limitation of microfoam volume to 5 mL or less (if possible).
5. Compression of the axial vein 5 cm caudal to the saphenofemoral or saphenopopliteal junctions and compression of perforator veins during microfoam injection.
6. Dorsiflexion and plantar flexion of the ipsilateral foot and ankle for 20 repetitions after microfoam injection.

Source: Adapted from Jimenez JC, Lawrence PF, Woo K, Chun TT, Farley SM, Rigberg DA, et al. Adjunctive Techniques to minimize Thrombotic Complications following Microfoam Sclerotherapy of Saphenous Trunks and Tributaries. J Vasc Surg Venous Lymphat Disord. 2021;9:904–909 (Elsevier).[18]

anatomy, and foam volume used may also influence the likelihood of thrombotic complications following PCF.

Cyanoacrylate Embolization of the Saphenous Veins

There is limited data available regarding the incidence of ARTE and DVT following cyanoacrylate embolization (CAE) (VenaSeal®, Medtronic, Minneapolis, MN) of the saphenous veins. However, the reported incidence in the current literature suggests severe ATEs are relatively infrequent and comparable to the rates following thermal ablation. O'Banion and colleagues reported an incidence of 1.9% of glue related ARTE and 0.3% for DVT in a review of 396 CAE procedures.[22] In the same study the rates of ARTE and DVT following RFA were 1.9% and 0.1%. In the randomized VeClose study, no patient in either the CAE group (n = 108) or the RFA group (n = 114) developed a DVT or pulmonary embolus.[23]

Mechanochemical Ablation

Mechanochemical ablation (MOCA) is a technique that utilizes a catheter with an oscillating wire tip to induce endothelial damage with simultaneous infusion of liquid sclerosant to occlude the refluxing truncal vein. Like other non-thermal techniques discussed, the incidence of ATEs is widely variable across different published studies. In the randomized MARADONA trial comparing truncal closure with either MOCA (n = 105) or RFA (n = 104), there was no ARTE or DVT reported in the MOCA group and one DVT reported in the RFA group.[24] Chen and colleagues performed 104 ablation procedures on 86 patients and reported an incidence of ARTE of 14.6%.[25] Thus, based on the existing literature, it is difficult to know the true frequency of ATEs following MOCA. Because this method of ablation requires simultaneous catheter pullback and injection of sclerosant, there is more user dependent technical variability between procedures and operators compared with thermal ablation. This may explain the increased range of ATEs currently reported.

RISK FACTORS FOR ADVERSE THROMBOTIC EVENTS FOLLOWING SAPHENOUS VEIN ABLATION

Because development of EHIT following thermal ablation is a low frequency event, precise categorization of risk factors is difficult and the data supporting them is inconsistent. Large vein diameter has been described as a potential risk factor for development of EHIT and ARTE following both thermal and non-thermal ablation.[4,19] In a study by Harlander-Locke from our institution, 1000 consecutive saphenous RFAs were performed.[26] The rate of EHIT was 1.8%, and no DVTs were reported. Multivariate analysis identified vein diameter >8 mm and a history of prior DVT to be risk factors. Additional studies have also suggested that larger target vein diameters may predispose to EHIT.[27,28]

History of prior DVT has been linked by numerous authors as a risk factor to the development of thrombotic complications following thermal ablation.[29–31] Other potential risk factors include concomitant phlebectomy,[30] increased age,[32] body mass index,[33] Caprini score,[34] deep venous reflux,[35] anatomy of the superficial epigastric vein,[36] and known hypercoagulable disorders.[37] Because of this limited and conflicting evidence, it is difficult to accurately predict which patients will experience EHIT. The literature identifying risk factors for ARTE following non-thermal ablation is even more limited. Thus, no formal risk stratification model or guidelines for medical thromboprophylaxis exist currently.

POST-PROCEDURE SURVEILLANCE AND TREATMENT OF ADVERSE THROMBOTIC EVENTS

Post-Procedure Ultrasound Screening for ARTE and DVT

Despite the risk of EHIT, non-thermal ARTE, and DVT following ambulatory varicose vein treatments, the incidence of clinically significant thrombotic complications (ie. pulmonary and paradoxical emboli) are very rare. Since the inception of ambulatory endovenous treatments for truncal vein insufficiency, various post-procedure surveillance and treatment protocols for ATEs have been proposed.

The most recent SVS, AVF, and AVLS guidelines provide evidence-based protocols for treating post-procedure thrombotic events[2] (Table 11.3). One new guideline that differs from the 2011 consensus document[38] is the recommendation that routine early post-procedural duplex ultrasound scanning to rule out ARTE and DVT is not required for asymptomatic patients undergoing thermal ablation of the saphenous vein. This recommendation is based on the low overall frequency of thromboembolic events in asymptomatic patients and the overall cost of routine ultrasound testing to the patient and healthcare system.[10]

However, there is insufficient evidence to extend this recommendation to patients who undergo non-thermal ablation of the saphenous vein. Because the rates of ARTE and DVT following MFA, MOCA, CAE, and PCF are not well-defined, we continue to perform routine post-procedural ultrasounds at 48–72 hours. Although it can be difficult to define patients at "high-risk" for post-procedural thromboembolic complications, providers should have a low index of suspicion for performing an ultrasound for patients, especially if they present with pain and swelling or if any evidence of possible thrombotic complication exists.

Table 11.3 Summary of Society for Vascular Surgery, American Venous Forum, and American Vein and Lymphatic Society Guidelines Pertaining to Treatment of Post-Procedural Adverse Thrombotic Events

11.3. Treatment of DVT and ARTE
11.3.1. For patients with acute isolated distal DVT, without severe symptoms or risk factors for extension we suggest serial imaging of the deep veins for 2 weeks.
GUIDELINE: Grade of recommendation: 2 (weak), Quality of Evidence: B (moderate)
11.3.2. For patients with isolated distal DVT and severe symptoms or risk factors for extension we suggest anticoagulation.
GUIDELINE: Grade of recommendation: 2 (weak), Quality of Evidence: C (low to very low)
11.3.3. For patients with acute proximal DVT we recommend anticoagulation with a direct oral anticoagulant (over a vitamin K antagonist)
GUIDELINE: Grade of recommendation: 1 (strong), Quality of Evidence: B (moderate)
11.3.4. For patients with symptomatic ARTE after endovenous ablation, we recommend anticoagulation with a direct oral anticoagulant (over a vitamin K antagonist)
GUIDELINE: Grade of recommendation: 1 (strong), Quality of Evidence: C (low to very low)
11.4.1. For patients with asymptomatic ARTE III and IV after endovenous ablation, anticoagulation with a direct oral anticoagulant (over a vitamin K antagonist) should be performed.
CONSENSUS STATEMENT
11.4.2. For patients who receive anticoagulation for ARTE following endovenous ablation, treatment either until the thrombus retracts or longer therapy according to standard DVT guidelines should be given.

Source: Adapted from Gloviczki P, Lawrence PF, Wasan SM, Meissner MH, Almeida J, Brown KR. The 2023 Society for Vascular Surgery, American Venous Forum, and American Vein and Lymphatic Society Clinical Practice Guidelines for the Management of Varicose Veins of the Lower Extremities. Part II, J Vasc Surg Venous Lymphat Disord. 2023. In Press (Elsevier).[2]

Treatment of Thrombotic Complications Following Varicose Vein Treatments

Medical anticoagulation is the mainstay of treatment for patients who develop clinically significant thrombotic complications following treatments for varicose veins. The most recent SVS, AVF, and AVLS guidelines recommend anticoagulation with direct oral anticoagulants (DOAC) for all patients with symptomatic ARTE and for asymptomatic patients with EHIT III and IV. This is also recommended for patients who develop an acute, proximal DVT following ablation and for symptomatic patients with isolated distal DVT. Patients at high risk for thrombus extension from an isolated distal DVT should also be anticoagulated.

Because EHIT tends to resolve with short-term periods of anticoagulation, the official recommendation based on the recent SVS/AVF/AVLS guidelines is to treat until the thrombus retracts into the truncal vein. The pathophysiology of ARTE compared with EHIT is not completely known. Thus, we recommend that duration of anticoagulation be determined on an individual patient basis for ARTE following non-thermal closure. In our clinical experience using commercially manufactured endovenous microfoam, for EHIT II and III, we recommend apixaban 5 mg po BID weekly until thrombus retraction is confirmed by duplex ultrasound.

For patients with occlusive DVT (EHIT IV), we recommend therapeutic anticoagulation with DOAC therapy for at least 3 months based on the most recent CHEST guidelines for treatment of VTE.[39] Although extensive post-procedure DVT is uncommon, patients who develop clinically significant and/or refractory thromboembolic complications should be referred to a hematologist for a formal hypercoagulable evaluation.

SUPERFICIAL VENOUS THROMBOSIS FOLLOWING TREATMENTS FOR VARICOSE VEINS

Superficial venous thrombosis (SVT) can occur when thrombus develops in a superficial truncal or tributary vein causing an inflammatory response. Common symptoms include localized pain, redness, and swelling of the affected area. A firm nodule or "lump" may develop, which may resolve or persist long-term.

Acute SVT of truncal and tributary veins has been reported following both thermal and non-thermal treatments for varicose veins and occur with more frequency than DVT. In a recent review of six studies and 1,256 thermal and non-thermal truncal ablations, there was no difference in the incidence of SVT between the two groups (thermal–8.4%, non-thermal–6.8%, $p = 0.38$).[40] In a recent comparison of MFA and RFA for thigh GSV and AASV symptomatic reflux, SVT was more common following MFA (MFA–15%, RFA–6%, $p = 0.06$).[41] Similar rates have been reported following MOCA.[42]

Aside from the typical superficial phlebitis that occurs following other varicose vein treatments, a distinct, prolonged phlebitis-like abnormal reaction (PLAR) has been reported following cyanoacrylate closure of the saphenous veins.[43] It is believed to be a type IV hypersensitivity reaction to the cyanoacrylate compound that mimics the pain, redness, and swelling associated with conventional SVT (Figure 11.2). Park and colleagues demonstrated that PLAR occurred in 25.4% of limbs treated with CAE in their study.[44] Formal protocols for prophylaxis and treatment have not yet been established but awareness, recognition, and prompt management by the venous specialist with antihistamines and oral steroids is important.

The most recent SVS, AVF, and AVLS guidelines address the management of SVT but not specifically for patients who have undergone superficial venous interventions.[2] The recent CHEST guidelines update address treatment of SVT and are presented in Table 11.4.[45] They

Table 11.4 Updated CHEST Guidelines Pertaining to Superficial Venous Thrombosis

Guidance Statements
18. In patients with superficial venous thrombosis (SVT) of the lower limb at increased risk of clot progression to DVT or PE (see text), we suggest the use of anticoagulation for 45 days over no anticoagulation (weak recommendation, moderate-certainty evidence).
19. In patients with SVT who are treated with anticoagulation, we suggest fondaparinux 2.5 mg daily over other anticoagulant treatment regimens such as (prophylactic- or therapeutic-dose) LMWH (weak recommendation, low-certainty evidence).
20. In patients with SVT who refuse or are unable to use parenteral anticoagulation, we suggest rivaroxaban 10 mg daily as a reasonable alternative for fondaparinux 2.5 mg daily (weak recommendation, low-certainty evidence).

Source: Adapted from Stevens SM, Woller SC, Kreuziger LB, Bounameaux H, Doerschug K, Geersing GJ, et al. Antithrombotic Therapy for VTE Disease: Second Update of the CHEST Guideline and Expert Panel Report. Chest. 2021;160(6):e545–e608 (Elsevier).[39]

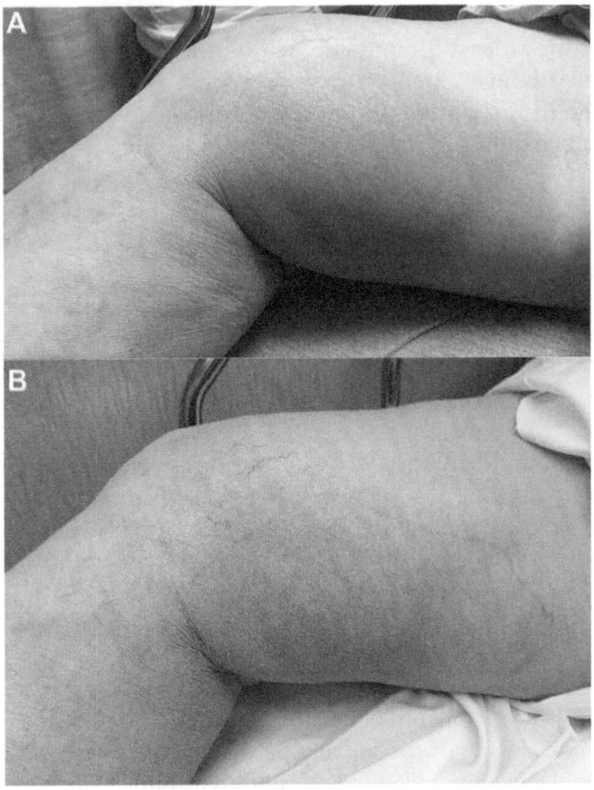

Figure 11.2 Phlebitic-like abnormal reaction (PLAR) noted immediately following cyanoacrylate closure. This resolved following treatment with oral steroids.

are also not specific to patients following varicose vein treatments. Appropriate treatment for most patients presenting with symptoms of SVT includes duplex ultrasound to rule out EHIT, ARTE and/or DVT, non-steroidal anti-inflammatory medications, warm compresses, leg elevation, and compression stockings (if tolerated). Most patients obtain symptomatic relief with these methods in 10–14 days. Occasionally, superficial phlebitis can result in an uncomfortable, palpable nodule or "lump," which can lead to overlying hyperpigmentation. We find that incision and drainage of "trapped blood" or phlebectomy under local anesthesia provides relief and can limit the duration and extent of the skin hyperpigmentation.

CONCLUSIONS

Although infrequent, ATEs may occur following surgical, thermal, and non-thermal varicose vein treatments. Venous specialists should be familiar with the most recent SVS/AVF/AVLS nomenclature and treatment guidelines for varicose veins of the lower extremities.[2] Diagnosis and appropriate medical management of ARTE, EHIT, SVT, and DVT following varicose vein procedures decreases patient morbidity and improves clinical outcomes.

REFERENCES

1. Pannucci CJ, Shanks A, Moote MJ, Bahl V, Cederna PS, Naughton NN, et al. Identifying patients at high risk for venous thromboembolism requiring treatment after outpatient surgery. Ann Surg. 2012;255:1093–1099.
2. Gloviczki P, Lawrence PF, Wasan SM, Meissner MH, Almeida J, Brown KR. The 2023 Society for Vascular Surgery, American Venous Forum, and American Vein and Lymphatic Society clinical practice guidelines for the management of varicose veins of the lower extremities. Part II. J Vasc Surg Venous Lymphat Disord. In Press.
3. Kabnick LS, Sadek M, Bjarnason H, Coleman DM, Dillavou ED, Hingorani AP, et al. Classification and treatment of endothermal heat-induced thrombosis: Recommendations from the American Venous Forum and the Society for Vascular Surgery. J Vasc Surg Venous Lymphat Disord. 2021;9:6–22.
4. Lawrence PF, Chandra A, Wu M, Rigberg D, DeRubertis B, Gelabert H, et al. Classification of proximal endovenous closure levels and treatment algorithm. J Vasc Surg. 2010;52:388–393.
5. Kabnick LS, Ombrellino M, Agis H, Mortiz M, Almeida J, Baccaglini U, et al. Endovenous heat induced thrombosis (EHIT) at the superficial deep venous junction: A new post-treatment clinical entity, classification and potential treatment strategies. Presented at the 18th Annual Meeting of the American Venous Forum; Miami; February 22–26, 2006.
6. Van Rij AM, Chai J, Hill GB, Christie RA. Incidence of deep vein thrombosis after varicose vein surgery. Br J Surg. 2004;91:1582–1585.
7. Puttaswamy V, Fisher C, Applebery M. Venous thromboembolism following varicose vein surgery: A prospective analysis. ANZ J Surg. 2000;70:150.
8. Wolkowski K, Wolkowski M, Urbanek T. Venous thromboembolism prophylaxis and thrombotic risk stratification in the varicose veins surgery-prospective observational study. J Clin Med. 2020;9:3970.
9. Hingorani AP, Ascher E, Markevich N, Schutzer RW, Kallakuri S, Hou A, et al. Deep venous thrombosis after radiofrequency ablation of the greater saphenous vein: A word of caution. J Vasc Surg. 2004;40:500–504.
10. Suarez LB, Alnahhal KI, Salehi PA, King EG, O'Donnell TF, Jr., Iafrati MD. A systematic review of routine post operative screening duplex ultrasound after thermal and non-thermal endovenous ablation. J Vasc Surg Venous Lymphat Disord. 2022;11(1):193–200.e6.
11. Healy DA, Kimura S, Power D, Elhaj A, Abdeldaim Y, Cross KS, et al. A systematic review and meta-analysis of thrombotic events following endovenous thermal ablation of the great saphenous vein. Eur J Vasc Endovasc Surg. 2018;56(3):410–424.
12. Healy DA, Twyford M, Moloney T, Kavanagh EG. Systematic review on the incidence and management of endovenous heat-induced thrombosis following endovenous thermal ablation of the great saphenous vein. J Vasc Surg Venous Lymphat Disord. 2021;9(5):1312–1320.e10.
13. Redondo P, Cabrera J. Microfoam sclerotherapy. Semin Cutan Med Surg. 2005;24:175–183.
14. King JT, O'Byrne M, Vasquez M, Wright D; VANISH-1 Investigator Group. Treatment of truncal incompetence and varicose veins with a single administration of a new polidocanol endovenous microfoam preparation improves symptoms and appearance. Eur J Vasc Endovasc Surg. 2015;50:784–793.
15. Todd KL, Wright DI; VANISH-2 Investigator Group. The VANISH-2 Study: A randomized, blinded, multicenter study to evaluate the efficacy and safety of polidocanol endovenous microfoam 0.5% and 1.0% compared with placebo for the treatment of saphenofemoral junction incompetence. Phlebology. 2014;29:608–618.
16. Gibson K, Kabnick L; Varithena ® 013 Investigator Group. A multicenter, randomized, placebo-controlled study to evaluate the efficacy and safety of Varithena® (polidocanol endovenous microfoam 1%) for symptomatic, visible varicose veins with saphenofemoral junction incompetence. Phlebology. 2017;32:185–193.

17. Deak ST. Treatment of superficial venous insufficiency in a large patient cohort with retrograde administration of ultrasound-guided polidocanol endovenous microfoam versus endovenous laser ablation. J Vasc Surg Venous Lymphat Disord. 2022;10:999–1006.e2.
18. Jimenez JC, Lawrence PF, Woo K, Chun TT, Farley SM, Rigberg DA, et al. Adjunctive techniques to minimize thrombotic complications following microfoam sclerotherapy of saphenous trunks and tributaries. J Vasc Surg Venous Lymphat Disord. 2021;9:904–909.
19. Chin AL, Talutis SD, Lawrence PF, Woo K, Rollo J, Jimenez JC. Factors associated with ablation related thrombus extension (ARTE) following GSV closure with endovenous microfoam ablation. Accepted for presentation: 38th Annual Meeting of the Western Vascular Society; Kauai; September 9–12, 2023.
20. Dannell O, Dorler M, Stockfleth E, Stucker M. Factors influencing superficial and deep vein thrombosis after foam sclerotherapy in varicose veins. J Dtsch Dermatol Ges. 2022;20:929–938.
21. De Aguiar ET, Dos Santos JB, Carvalho DD. Venous thromboembolism after ultrasound guided foam sclerotherapy. Phlebology. 2021;36:233–239.
22. O'Banion LAA, Siada S, Cutler B, Kochuney M, Collins T, Ali A, et al. Thrombotic complications after radiofrquency and cyanoacrylate endovenous ablation: Outcomes of a multicenter real-world experience. J Vasc Surg Venous Lymphat Disord. 2022;10:1221–1228.
23. Morrison N, Gibson K, McEnroe S, Goldman M, King T, Weiss R, et al. Randomized trial comparing cyanoacrylate embolization and radiofrequency ablation for incompetent great saphenous veins (VeClose). J Vasc Surg. 2015;61:985–994.
24. Holewijn S, van Eekeren RRJP, Vahl A, de Vries JPPM, Reijnen MMPJ. Two-year results of a multicanter randomized controlled trial comparing mechanochemical endovenous ablation to radiofrequency ablation in the treatment of primary great saphenous vein incompetence (MARADONA trial). J Vasc Surg Venous Lymphat Disord. 2019;7:364–374.
25. Chen AJ, Ulloa JG, Torrez T, Yeh SL, de Virgilio CM, Gelabert HA, Rigberg DA, et al. Mechanochemical endovenous ablation of the saphenous vein: A look at contemporary outcomes. Ann Vasc Surg. 2022;82:7–12.
26. Harlander-Locke M, Jimenez JC, Lawrence PF, Derubertis BG, Rigberg DA, Gelabert HA. Endovenous ablation with concomitant phlebectomy is a safe and effective method of treatment for symptomatic patients with axial reflux and large incompetent tributaries. J Vasc Surg. 2013;58:166–172.
27. Bontinis V, Bontinis A, Koutsoumpelis A, Potouridis A, Giannopoulos A, Rafailidis V, et al. Endovenous thermal ablation in the treatment of large great saphenous veins of diameters > 12 mm: A systematic review meta-analysis and meta-regression. Vasc Med. 2023. In Press.
28. Skeik N, Murray B, Carlson C, Jayarajan SN, Manunga J, Mirza A, et al. Determining risk factors for endovenous heat induced thrombosis after radiofrequency ablation. Ann Vasc Surg. 2021;71:1–8.
29. Ryer EJ, Elmore JR, Garvin RP, Cindric MC, Dove JT, Kekulawela S, et al. Value of delayed duplex ultrasound assessment after endothermal ablation of the great saphenous vein. J Vasc Surg. 2016;64:446–451.
30. Hicks CW, DiBrito SR, Magruder JT, Weaver ML, Barenski C, Heller JA. Radiofrequency ablation with concomitant stab phlebectomy increases risk of endovenous heat-induced thrombosis. J Vasc Surg Venous Lymphat Disord. 2017;5:200–209.
31. Sufian S, Arnez A, Labropoulos N, Lakhanpal S. Incidence, progression, and risk factors for endovenous heat-induced thrombosis after radiofrequency ablation. J Vasc Surg Venous Lymphat Disord. 2013;1:159–164.
32. Kibrik P, Chait J, Arustamyan M, Alsheekh A, Rajee S, Marks N, et al. Safety and efficacy of endovenous ablations in octogenarians, nonagenarians, and centenarians. J Vasc Surg Venous Lymphat Disord. 2020;8:95–99.
33. Pasenidou K, Tang TY, Juszczak M, Tiwari A. Factors affecting residual stump length following endovenous laser ablation. Vasc Endovascular Surg. 2023;57:339–343.
34. Rhee SJ, Cantelmo NL, Conrad MF, Stoughton J. Factors influencing the incidence of endovenous heat-induced thrombosis (EHIT). Vasc Endovascular Surg. 2013;47:207–212.

35. Satam K, Aurshina A, Zhuo H, Zhang Y, Cardella J, Aboian E, et al. Incidence and significance of deep venous reflux in patients treated with saphenous vein ablation. Ann Vasc Surg. 2023;91:182–190.
36. Kitagawa A, Yamada Y, Nagao T. The proximity of the superficial epigastric vein to the saphenofemoral junction is associated with endovenous heat-induced thrombosis after radiofrequency ablation for varicose veins. J Vasc Surg Venous Lymphat Disord. 2021;9:669–675.
37. Korepta LM, Watson JJ, Mansour MA, Chambers CM, Cuff RF, Slaikeu JD, et al. Outcomes of a single-center experience with classification and treatment of endothermal heat-induced thrombosis after endovenous ablation. J Vasc Surg Venous Lymphat Disord. 2017;5:332–338.
38. Gloviczki P, Comerota A, Dalsing MC, Eklof BG, Gillespie DL, Gloviczki ML, et al. The care of patients with varicose veins and associated chronic venous diseases: Clinical practice guidelines of the Society for Vascular Surgery and the American Venous Forum. J Vasc Surg. 2011;53:2S–48S.
39. Stevens SM, Woller SC, Kreuziger LB, Bounameaux H, Doerschug K, Geersing GJ, et al. Antithrombotic therapy for VTE disease: Second update of the CHEST guideline and expert panel report. Chest. 2021;160(6):e545–e608.
40. Hassanin A, Aherne TM, Greene G, Boyle E, Egan B, Tierney S, et al. A systematic review and meta-analysis of comparative studies comparing nonthermal versus thermal endovenous ablation in superficial venous incompetence. J Vasc Surg Lymphat Disord. 2019;7:902–913.
41. Talutis SD, Chin AL, Lawrence PF, Woo K, Jimenez JC. Comparison of outcomes following polidocanol microfoam and radiofrequency ablation of incompetent thigh great and accessory saphenous veins. J Vasc Surg Venous Lymphat Disord. 2023;11:916–920.
42. Baccellieri D, Apruzzi L, Ardita V, Favia N, Saracino C, Carta N, et al. Early results of mechanochemical ablation for small saphenous vein incompetency using 2% polidocanol. J Vasc Surg Venous Lymphat Disord. 2021;9:683–690.
43. Nasser H, Ivanics T, Shakaroun D, Lin J. Severe phlebitis-like abnormal reaction following great saphenous vein cyanoacrylate closure. J Vasc Surg Venous Lymphat Disord. 2019;7:578–582.
44. Park I, Jeong MH, Park CJ, Park WLL, Park DW, Joh JH. Clinical features and management of "Phlebitis-like Abnormal Reaction" after cyanoacrylate closure for the treatment of incompetent saphenous veins. Ann Vasc Surg. 2019;55:239–245.
45. Stevens SM, Woller SC, Kreuziger LB, Bounameaux H, Doerschug K, Geersing GJ, et al. Executive summary: Antithrombotic therapy for VTE disease: Second update of the CHEST guideline and expert panel report. Chest. 2021;160:2247–2259.

Chapter 12

Pathophysiology and Management of Chronic Venous Stasis Ulcers

Antalya Jano and Eric S. Hager

INTRODUCTION

Chronic venous stasis ulcers (VSUs) are open skin lesions that occur in the lower extremities and are commonly seen in late stages of chronic venous insufficiency (CVI).[1,2] They most often occur from venous hypertension arising from either proximal venous obstruction or valvular reflux. Factors such as obesity, heart failure, retroperitoneal fibrosis, and inadequate calf muscle pump function all contribute to increasing venous pressures.[3,4] Venous hypertension causes a local inflammatory change, leading to the deposition of fibrin that forms a "cuff," inhibiting oxygen and nutrient diffusion across capillary beds and leading to impaired wound healing as a result.[3]

Clinically, VSUs present with irregular shape and well-circumscribed borders, typically along the medial and lateral aspects of the distal ankle.[5,6] Accompanying symptoms can include pain, inflammation, and significant drainage. VSUs represent late findings in the spectrum of venous disease, which includes edema, stasis dermatitis, dermal hyperpigmentation, and subcutaneous fibrosis.[6,7] VSUs tend to have a chronic course with significant morbidity, mortality, and socioeconomic burden.[8,9] Given their overall prevalence of 1–3% in the United States, there is significant interest in rapid identification and initiation of treatment to accelerate healing and prevent recurrence.[2]

The mainstay of management involves compression therapy via garments or bandages to control edema and drainage.[1] Some data suggests that systemic medications such as pentoxifylline or aspirin may be used as adjuvants, but these therapies remain controversial.[11] In addition to compression and drainage management, proper wound care consisting of debridement and infection control is of utmost importance.[10,11] Overall, conservative management has excellent early results, with closure rates approaching 97% at 6 months.[12] However, recurrence rates within 2 years range from 70–100% in non-compliant patients and 30–40% in those who consistently maintain exceptional skin care and compression.[13] Treatment of venous insufficiency via endovenous ablation techniques seeks to speed healing and reduce recurrence rates by either removing obstruction or eliminating reflux and has been shown to increase ulcer-free time by up to 29 days within the first year after intervention.[14]

EPIDEMIOLOGY AND SOCIOECONOMIC BURDEN

In the United States, chronic venous stasis ulcers pose significant clinical, financial, and social burdens for patients, providers, and the healthcare system. VSUs comprise 70–90% of lower leg ulcers and have high rates of recurrence even with maximal medical therapy.[15,16] About 600,000 individuals develop a VSU annually.[17] Prevalence increases with age, with VSUs affecting up to 5% of American individuals over the age of 65 years.[18] For patients, the incurred annual medical costs have been calculated as $6,391 and $7,030 in those with

DOI: 10.1201/9781003316626-14

Medicare and private insurance, respectively.[9] Avoiding these costs does not come without consequence; untreated ulcers lead to morbidity resulting from pain, discomfort, and fluid discharge, with possible development of secondary amyloid disease, anemia, hypoproteinemia, or malignant change.[19,20] In addition to the medical and economic burden, the psychosocial effects on patients with VSUs is not to be understated. Frequent wound care visits can lead to loss of productivity in younger patients and increased disability in elderly patients.[5] About 4.6 million workdays per year are lost secondary to CVI. The pain, bulky dressings, and recurrent hospitalizations may push patients into social isolation, which further impacts quality of life.[5] Lastly, the Medicare and commercial annual costs to the US healthcare system are $18,986 and $13,653, respectively, representing an annual US payer burden of $14.9 billion.[9]

PATHOPHYSIOLOGY OF CHRONIC VENOUS STASIS ULCERS

The mechanism behind chronic VSU formation results from the interplay between genetic predisposition and venous hypertension. Normally, the lower extremity venous outflow occurs from superficial to deep via perforating veins.[7] The superficial system consists largely of the great and small saphenous veins. Deep veins include three sets of paired tibial veins, the popliteal vein, the femoral vein in the thigh, and the deep and common femoral veins.[7] Valves are found throughout the venous systems and are responsible for maintaining unidirectional blood flow from the superficial to deep veins.[19] Blood reaches the heart via leg muscle contraction, which compresses the deep veins and leads to a transient pressure increase within the deep system that pushes blood cephalad to the heart.[7,17] Here, the valves prevent reflux and transmission of elevated deep venous pressures to the superficial veins and capillaries.[17] Once the deep venous pressures have fallen, the valves open to drive flow from the superficial to deep system again.

Venous hypertension, then, arises primarily from two processes: reflux and obstruction. When a patient has an underlying pathology such as iliac vein stenosis or occlusion, venous outflow is impaired and causes significant venous hypertension. Venous reflux develops as a consequence of valvular incompetence, most often in the superficial system.[7,17]

The pathogenic steps from venous hypertension to development of chronic VSUs have been widely debated. It has been posited that sustained venous hypertension is transmitted to the capillaries, leading to distension of capillary walls and widening of endothelial pores.[21] Macromolecules such as fibrinogen then leak into the interstitial fluid within the dermis and subcutaneous tissue of the calf, doing so at a faster rate in those with venous disease than without.[21–23] Because fibrinogen is insoluble in the interstitial space, it polymerizes into a fibrin cuff that physically impedes oxygen and nutrient diffusion, causing cell death and ulceration.[7,17,21] Additional research suggests that fibrinogen, as well as other large molecules extravasating from damaged capillaries, may function to "trap" or inhibit growth factors, thereby preventing them from maintaining tissue integrity and facilitating wound healing.[7,17,24]

Leukocyte trapping may also contribute to formation of the fibrin cuff. Venous hypertension reduces the capillary perfusion pressure and thus the capillary flow rate, leading to "trapped" leukocytes.[25] These leukocytes release toxic oxygen metabolites (free radicals) and proteolytic enzymes that injure capillaries, thereby increasing their permeability to large molecules and perpetuating further white blood cell trapping.[25] Trapped leukocytes prevent further circulation, leading to ischemia in affected capillaries, poor perfusion, and ulcer formation.[25]

Moreover, leukocyte activation has been shown to increase elastase levels, which induces epithelial and vascular injury, and prompts release of TNF-α, which decreases fibrinolytic activity, thus promoting fibrin cuff formation via direct and indirect methods, respectively.[17,26]

Not only may local fibrinolytic abnormalities play a role in ulcer formation, but systemic fibrinolytic and coagulation irregularities may, too. Patients with venous disease and ulcers have demonstrated increased plasma fibrinogen, protein C, D-dimer, and fibrin-related antigen levels.[7,27–29] They have also been found to have decreased factor XIII activity, which may indicate factor consumption as excess fibrin is deposited.[7,30,31]

Unfortunately, the theory of the fibrin cuff that many of the aforementioned hypotheses fall back on is not without its weaknesses. It was discovered that fibrin cuffs were discontinuous and irregular around dermal capillaries impacted by venous hypertension, making them less likely to act as physical barriers.[24] Furthermore, fibrin cuffs were discovered to persist along the venous ulcer border even after the wound has healed.[25]

DIAGNOSIS OF CHRONIC VENOUS STASIS ULCERS

Clinical History

Patients with chronic VSUs often have preceding symptoms associated with chronic venous insufficiency. These include lower extremity heaviness, fatigue, and edema that tend to worsen with standing, progress throughout the day, and improve with rest and elevation. Hemosiderosis and lipodermatosclerosis are characteristic as well.[2,19] Patients with a history of obesity, deep vein thrombosis, sedentary lifestyle, female gender, and multiparity are at increased risk for developing chronic VSUs. There is a genetic component that predisposes to significant venous disease and includes hypercoagulability, May-Thurner syndrome, and Klippel-Trenaunay syndrome.[2,3,6,7]

Physical Exam

On exam, chronic VSUs present as shallow wounds with irregular, well-defined margins, and a granulated base (Figure 12.1).[7] Malodorous exudate may be observed. The ulcers are typically located in the distal third of the calf, superior to or over bony prominences such as the medial malleolus.[6] Depending on VSU and CVI stage, surrounding skin may be edematous, eczematous, hyperpigmented, or indurated and fibrotic, which leads to the "inverted champagne bottle" appearance characteristic of advanced lipodermatosclerosis.[6,7] Other evidence of CVI may be present as well: telangiectasias, reticular veins, varicosities, corona phlebectatica, and atrophie blanche.[3,6] CEAP classification may be used to catalogue VSUs (Figure 12.1a and 12.1b).

Testing

Initial testing in patients with suspected VSUs involves non-invasive imaging via venous duplex ultrasound, arterial pulse exam, and measurement of the ankle brachial index (ABI).[1,2] Color duplex ultrasound may be used to assess for reflux and obstruction particularly within superficial veins.[1,2,32] Reflux defined by the Society of Vascular Surgery as valve closure time >0.5 ms in saphenous, tibial, deep femoral, and perforating veins and >1 sec in femoral and popliteal veins, in addition to the presence of deep vein thrombosis, can also be assessed (Figure 12.2).[1]

(a)

(b)

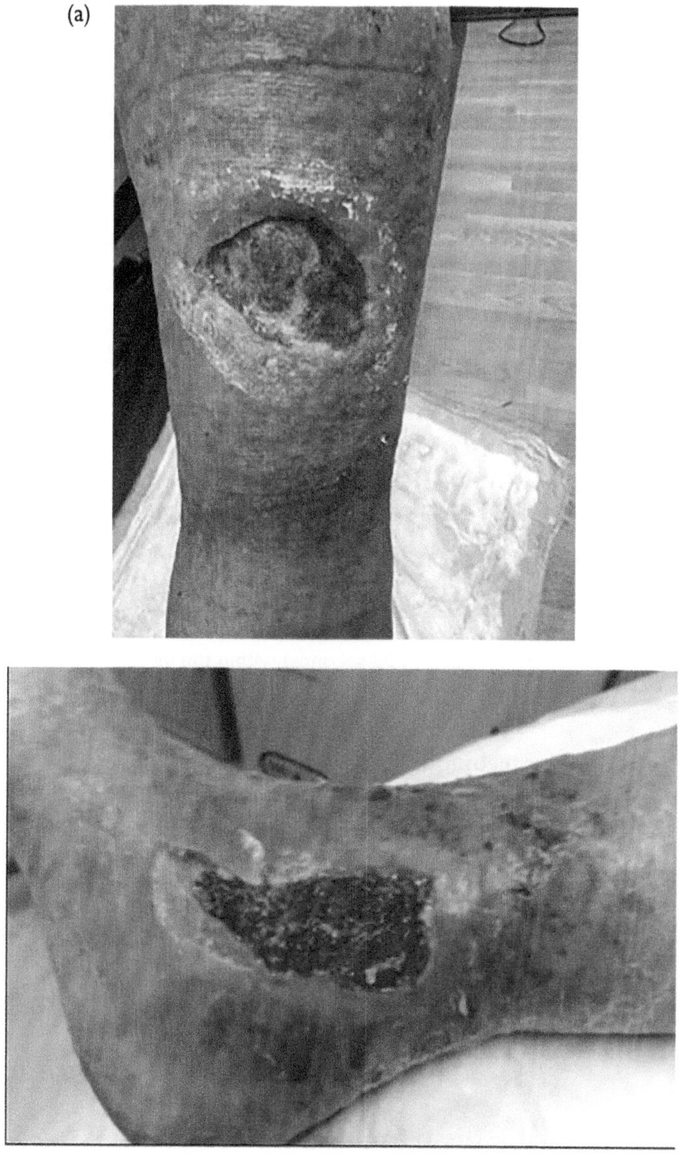

Figure 12.1 (a) Long, deep, red-pink-colored wound with scab-like tissue and yellow crusting located below inner ankle bone with surrounding redness and peeling of the skin, also representing a chronic venous stasis ulcer with granulated base. (b) Chronic venous stasis ulcers with granulated base superior to anterior ankle (a) and inferior to medial malleolus (b).

The proper technique for duplex scanning a patient for reflux most commonly involves using 4–7 MHz linear array transducers for deeper veins and higher frequency probes for those that are more superficial.[33] The patient should be instructed to assume a standing or upright position with the leg rotated outward and the heel on the ground.[1] The opposite leg should bear most of the patient's weight.

The diagnosis of common iliac stenosis by DUS is low, with a sensitivity of 47% with common iliac vein lesions and 79% with external iliac vein lesions.[34] This is due to obesity,

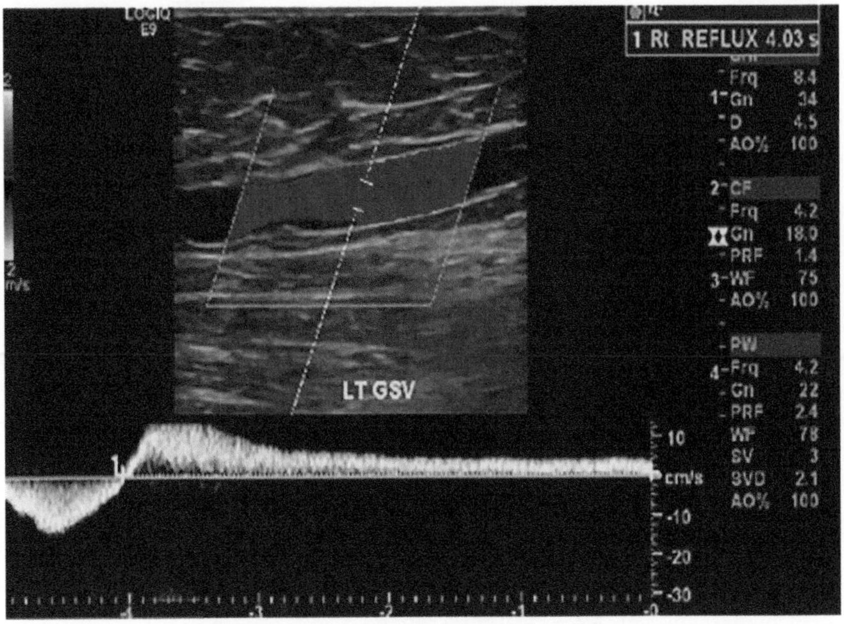

Figure 12.2 Duplex ultrasound showing reflux (4.03 seconds) within the left great saphenous vein.

overlying bowel gas, and poor technique.[34,35] There are several surrogate markers that can be used to suggest proximal stenosis, including the loss of respiratory phasicity in the common femoral vein, turbulent flow via color flow analysis, and loss of normal Valsalva response (Figure 12.3).[36]

In some cases, if the duplex is inadequate or is suggestive of proximal venous stenosis or occlusion, a CT or MRI may be used to visualize the deep venous system. If the ABI is abnormal and the patient has comorbidities that place them at risk for ischemia, evaluation of arterial blood flow must be performed, as VSU treatment may cause injury.[2] Lastly, biopsy of the VSU may be indicated if there is suspicion for malignant transformation to squamous cell carcinoma.[2]

TREATMENT OF CHRONIC VENOUS STASIS ULCERS

Compression Therapy

In patients without arterial disease, compression and wound care have been the gold standard of initial and long-term treatment of chronic VSUs. Compression is believed to improve venous drainage via increase of venous pump and lymphatic drainage.[7,37] It also alleviates edema by increasing local hydrostatic pressure and decreasing superficial venous pressure, thereby reducing fluid and macromolecule leakage into the interstitial space.[7,37] The reduction in edema ultimately leads to increased cutaneous blood flow and improved healing. It is important to note that compression therapy is contraindicated in uncompensated congestive heart failure. Patients with an ABI <0.5 can be carefully compressed, but frequent wound checks are critical as the patient may be in danger of exacerbating the ulceration

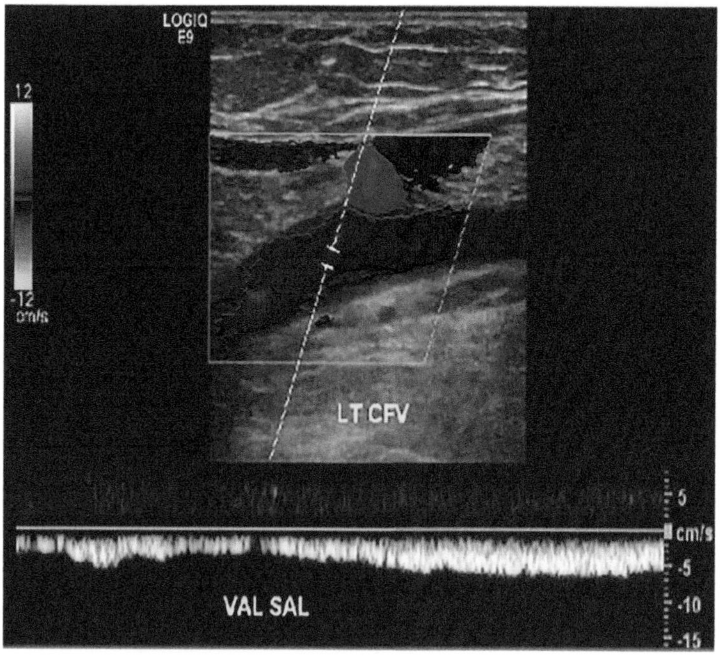

Figure 12.3 Duplex ultrasound showing continuous flow in the left femoral vein with loss of phasicity and abnormal response to Valsalva maneuver.

secondary to ischemia. In these situations, referral to a vascular surgeon or interventionalist is recommended.[7,38]

Selecting an appropriate compression strength depends on treatment stage: the decongestion phase, which targets CVI, reduces edema, and aids with ulcer healing, and the maintenance phase, which prevents edema and ulcer recurrence.[38] The objective of the former phase is to offer high working pressures during muscle contraction and lower resting pressures upon relaxation. Rigid inelastic, short-stretch bandages exhibit these properties and are applied at pressures of 40–60 mmHg. However, they can only be used in ambulatory patients, as they do not mold to accommodate changes in leg volume due to edema.[7,37,38] Elastic, long-stretch bandages provide higher resting pressures, better conform to the leg, and allow for frequent dressing changes.[7] These bandages are categorized based on indication: Class I (lightweight for dressing retention), Class II (support for ankle strain, sprains), Class IIIa (light compression, <20 mmHg), IIIb (moderate, ≥20–40 mmHg), IIIc (high, ≥41–59 mmHg), and IIId (very high, ≥60 mmHg).[7,37,38] Multilayered bandages featuring 2–4 layers of padding and pneumatic compression devices may also be considered when chronic VSUs do not respond to standard compression (Figure 12.4).[7] For the maintenance phase, elastic graded compression stockings with maximum pressure at the ankles and minimal pressure at the thighs are utilized. These stockings are divided into classes as well: Class I (10–22 mmHg for varicose veins, mild edema, leg fatigue), Class II (23–33 mmHg for severe varicosities, moderate edema, moderate venous insufficiency), and Class III (34–46 mmHg) and Class IV (≥49 mmHg), both for severe edema and venous insufficiency.[1,7]

With respect to outcomes based on a 2014 Cochrane systematic review, ulcer healing was improved when patients received compression vs. no compression; multilayer compression

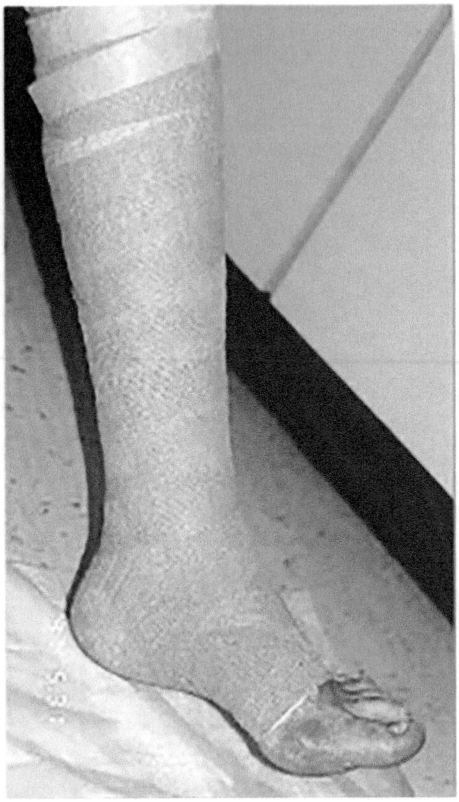

Figure 12.4 Multilayered compression bandage extending from mid-foot to below knee.

is more effective than single layer systems for complete healing at 6 months; 2- and 3-layer compression with elastic components heal more ulcers than those without elasticity at 1 year and 3–4 months, respectively; and faster healing is seen with 4-layer bandages vs. short-stretch bandages.[39] Furthermore, ulcer recurrence rates are higher in patients who were non-complaint vs. compliant with compression (65% vs. 32–34%).[12,40]

Wound Care

In addition to compression therapy, it is generally accepted that chronic VSUs should be covered to maintain a moist environment and accelerate wound healing. However, no evidence exists to support the effectiveness of one type of dressing over another when applied under the gold standard multilayer compression bandage.[40] Options for occlusive dressings include hydrogels, alginates, hydrocolloids, foams, and films. Dressing selection depends on wound location, size, depth, moisture balance, presence of infection, allergies, comfort, odor management, ease and frequency of dressing changes, cost, and availability.[2,7] Chemical debridement of necrotic tissue via topical application of proteolytic enzymes such as collagenase, papain, trypsin, and tissue plasminogen activator may be anecdotally effective but does not have strong evidence from large-scale randomized control studies.[7] Clinical efficacy of mechanical debridement via wet-to-dry dressings, hydrotherapy, irrigation, and dextranomers in chronic VSUs is similarly unclear.[7]

While concomitant use of topical antibiotics and antiseptics is not typically recommended, cadexomer-iodine preparations are relatively safer, have antimicrobial properties, and have been shown to be effective in debridement, stimulation of granulation tissue, and overall wound healing.[7,41] For example, ulcer size may be reduced by 90–94% within 12 weeks of cadexomer-iodine use as compared to 68% with standard compression alone.[42] The percentage of patients with complete wound healing at the end of 12 weeks is also significantly higher than in those with standard care alone (58–65% vs. 20%, respectively).[42]

Adjuvant systemic therapy has also been studied. Systemic antibiotics have not been shown to improve the healing rates of venous ulcers and should only be utilized in cases with observed cellulitis.[7,43] Stanazol, an anabolic steroid and derivative of testosterone, helps alleviate lipodermatosclerosis but does not increase the rate of healing of VSUs and does have side effects of temporary elevation of liver transaminases and depression of HDL levels.[44] Pentoxifylline has fibrinolytic activity and may work by reducing leukocyte adhesion to the vascular endothelium.[7,45] When pentoxifylline was administered orally alongside compression therapy, complete wound healing was decreased by 2 months in the intervention group and saw significant decrease in size at 3 months of treatment.[46] Moreover, increased rates of venous ulcer healing may be seen with oral enteric-coated aspirin (300 mg/daily) and compression therapy, but existing evidence is not compelling.[47]

Lastly, large venous ulcers greater than 25 cm^2 in size should be primarily treated with skin grafting, as healing is often unlikely otherwise. Skin grafting may also be used for ulcers that do not heal with standard care.[2] Autologous split-thickness skin grafting has been shown to have a success rate of up to 90% at 5 years.[16]

Surgical Intervention

As reviewed earlier, the mainstay of treatment for venous ulceration is compression therapy and wound care. While such conservative management has been shown to heal up to 97% of wounds at 6 months, it fails to address the underlying cause of ulceration and may lead to high rates of recurrence; within 3 months of healing, these rates have been reported at approximately 70%.[48] Traditional open surgical approaches targeted superficial vein reflux and demonstrated a reduction in recurrence rates when compared to compression alone. The ESCHAR trial found that 24-week healing rates were similar in patients who were treated with compression and ablative superficial venous surgery vs. compression alone. However, 12-month ulcer recurrence rates were significantly reduced in the compression and surgery group (12% vs. 28%).[49] Long-term results reflect this pattern as well; at 4 years, rates of ulcer recurrence were 51% for the compression group and 31% for the compression plus surgery group.[50] Furthermore, Marston et al. reported that patients with chronic venous ulceration treated with saphenous stripping had less ulcer recurrence compared to those treated with compression (15% vs. 34%).[51–53] More importantly, his study did not observe a statistically significant difference in ulcer healing in compression plus venous ligation and stripping procedures vs. compression alone (82% vs. 76%).[51] Traditional vein stripping is rarely performed in contemporary venous practice and has been replaced by minimally invasive endovenous techniques.

Endovenous techniques that help alleviate venous hypertension have evolved along with our understanding of the pathophysiology of venous ulcerations. These techniques include superficial axial vein ablation, perforator vein ablation, and iliac stenting.

Ablation of Superficial Axial Reflux

Endovenous ablation of superficial venous reflux has been found to reduce ulcer recurrence rates, especially if done early in the disease course. The 2018 EVRA trial compared two treatment groups: group 1 received compression therapy and early endovenous ablation (within 2 weeks) of randomization vs. group 2 that received compression therapy alone with ablation deferred until after the ulcer healed or until 6 months after randomization if it did not heal.[14] Methods of ablation included endovenous laser or radiofrequency, ultrasound-guided foam sclerotherapy, or non-thermal (cyanoacrylate glue or mechanochemical) performed either alone or together.

Patients with early intervention demonstrated quicker ulcer closure and shorter healing times than those with deferred intervention, at 56 days vs. 82 days, respectively.[14] The rate of ulcer healing at 24 weeks was 85.6% and 76.3% in early and deferred intervention groups, respectively. Lastly, those with early ablation experienced more free time from ulcers than those with deferred ablation (306 vs. 278 days).[14]

Older studies also point to the importance of ablation in chronic VSUs that have failed conventional compression therapy. Harlander-Locke et al. looked at patients with CEAP 6 ulcers who did not show improvement after more than 5 weeks of compression therapy and subsequently underwent ablation of at least one competent vein.[53] After ablation was successfully performed, ulcer healing time improved from +1.0 ± .1 cm^2/month to −4.4 ± .1 cm^2/month.[53] In addition, following an observation period of at least 6 months, 76.3% of patients healed in 142 ± 14 days. Of these, four patients with 6 ulcers recurred (7.1%), with two rehealing.[53] In addition, Viarengo et al. found that patients with CEAP C4, C5, or C6 ulcers followed over a period of 12 months, 81.5% of wounds in those who had undergone endovenous laser (EVL) ablation of the great and/or small saphenous vein plus elastic or inelastic compression therapy healed, while only 24% healed in those receiving compression therapy only.[54] Recurrence rate in the EVL group was 0% vs. 44.4% in compression-only group.[54] There was a significant difference in mean wound area decrease between the groups as well; wound area decreased from 22.26 to 2.7 cm^2 in the EVL group and from 17.48 to 12.76 cm^2 in the compression-only group.[54]

Ablation of Perforating Veins

Patients who have had refluxing saphenous veins ablated and have patent and refluxing perforating veins as per American Venous Forum guidelines (outward flow of >500 ms duration, with a diameter of >3.5 mm) should undergo perforator ablation (Figure 12.5).[1] Lawrence et al. examined patients with persisting venous ulcers after at least 3 months of conservative management (compression therapy, debridement, topical and systemic antibiotic treatment, topical growth factors, and skin substitutes) who underwent endovenous radiofrequency perforator ablation.[55] Ablation was successful in 71% of patients. VSUs healed in patients with successful ablation of at least one perforator vein in 90% of patients at a mean of 138 days.[55]

Furthermore, in a more recent 2020 study by Lawrence et al., patients who received both superficial and perforator ablation had a 17% improvement in healing at 36 months compared to patients who underwent truncal vein ablation alone (68% vs. 51%, respectively).[56] However, no difference in ulcer recurrence rates was found. Similarly, performing ultrasound-guided foam sclerotherapy (UGFS) of the pathologic perforating vein concomitantly with radiofrequency ablation (RFA) of saphenous vein reflux leads to improved VSU healing;

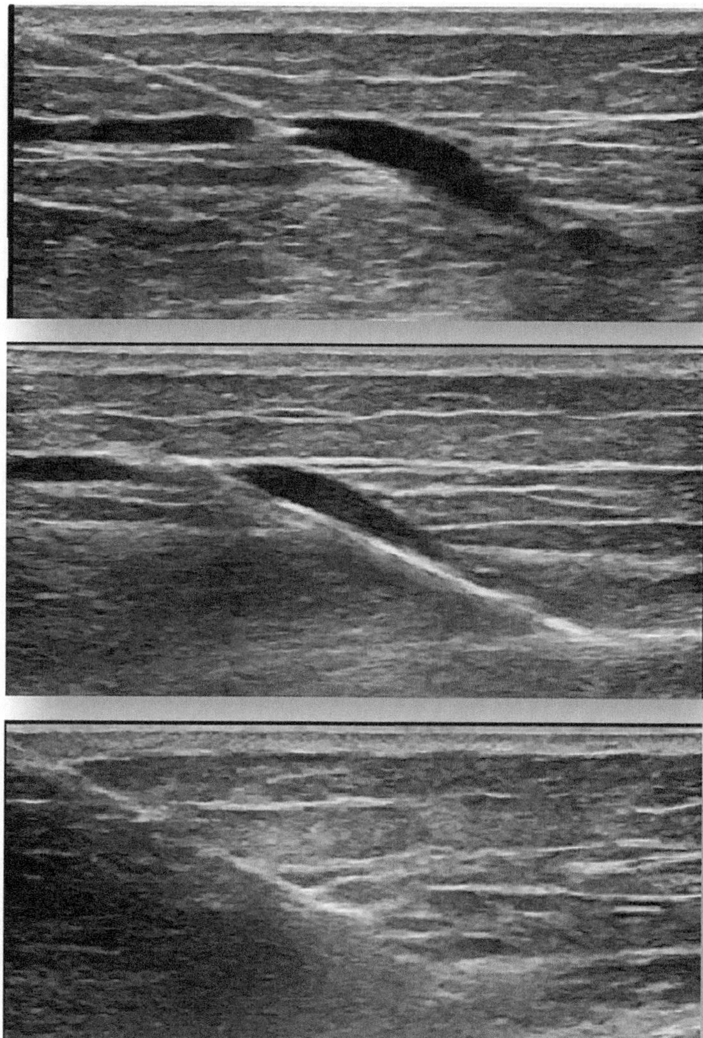

Figure 12.5 Duplex ultrasound images of a laser ablation of a pathologic perforating vein.

median time to healing is significantly longer in the RFA-only group compared to the RFA and UGFS group (172 days vs. 116 days, respectively).[57] At 1 year after RFA, the ulcer healing rate in the RFA-only group was also significantly lower than the RFA and UGFS group (56.9% vs. 100%, respectively).[57] Of four different factors (deep vein reflux, diabetes mellitus, concomitant UGFS, and concomitant phlebectomy), UGFS of perforating vein at time of RFA was the only one that was significantly associated with ulcer healing (HR, 2.84; 95% CI, 1.07–7.55; $p = 0.037$).[57]

In terms of ablation modality, Reitz et al. found no difference in healing rates of VLUs when comparing treatment with chemical ablation via ultrasound-guided foam sclerotherapy or thermal ablation via endovenous laser therapy or radiofrequency ablation.[58]

Stenting of Iliac Veins

In patients with chronic VSUs that have failed to heal after superficial and/or perforator ablation, interrogation of the iliac veins may be helpful in identifying potential outflow obstruction. Alleviating venous hypertension by improving deep vein outflow via iliac vein stenting has been effective in venous ulcer closure.

The gold standard for evaluation of a patient with suspected iliac vein stenosis or occlusion is intravascular ultrasound, although magnetic resonance venography and computed tomography angiography with venous filling phase can be exceedingly helpful. When iliac vein stenosis or occlusion is identified, there is a preponderance of data to support stenting to reduce venous hypertension.

In 2014, George et al. evaluated patients with C6 VSUs who had failed compression therapy or superficial venous intervention for deep vein lesions.[59] A group of 44 limbs with venous ulcers, 31 of which were post-thrombotic lesions and 13 non-thrombotic, was treated with iliac vein stenting. Sustained ulcer healing was achieved in 60% of limbs.[59] An additional 20% of ulcers had reduced in size. Ulcers recurred in 13% of limbs, with half healing after intervention for new incompetence in superficial veins.[59] Overall, it has been shown that endovascular iliocaval and infrainguinal venous stenting helps improve clinical symptoms, 1-year patency rate, and healing of recalcitrant venous ulcers.[52,59]

CONCLUSIONS

Chronic venous stasis ulceration is a challenging pathology to treat with a complex pathophysiology and significant socioeconomic burden. Local wound care with gentle debridement of devitalized tissue, ulcer coverage, and lower extremity compression are mainstays of treatment. The identification of venous reflux or obstruction is important for selecting targeted therapy toward pathologic veins. There is a preponderance of data to suggest that ablation of axial refluxing veins, pathologic perforating veins, and/or stenting of iliac vein occlusion can speed ulcer healing and reduce recurrence rates. Successful treatment of chronic venous ulceration often requires a multimodality approach which, over time, can heal ulceration in most patients.

REFERENCES*

*For articles without PMCIDs, PMIDs were provided. For those without PMIDs, DOIs were provided.

1. Thomas F. O'Donnell, et al. Management of venous leg ulcers: Clinical practice guidelines of the Society for Vascular Surgery® and the American Venous Forum. *Journal of Vascular Surgery* (2014); 60(2 Suppl):3S–59S. PMID: 24974070.
2. Susan Bonkemeyer Millan. Venous Ulcers: Diagnosis and Treatment. *American Family Physician* (2019); 100(5):298–305. PMID:31478635.
3. Biju Vasudevan. Venous leg ulcers: Pathophysiology and classification. *Indian Dermatology Online Journal* (2014); 5(3):366–70. PMC4144244.
4. Shinya Takase, et al. Venous hypertension, inflammation and valve remodeling *European Journal of Vascular and Endovascular Surgery* (2004); 28(5):484–93. PMID: 15465369.
5. Brajesh K. Lal. Venous ulcers of the lower extremity: Definition, epidemiology, and economic and social burdens. *Seminars in Vascular Surgery* (2015); 28(1):3–5. PMID: 26358303.

6. Cathy Thomas Hess. Venous ulcer assessment and management: Using the updated CEAP classification system. *Advances in Skin & Wound Care* (2020); 33(11):614–15. PMID: 33065684.
7. Isabel C. Valencia, et al. Chronic venous insufficiency and venous leg ulceration. *Journal of the American Academy of Dermatology* (2001); 44(3):401–21. PMID: 11209109.
8. Raghu Kolluri, et al. An estimate of the economic burden of venous leg ulcers associated with deep venous disease. *Society for Vascular Medicine* (2022); 27(1):63–72. PMID: 34392750.
9. J. Bradford Rice, et al. Burden of venous leg ulcers in the United States. *Journal of Medical Economics* (2014); 17(5):347–56. PMID: 24625244.
10. Ting Xie, et al. The venous ulcer continues to be a clinical challenge: An update. *Burns & Trauma* (2018); 6:18. PMC6003071.
11. Adam J. Singer, et al. Evaluation and management of lower-extremity ulcers. *New England Journal of Medicine* (2017); 377(16):1559–67. PMID: 29045216.
12. JC Mayberry, et al. Fifteen-year results of ambulatory compression therapy for chronic venous ulcers. *Surgery* (1991); 109(5):575–81. PMID: 2020902.
13. E. Andrea Nelson, Sally E M Bell-Syer. Compression for preventing recurrence of venous ulcers. *Cochrane Database of Systemic Reviews* (2014); 2014(9):CD002303. PMC7138196.
14. Manjit S. Gohel, et al. A randomized trial of early endovenous ablation in venous ulceration. *New England Journal of Medicine* (2018); 378(22):2105–14. PMID: 29688123.
15. Chandan K. Sen, et al. Human skin wounds: A major and snowballing threat to public health and the economy. *Wound Repair and Regeneration* (2009); 17(6):763–71. PMC2810192.
16. Kathleen J. Finlayson, et al. Predicting the likelihood of venous leg ulcer recurrence: The diagnostic accuracy of a newly developed risk assessment tool. *International Wound Journal* (2018); 15(5):686–94. PMC7949606.
17. Luciana P. Fernandes Abbade, Sidnei Lastória. Venous ulcer: Epidemiology, physiopathology, diagnosis and treatment. *International Journal of Dermatology* (2005); 44(6):449–56. PMID: 15941430.
18. E. Andrea Nelson, Una Adderley. Venous leg ulcers. *BMJ Clinical Evidence* (2016); 2016:1902. PMC4714578.
19. Stephen C. Nicholls. Sequelae of untreated venous insufficiency. *Seminars in Interventional Radiology* (2005); 22(3):162–68. PMC3036289.
20. Jenni E. Salenius, et al. Long-term mortality among patients with chronic ulcers. *Acta Dermato-Venereologica* (2021); 101(5):adv00455. PMC9367040.
21. NL Browse, K G Burnand. The cause of venous ulceration. *Lancet* (1982); 2(8292):243–45. PMID: 6124673.
22. DE Speiser, A Bollinger. Microangiopathy in mild chronic venous incompetence (CVI): Morphological alterations and increased transcapillary diffusion detected by fluorescence videomicroscopy. *International Journal of Microcirculation, Clinical and Experimental* (1991); 10(1):55–66. PMID: 2019484.
23. A. Bollinger, et al. Transcapillary and interstitial diffusion of Na-fluorescein in chronic venous insufficiency with white atrophy. *International Journal of Microcirculation, Clinical and Experimental* (1982); 1(1):5–17. PMID: 7188441.
24. Vincent Falanga, et al. Dermal pericapillary fibrin in venous disease and venous ulceration. *Archives of Dermatology* (1987); 123(5):620–23. PMID: 3555351.
25. Vincent Falanga, W H Eaglstein. The "trap" hypothesis of venous ulceration. *Lancet* (1993); 341(8851):1006–8. PMID: 7682272.
26. Alain L. Claudy, et al. Detection of undegraded fibrin and tumor necrosis factor-alpha in venous leg ulcers. *Journal of the American Academy of Dermatology* (1991); 25(4):623–27. 1791219.
27. JB Pardes, et al. Skin capillaries surrounding chronic venous ulcers demonstrate smooth-muscle cell hyperplasia and increased laminin and type-IV collagen. *Journal of Investigative Dermatology* (1990); 94:563.
28. Vincent Falanga, et al. Protein C and protein S plasma levels in patients with lipodermatosclerosis and venous ulceration. *JAMA Archives of Dermatology* (1990); 126(9):1195–97. PMID: 2144413.

29. Vincent Falanga, et al. Fibrin- and fibrinogen-related antigens in patients with venous disease and venous ulceration. *JAMA Archives of Dermatology* (1991); 127(1):75–78. PMID: 1986710.
30. M Paye, et al. Factor XIII of blood coagulation modulates collagen biosynthesis by fibroblasts in vitro. *Pathophysiology of Haemostasis and Thrombosis* (1989); 19(5):274–83. PMID: 2777140.
31. Martijn Van de Scheur, V Falanga. Pericapillary fibrin cuffs in venous disease. A reappraisal. *Dermatologic Surgery* (1997); 23(10):955–59. PMID: 9357508.
32. Angela A. Kokkosis, et al. Investigation of venous ulcers. *Seminars in Vascular Surgery* (2015); 28(1):15–20. PMID: PMID: 26358305.
33. Nicos Labropoulos, et al. Criteria for defining significant central vein stenosis with duplex ultrasound. *Journal of Vascular Surgery* (2007); 46(1):101–7. PMID: 17540535.
34. Evan J. Zucker, et al. Imaging of venous compression syndromes. *Cardiovascular Diagnosis and Therapy* (2016); 6(6):519–32. PMC5220205.
35. Katelyn N. Brinegar, et al. Iliac vein compression syndrome: Clinical, imaging and pathologic findings. *World Journal of Radiology* (2015); 7(11):375–81. PMC4663376.
36. M-Grace Knuttinen, et al. May-Thurner: Diagnosis and endovascular management. *Cardiovascular Diagnosis and Therapy* (2017); 7(Suppl 3):S159–64. PMC5778514.
37. H Partsch. Compression therapy of the legs. A review. *Journal of Dermatologic Surgery and Oncology* (1991); 17(10):799–805. PMID: 1918586.
38. MJ Callam, et al. Arterial disease in chronic leg ulceration: An underestimated hazard? Lothian and forth valley leg ulcer study. *BMJ Clinical Research Edition* (1987); 294(6577):929–31. PMC1245996.
39. Karen F. Mauck, et al. Systematic review and meta-analysis of surgical interventions versus conservative therapy for venous ulcers. *Journal of Vascular Surgery* (2014); 60(2 Suppl):60S–70S. PMID: 24835693.
40. Peter J. Franks, et al. Risk factors for leg ulcer recurrence: A randomized trial of two types of compression stocking. *Age and Ageing* (1995); 24(6):490–94. PMID: 8588538.
41. Sophia Tate, et al. Dressings for venous leg ulcers. *BMJ* (2018); 361:k1604. PMID: 29720376.
42. B. Gilchrist. Should iodine be reconsidered in wound management? European Tissue Repair Society. *Journal of Wound Care* (1997); 6(3):148–50. PMID: 9256712.
43. Radhakrishnan Raju, et al. Efficacy of cadexomer iodine in the treatment of chronic ulcers: A randomized, multicenter, controlled trial. *Wounds: A Compendium of Clinical Research and Practice* (2019); 31(3):85–90. PMID: 30720444.
44. Alberto Alinovi, et al. Systemic administration of antibiotics in the management of venous ulcers. A randomized clinical trial. *Journal of the American Academy of Dermatology* (1986); 15(2 Pt 1):186–91. PMID: 3528240.
45. Polly Carson, et al. Liver enzymes and lipid levels in patients with lipodermatosclerosis and venous ulcers treated with a prototypic anabolic steroid (stanozolol): A prospective, randomized, double-blinded, placebo-controlled trial. *International Journal of Lower Extremity Wounds* (2015); 14(1):11–8. PMID: 25652757.
46. E. Franzini, et al. Effects of pentoxifylline on the adherence of polymorphonuclear neutrophils to oxidant-stimulated human endothelial cells: Involvement of cyclic AMP. *Journal of Cardiovascular Pharmacology* (1995); 25(Suppl 2):S92–95. PMID: 8699872.
47. Hossien Parsa, et al. The effect of pentoxifylline on chronic venous ulcers. *Wounds: A Compendium of Clinical Research and Practice* (2012); 24(7):190–94. PMIID: 25874541.
48. Sebastian Probst, et al. The effect of pentoxifylline on chronic venous ulcers. *Journal of Tissue Viability* (2020); 24(7):190–94. PMID: 31974010.
49. Jamie R. Barwell, et al. Comparison of surgery and compression with compression alone in chronic venous ulceration (ESCHAR study): Randomised controlled trial. *Lancet* (2004); 363(9424):1854–59. PMID: 15183623.
50. Manjit S. Gohel, et al. Long term results of compression therapy alone versus compression plus surgery in chronic venous ulceration (ESCHAR): Randomised controlled trial. *BMJ* (2007); 335(7610):83. PMC1914523.

51. William A. Marston, et al. Incidence of venous leg ulcer healing and recurrence after treatment with endovenous laser ablation. *Journal of Vascular Surgery: Venous and Lymphatic Disorders* (2017); 5(4):525–32. PMID: 28623990.
52. Shi-Yan Ren, et al. Strategies and challenges in the treatment of chronic venous leg ulcers. *World Journal of Clinical Cases* (2020); 8(21):5070–85. PMC7674718.
53. Michael Harlander-Locke M, et al. The impact of ablation of incompetent superficial and perforator veins on ulcer healing rates. *Journal of Vascular Surgery* (2012); 55(2):458–64. PMID: 22133452.
54. Luiz Marcelo Aiello Viarengo, et al. Endovenous laser treatment for varicose veins in patients with active ulcers: Measurement of intravenous and perivenous temperatures during the procedure. *Dermatologic Surgery* (2007); 33(10):1234–42. doi:10.1111/j.1524–4725.2007.33259.x
55. Peter F. Lawrence, et al. Endovenous ablation of incompetent perforating veins is effective treatment for recalcitrant venous ulcers. *Journal of Vascular Surgery* (2011); 54(3):737-42. PMID: 21658887.
56. Peter F. Lawrence, et al. Treatment of superficial and perforator reflux and deep venous stenosis improves healing of chronic venous leg ulcers. *Journal of Vascular Surgery: Venous and Lymphatic Disorders* (2020); 8(4):601–9. PMID: 32089497.
57. Nuttawut Sermsathanasawadi, et al. Factors that influence venous leg ulcer healing and recurrence rate after endovenous radiofrequency ablation of incompetent saphenous vein. *Journal of Vascular Surgery: Venous and Lymphatic Disorders* (2020); 8(3):452–57. PMID: 31843485.
58. Katherine M. Reitz, et al. Complete venous ulceration healing after perforator ablation does not depend on treatment modality. *Annals of Vascular Surgery* (2021); 70:109-115. PMC7744434.
59. R George, et al. The effect of deep venous stenting on healing of lower limb venous ulcers. *European Journal of Vascular and Endovascular Surgery* (2014); 48(3):330–36. PMID: 24953000.

Chapter 13

Lymphedema

Diagnosis and Contemporary Management

Jordan F. Stafford, Drayson Campbell, and Steven M. Dean

INTRODUCTION

Lymphedema is a broad term used to describe swelling in the head, trunk, or, more commonly, the extremities as a result of impaired lymphatic flow. The lymphatic system is a complex network of vessels whose primary purpose is to return interstitial fluid from the periphery to circulation. When obstructed, protein-rich interstitial fluid accumulates leading to a pathological increase in subcutaneous tissues, skin fibrosis, increased risk of infection, significant disability, and psychosocial impairment.

CLINICAL FEATURES

Clinical Classification

Primary

Primary lymphedema is most commonly caused by lymphatic "obstruction" as a result of hypoplasia or aplasia of lymphatics. A smaller subset of primary lymphedema is a result of "reflux" or "hyperplasia" of megalymphatic vessels. The timing of swelling onset is often used to classify primary lymphedema: including from birth to age 2 years (congenital – Milroy disease), at puberty (lymphedema praecox – Meige disease), or post-adolescence (lymphedema tarda – typically after age 35).(1) Though these terms further categorize lymphedema, they generally do not impact therapy. Multiple genetic mutations are associated with primary syndromic lymphedema, including Turner, Emberger, Klinefelter, Noonan, Hennekam, yellow nail (Figure 13.1), and Aagenaes syndrome.

Secondary

Secondary lymphedema results from external sources causing obstruction of lymphatics. Filarial worm infection remains a common cause worldwide. Although malignancy and iatrogenesis from cancer therapies are usually referenced as the dominant cause of secondary lymphedema in the United States, contemporary evidence suggests chromic venous insufficiency is likely the dominant secondary etiology.(2) Others have recently posited that a constitutional lymphatic weakness is the most common cause of lymphedema and may affect up to one in five individuals.(3) Lower extremity cancer-related secondary lymphedema is commonly seen in gynecological cancers, sarcoma, metastatic melanoma, and genitourinary cancers.(4–6) Secondary lymphedema can also be seen after local or vascular trauma, burns, dermatitis, pregnancy, Class III obesity, and rheumatoid arthritis.

DOI: 10.1201/9781003316626-15

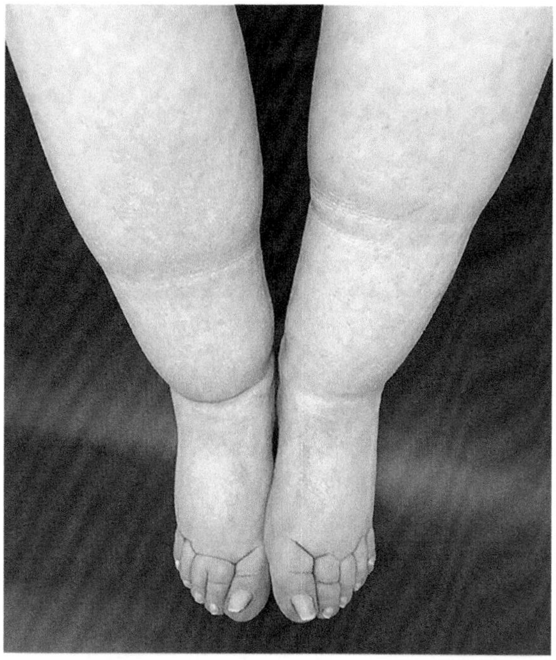

Figure 13.1 Yellow nail syndrome manifested by a triad of lymphedema, yellow nails, and bronchiectasis.

Table 13.1 The International Society of Lymphology (ISL) – Stages of Lymphedema[7]

Stage 0	No visible swelling despite lymphatic disruption, subjective symptoms may exist.
Stage I	Early proteinaceous fluid accumulation when the limb is dependent, that completely subsides with elevation. Limb is soft with pitting.
Stage II	Limb elevation rarely reduces swelling, and pitting is generally present early. Later stage II disease may no longer pit, as fibrosis and subcutaneous fat deposition is more prevalent.
Stage III	Pitting is generally absent with development of elephantiasic skin changes with severe hyperkeratosis and warty overgrowths. Elevation does not commonly effect swelling, as fibrofatty deposition is pronounced.

Presentation

History remains an essential diagnostic tool when evaluating a patient for lymphedema. Lymphatic deficiency typically begins with limb heaviness and development of swelling during dependency. Mild limb swelling of early disease may elude patients, though the subsequent increase in limb volume becomes clinically evident. Nearly one-half of patients suffer from chronic or recurrent cellulitis, due to the local immunocompromised district. Thus, lymphedema should be suspected in patients with swelling and chronic/recurrent cellulitis.

Several physical exam findings support the diagnosis of lymphedema. A positive Stemmer sign, or the inability to pinch the dorsum of the dorsal foot/toe or hand/finger, has been positively correlated with lymphoscintigraphic evidence of lymphedema, though this is commonly seen only when fibrosis and skin changes develop (ISL stage II or III).[8] Preferential swelling of the dorsum of the foot can create a "buffalo hump," and the toes may display

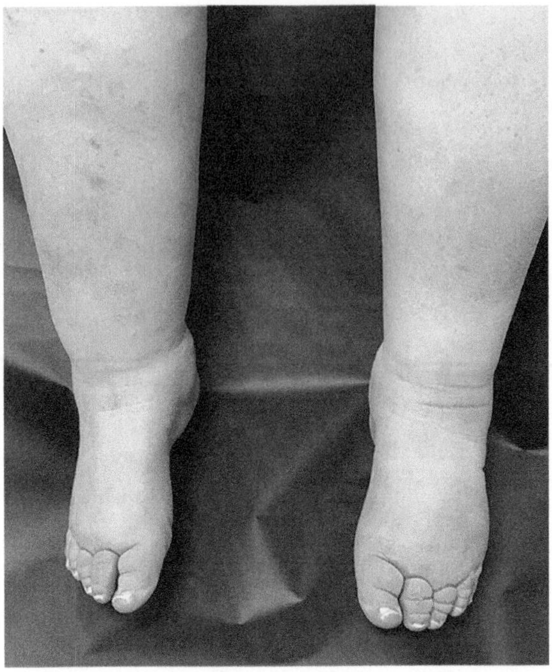

Figure 13.2 Bilateral lower extremity primary lymphedema (ISL Stage II) with characteristic clinical features including a pronounced left pedal "buffalo hump," exaggerated deep dorsal skin creases in the toes, and hypoplastic/upturned toenails.

a blunt "squared off" appearance with deep dorsal skin creases (Figure 13.2). Additionally, cutaneous manifestations include a *peau d'orange* appearance, hyperkeratosis, papulonodules, and rarely ulcerations (Figure 13.3).

Diagnosis

The diagnosis of peripheral lymphedema is largely clinical, based on history and physical examination. However, when the diagnosis or etiology is in question, several imaging strategies have evolved to evaluate for the presence and severity of lymphatic dysfunction.

Lymphoscintigraphy and Computerized Tomography

Radionuclide lymphoscintigraphy is performed by interstitial injection of Technetium-99m (Tc99m) labeled colloid molecules, then tracking flow through the lymphatic system using a gamma camera[9] (Figure 13.6). This imaging modality is commonly used in both static and dynamic testing, as tracer molecules of various sizes are used for lymphedema assessment and sentinel lymph node (SLN) mapping. Radionucleotide lymphoscintigraphy is described as the gold standard imaging technique for the diagnosis of lymphedema, with a reported high sensitivity (96%) and specificity (100%).[10, 11] Many criticisms of lymphoscintigraphy focus on interfacility protocol variability and poor image resolution, as a nuclear scan hindered by scatter.[12] However, lymphoscintigraphy plays an important role in objectively identifying the presence and clinical stage of lymphedema and can assist surgical decision-making.[12–14]

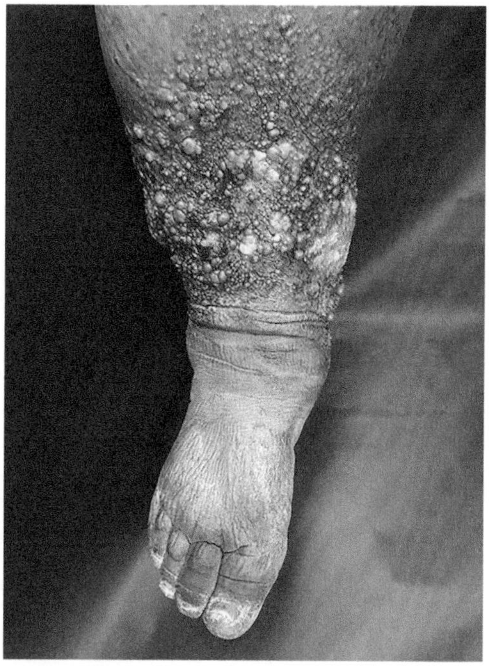

Figure 13.3 ISL Stage III primary lymphedema with an array of representative skin findings including hyperpigmentation, hyperkeratosis, papulonodules, and distal medial shallow fibrinous ulceration. Also note the squaring of the toes and hypoplastic, upturned toenails.

Table 13.2 Differential Diagnosis

Chronic Venous Insufficiency	Hyperpigmentation, ectatic veins, xeroderma with eczema and/or ulcerations within the mid and distal "gaiter" distribution of the calf; feet are typically spared unless secondary lymphedema or "phlebolymphedema" exists (Figure 13.4).

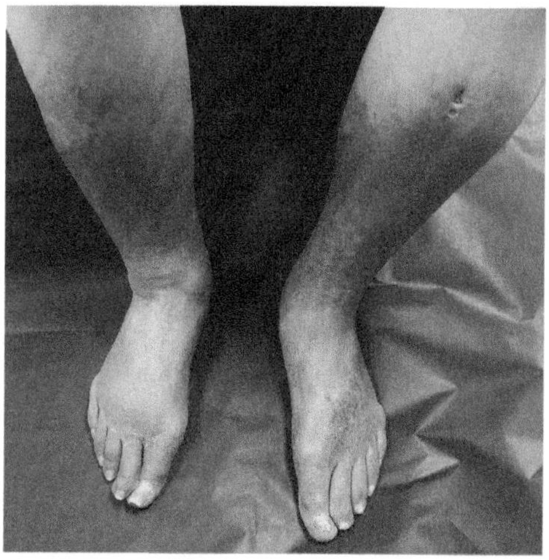

Figure 13.4 Phlebolymphedema is the constellation of chronic venous insufficiency complicated by secondary lymphedema. In contrast to the marked dorsal pedal and toe swelling of primary lymphedema, the foot and toe swelling in phlebolymphedema is typically modest.

Deep Venous Thrombosis	Typically acute, painful/tender and unilateral; larger thrombus burden yields an erythrocyanotic appearance with dilated superficial collateral veins and increased heat.
Lipedema	Abnormal accumulation of painful inflammatory adipocytes, most commonly seen in the pelvis through both ankles but usually spares the feet (unless associated with secondary lymphedema). The Stemmer sign is typically absent. Adipose tissue is usually tender and bruises easily (Figure 13.5).

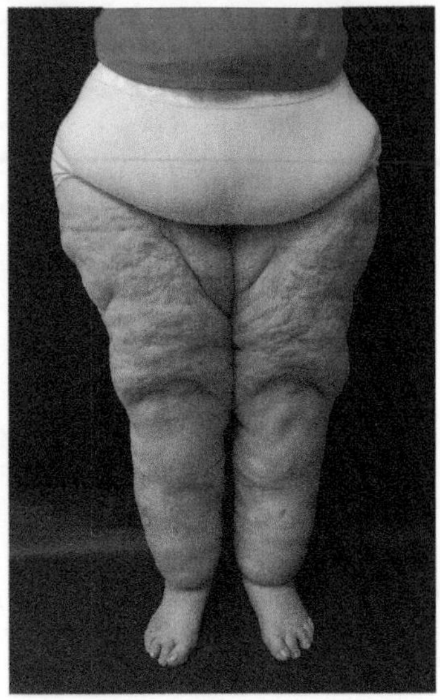

Figure 13.5 Lipedema is distinguished from lymphedema by distinctive symmetrical painful/tender diet-resistant leg swelling which spares the feet and toes. Other notable features include the ankle cuff sign and a "pear-shaped" body with a distinctive mismatch in the size of the torso when compared to the hips and thighs.

Pretibial Myxedema	Abnormal accumulation of mucinous, hyaluronic acid-rich substances into the skin and subcutaneous tissues, usually associated with Graves' disease. Classically characterized by the triad of non-pitting pretibial discoloration, nodules, or plaques with ophthalmopathy and acropachy.
Factitious Edema	Self-injurious behavior where a cuff or tourniquet is applied to mechanically obstruct proximal venous/lymphatic drainage. Upon close inspection, a demarcation from the constricting device will typically be present.
Systemic Fluid Overload	Bilateral, pitting edema in the setting of renal, hepatic, or cardiac dysfunction. No skin changes.

Near-Infrared Lymphography

Near-Infrared Lymphography (NIR) is performed with intracutaneous introduction of fluorescent dye (most commonly indocyanine green due to its affinity for albumin binding and near-infrared fluorescence wavelength; ICG), which is detected by a coupled-charged detector camera within superficial lymphatic beds.[9,15,16] NIR lymphography is able to delineate more precise superficial lymphatic anatomy (used up to 2 cm depths) compared

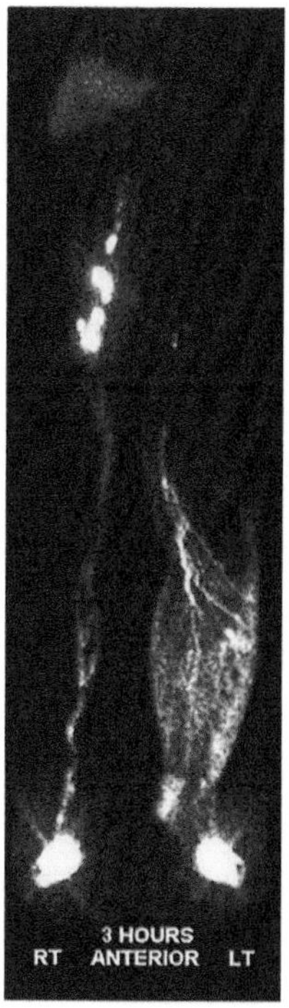

Figure 13.6 Abnormal left leg lymphoscintigraphy in a patient with longstanding ISL Stage II primary lymphedema. Specific abnormalities include marked dermal backflow within the calf, tortuous lymphatic collaterals, absent lymphatic trunks, and non-existent inguinal lymph nodes.

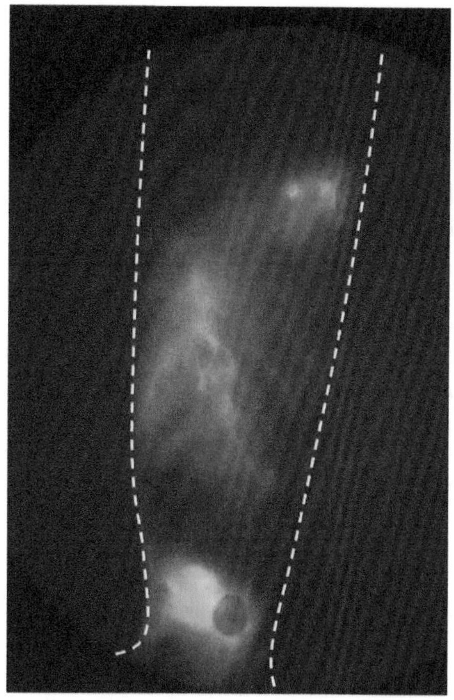

Figure 13.7 Abnormal right leg near-infrared lymphography in a patient with ISL Stage II primary lymphedema. Characteristic defects include a stardust pattern with patchy dermal infiltration with backflow combined with a very limited linear pattern. The visible lymphatic vessels are abnormal with dilatation with segmentation. (Image courtesy of John Rasmussen, PhD.)

to lymphoscintigraphy related to low light scatter in the NIR range compared to gamma emission.(9) This allows for visualization of collecting system contractility and identification of backflow patterns of dermal lymphatics, which are correlated to the severity of lymphatic dysfunction and clinical symptoms.(17–20) Compared to normal, linear lymphatic flow, backflow patterns can be described as "Splash" if there is slowed flow (illustrated by focused, but nonlinear dermal patches interspersed among faint linear patterns), "Stardust" if flow is severely limited (patchy dermal infiltration with very limited linear pattern [Figure 13.7]), and "Diffuse" in the absence of lymphatic flow (tracer does not extend past injection site).(20)

NIR lymphography has also been used to assess both conservative and surgical lymphedema treatment. Koelmeyer and colleagues have demonstrated improved conservative management in upper extremity lymphedema while using NIR as an adjunct to target more effective manual lymphatic drainage.(21) Additionally, NIR is increasingly used in preoperative microsurgical mapping. Hara and Mihara found in a prospective study that they were able to identify higher numbers of patent and functional lymphatic channels to be used in lymphovenous anastomosis (LVA), compared to lymphoscintigraphy.(22)

Magnetic Resonance Imaging

Magnetic resonance lymphography (MRL) has been described in clinical practice for evaluating the lymphatic system for over 20 years, as dilated lymphatic channels can be visualized adequately without contrast. Heavily T2-weighted non-contrast MR sequences have been found to highlight stagnant lymphatic fluid while depressing surrounding tissue signal to identify lymphatic leak and dilated lymphatic channels in extremities, which supports lymphatic as opposed to venous causes of swelling.[23, 24] For surgical planning, however, interstitially-injected gadolinium contrast on T1-weighted images illustrate the dilated lymphatic vasculature, while also better identifying surrounding aberrant tissue anatomy that may alter target vessel planning or detect additional secondary causes of lymphedema.[25–28]

Compared to lymphoscintigraphy or NIR, MRL offers significantly improved spatial resolution and characterization of both lymphatic channels as well as adjacent blood vessels.[26] Limitations to MRL include adjacent arteriovenous enhancement with contrast making lymphatic vessel identification difficult, expensive and time-consuming testing, limited availability, and no lymphatic specific tracers currently available.[9]

Direct Contrast Lymphography

Direct contrast lymphangiography has largely been displaced in the diagnosis and preoperative planning in lymphedema. Techniques involve direct visualization of deep lymphatic structures with inoculation of contrast dyes and plain X-ray to visualize channels. As a diagnostic tool, this is limited as technically challenging and higher exposure to radiation compared to other modern imaging modalities. Indirect contrast injection, however, is sometimes used intraoperatively to better visualize specific drainage basins and assist with LVA.[11]

MANAGEMENT OF LYMPHEDEMA

A multifaceted approach is often necessary to manage lymphedema, including lifestyle modification, psychotherapy, physiotherapy, pharmacotherapy, and surgical intervention. The principal goal of lymphedema management is to improve patients' quality of life and reduce disability through a reduction in limb girth, symptomatic relief, and the limitation of progression and complications. Optimal treatment must be made on an individual basis, and no systematic review or meta-analysis has identified a single best approach.

Conservative Approaches

Physiotherapy is critical at all stages of lymphedema and should begin with complex decongestive therapy (CDT), which is often regarded as the "gold standard" for lymphedema treatment.[5,29–31] Moreover, it is critical to minimize factors that aggravate existing lymphedema.

Complex Decongestive Therapy (CDT)

CDT incorporates multiple techniques such as manual lymphatic drainage (MLD), compression bandaging, and exercise to restore functional limb use through the reduction of interstitial fluid volume. CDT has well documented efficacy, achieving a >50% volume reduction in both upper and lower extremity lymphedema.[32] Early implementation of CDT (i.e., before significant disability) is likely beneficial, and a recent report noted a two-fold reduction of limb volume compared to a control.[33]

Manual Lymphatic Drainage (MLD)

MLD is a safe and beneficial technique that is designed to enhance anterograde flow of lymph through gentle massage. An initial massage of the contralateral limb and trunk helps to clear lymph buildup downstream of the affected limb which maximizes MLD's efficacy in the affected limb. Importantly, MLD may be more effective for mild-moderate lymphedema than moderate-severe disease due to the development of fibrosis.[34]

Compression

External compression devices are used in the initial volume reduction and the maintenance phases of CDT. Compression devices are primarily a volume reduction tool, although they also act as a skin protectant barrier.

In the initial stages of lymphedema volume reduction, short-stretch bandages and padding material are oriented to create external pressure that aids natural lymphatic flow during muscular contraction. Pressure can be modified by different strength bandages and the incorporation of stiff foam pads. Importantly, wraps are initially worn by patients constantly, with exceptions only made for bathing and MLD.

When MLD and compression bandaging achieve maximal volume reduction, patients transition to a maintenance phase of therapy, which uses elastic or inelastic compression garments to maintain limb size. Daytime wear is typically sufficient to preserve the volume reduction achieved with intense MLD and bandaging, but some patients may require nocturnal compression. Still, strict compliance with daily wear should be emphasized to avoid volume re-expansion.

Elastic garments are typically preferred unless significant impairment (e.g., obesity, limb disfigurement, poor manual dexterity, discomfort, and/or time constraints) prevents their application.[35] Pressures range from 20–60 mmHg, with higher pressures needed for more advanced disease.

Inelastic compression devices tend to be secured with Velcro and allow for more flexibility (e.g., approximately 20% of diameter variability). While this offers patients the ability to gradually tighten the garment, patients must be properly consulted to avoid inadequate pressure and subsequent regression.

Pneumatic compression pumps (PCPs) are an adjunct to CDT, though they have yet to demonstrate significant clinical efficacy compared to CDT alone.[36] PCPs can be designed to include a single, ascending pressure or have a pressure gradient (i.e., higher distal pressures to mimic the muscle pump that normally advances lymphatic flow). Notable contraindications for use include acute deep venous thrombosis, acute congestive heart failure, and somewhat controversial, active malignancy due to metastatic concerns.[33, 37]

Lifestyle Modification

Limitation of surgical resection (e.g., sentinel lymph node biopsy over lymph node dissection), radiotherapy, and cellulitis is paramount to minimizing the severity of secondary lymphedema, but lifestyle factors play a significant role in the control of lymphedema.[33, 37–40] Poor lifestyle management can result in regression of improvements made by past measures such as CDT.

Weight

Obesity can both aggravate existing lower extremity lymphedema and contribute to its development, with one study documenting a 74% prevalence of lymphedema in morbidly obese patients.[41] In addition to a contribution to lymphatic dysfunction, the inflammation that results from obesity can cause structural changes in lymphatic vessels as observed in mouse models.[42–46] Thus, weight loss should be a primary goal for any obese patient struggling with lymphedema.

Exercise and Physical Therapy

Historically, patients with lower extremity lymphedema were advised to avoid exercise, but this suggestion has been debunked in the past few decades. Exercise can play a role in weight loss and contribute to decrease in severity of lymphedema through direct improvements in interstitial flow and protein resorption, reduced fibrosis formation, increased sympathetic tone, and strengthening of skeletal muscle.[37, 47–49] However, exercise should be conducted in a staged manner, as rapid changes to regimens can increase fluid load, aggravating swelling.

Patients should undergo physical therapy, which can offer an excellent introduction to appropriate exercises and positioning techniques that are too numerous to describe here. The elevation of affected limb(s) is a logical and cost-effective technique that utilizes gravity to decrease capillary leak and increase proximal lymph flow. Elevation at night and during prolonged rest should be advised, as these are two periods where muscular propulsion of lymph is minimal.

Skin Care

Skin care is critical to the prevention of ulcers and infections, two conditions that greatly aggravate the disability experienced by patients with lymphedema. Regular inspection, cleansing with soap and water, and moisturization of affected areas with an alcohol-free moisturizer are equally important. Patients should be advised to check for scaling and cracking, which can indicate a loss of the protective function of healthy skin. If left unmanaged, these can be common precursors to cellulitis or dermatolymphangioadenitis. Similarly, tinea pedis can arise from the moisture that is trapped between swollen digits, especially toes. Patients should take meticulous care of their nails and cuticles. Injuries here, such as ingrown toenails, can quickly lead to infection due to the preexisting limited blood and lymph flow.[33, 37, 39] Those who choose to rid affected areas of hair must use electric razors instead of other more abrasive methods (e.g., safety razor, depilatories, abrasive mitts).

Any sudden environmental aggravator can increase the risk for infections. Sunscreen should be a part of daily skin care, as the inflammation associated with a sunburn will increase interstitial lymphedema load. Similarly, prolonged exposure to extreme heat or cold can drastically change superficial blood flow, further aggravating patients' symptoms.

Social Support

An often under discussed lifestyle modification is social support. Patients with lymphedema experience disability and discomfort due to disfigurement, and the accompanying isolation can contribute to further deterioration of quality of life. Social support groups, whether in-person or over virtual platforms (e.g., Facebook groups), can help to normalize patients' condition and reduce feelings of isolation.[33, 50] Improved psychological well-being is especially important to maintain the motivation needed to manage lymphedema as patients can spend hours of their day with selfcare.

Pharmacotherapy

Pharmacotherapy may serve as an adjunct to conservative management of lymphedema, but medication has not demonstrated significant efficacy for management alone and is not curative. Historically, diuretics have been used, though no conclusive evidence-based data exists to support its independent use in lymphedema. Recent human studies have found some clinical improvement with specific non-steroidal anti-inflammatory drugs and benzopyrones; though efficacy is limited and may not be generalizable to all patients.[51–53] Additionally, benzopyrones are not available in the United States. At this time, antibiotics are the only medications with consistent long-term data supporting their use in both prophylaxis and acute infectious treatment of lymphedema.

Non-Steroidal Anti-Inflammatory Drugs (NSAIDs)

A small RCT in 2018 used ketoprofen, an NSAID, as an adjunct to compressive garments for 4 months in patients with both primary and secondary lymphedema. The study found a significant reduction in skin thickness after treatment (from 49.4 mm ± 5.7 mm reduced to 41.4 mm ± 5.8 mm, $p = 0.01$), with no difference noted in the compression garment alone group.[51] However, there was no difference in limb volume.

Antibiosis

Despite well-adhered conservative measures, chronic or recurrent cellulitis causes further damage to dermal lymphatics, can worsen skin quality, and aggravates edema. At the onset of local or systemic signs of soft tissue infection, antibiotic therapy with Streptococcus A and tinea pedis coverage should be initiated promptly to minimize additional lymphatic damage. Long-term antibiotic prophylaxis with penicillin or erythromycin have been shown to be effective in patients with recurrent cellulitis and dermatolymphangioadenitis.[54, 55] One trial tested IV benzathine penicillin compared to placebo over 38 months, noting significantly decreased incidence of soft tissue infection among the treated group throughout this treatment period (annual incidence decreased from 6.2% ± 3.6% to 1.7% ± 1.0% per patient, $p < 0.001$) (54). Additionally, a 2014 systematic review and meta-analysis of five randomized controlled trials (n = 535 patients) assessed antibiotic prophylaxis for up to 18 months,[55] finding reduced incidence of cellulitis in the prophylaxis group compared to the placebo group (8% vs. 18%, RR 0.46; 95% CI: 0.26–0.79). Both the 2014 review and the recent Polish trial, interestingly noted no severe adverse effects of antibiotic use.[54, 55] However, guidelines have not yet specified which patients should be initiated on antibiotics, nor the duration of treatment, drug of choice, or dosage. The study in Poland did note they initiated treatment for patients with an average of 3.3 ± 3.2 episodes soft tissue infections per year, which may be an appropriate baseline for practice, though should be individualized.

Surgery

Surgical treatment of lymphedema can be considered after a 6-month trial of conservative management and may prevent secondary irreversible tissue changes (fibrosis, subcutaneous adipose hypertrophy). Surgical treatment options are often classified as physiologic (reconstructive) or reductive (excisional).[56] Excisional procedures, including liposuction to remove accumulated adipose tissue deposits and direct excision for lymphofibrotic lesions, have shown some palliative success, but advances in microsurgical techniques have allowed for restoration of lymphatic physiology.

Preoperative evaluation utilizes MR lymphography and lymphoscintigraphy. T1-weighted MR lymphography with subdermal contrast highlights lymphatic vessels and abnormalities effectively, while lymphoscintigraphy may better highlight physiologically intact lymph nodes.[57]

Physiologic Procedures

Autologous Lymphatic Grafting (Vascularized Lymph Node Transfer)

Autologous lymphatic grafting, or vascularized lymph node transfer (VLNT), is commonly pursued in unilateral extremity disease secondary to surgical, radiation, or oncologic sequelae. VLNT may also be considered in select primary lymphedema patients caused by localized lymphatic destruction or unilateral atresia. VLNT has demonstrated its efficacy in ISL stage I, II, or III disease, when dermal backflow is noted on NIR lymphography or no functional lymphatic vessels are identified on imaging.[58, 59]

The lymphatic vessels are first harvested in bundles with surrounding lymph node clusters, then channels are anastomosed with recipient vessels and nodes. Commonly harvested lymph nodes are the lateral thoracic, inguinal, supraclavicular, and gastroepiploic nodes. For lower extremity transfer, the ventromedial thigh in the unaffected limb is often selected as the donor site. Bundles of lymph nodes and channels are ligated with either suture ligation or coagulation and dissected out with a pad of surrounding adipose tissue. If the graft vessel is transpositioned to the contralateral groin, the bundle is tunneled superior to the pubic symphysis. For arm edema, free-graft transfer is often achieved with supraclavicular or lower cervical lymphatic channels tunneled to the ipsilateral axilla.

Lymphatic transfer has demonstrated significant volume reduction and subjective improvement with decreased conservative therapy needs.[58, 60] One feared complication is secondary lymphedema due to the lymphatic disruption of the surgery to the donor limb. One group, evaluating reverse lymphatic mapping using dyes and radiotracer in the distal ipsilateral limb to visually maintain lymphatic anatomy of the donor limb, has reported success with avoiding iatrogenesis, though this preliminary data is not yet consistent among healthcare systems.[61]

Lymphovenous Anastomosis

Traditionally, lymphovenous anastomosis (LVA) has been used in early-stage disease, as fibrosis in later stage lymphedema causes lymphatic insufficiency.[56] However, more recent data in advanced-stage patients has demonstrated efficacy in treating advanced disease when ICG velocities remain high on lymphoscintigraphy (indicating sufficient proximal patency).[62, 63] The primary contraindications that remain include proximal venous occlusive disease and chronic venous insufficiency. Generally, a superficial lymphatic bundle is exposed in the anteromedial thigh or medial upper arm. Following exposure of the recipient venous tributaries, a tension-free end-to-end anastomosis is performed.

Results for LVA have demonstrated mixed efficacy. The largest study to date tracked 446 patients following LVA, finding 85% of patients treated in early-stage disease (ISL stage I) could discontinue conservative measures, maintain volume reduction of 69%, and reduce incidence of cellulitis by 87% over 7-year follow-up period.[64] More recently, a retrospective study of 42 patients following LVA for late-stage lower extremity lymphedema (stage II or III) reduced incidence of cellulitis and noted a 15% limb volume reduction at 1 year.[63] Upper extremity response is more variable, though, with a systematic review of 16 studies showing a range of 0 to 100% objective clinical improvement (limb circumference, volume measurement, or volume differential) and 50–100% subjective improvement as reported by patients.[65]

Reductive Procedures

In later stage disease, fibrosis and lipodystrophy can be palliatively excised with direct excision or liposuction to prevent secondary sequelae of chronic lymphedema.

Suction-Assisted Lipectomy (Liposuction)

To reduce the volume of fibrotic, hypertrophied adipose tissue, suction-assisted lipectomy, or liposuction, has been described with positive results. Multiple 2–4 mm skin incisions are made circumferentially in the affected limb, pathologic adipose tissue superficial to the deep fascia is excised. Liposuction has been used for decades with success and improved patient satisfaction. Brorson and colleagues in 2003, noted that patients undergoing liposuction had significant reduction in total arm volume over 1-year follow-up compared to conservative CDT alone, and recent studies have found a decreased incidence of cellulitis compared to conservative therapy alone.[66, 67]

Subcutaneous Excision with Flap Coverage

Lymphofibrotic subcutaneous tissue of the affected limb is excised circumferentially, then covered with intact dermal flaps or skin grafting. While some are modifying this procedure for upper extremity disease, the majority of data is centered on advanced-stage lower extremity lymphedema.[68] Due to the extensive nature of this procedure, it is performed in stages, first with excision of the medial lower limb and then laterally.

An incision is made 1cm posterior to the medial malleolus and extended proximally to the medial mid-thigh. All subcutaneous tissue (including fibrotic deep fascia) beneath the flaps is then excised, with preservation of the sural nerve and peri-joint fascia. The second stage is commonly performed 3–6 months following the first stage in the lateral lower limb, carefully preserving the peroneal nerve and its branches.[68]

Miller and colleagues reported significant reduction in affected limb volume in long-term follow up and near-elimination of cellulitis.[68] Subcutaneous excision has had positive results in patient quality of life, though it does carry risk of wound complications, nerve damage, scarring, and prolonged hospitalization.

Combined Surgical Approaches

More recently, groups have been combining the aforementioned approaches with some success. Bolletta and colleagues were able to use VLNT followed by liposuction to reduce the mean limb circumference by >50% over a 3-year period and decrease incidence of cellulitis in patients with advanced-stage lower limb lymphedema ($p < 0.05$).[69] Unfortunately, they did not find a similar results in upper extremity disease. Similar results have also been reported following combined subcutaneous excision and VLNT with improved clinical and quality of life in patients suffering from lymphedema.[70, 71]

CONCLUSIONS

The mainstays of treatment for peripheral lymphedema are conservative measures and exacerbation reduction. Pharmacological adjuncts have largely had mixed success, though antibiotic prophylaxis has been shown to decrease infectious sequelae and improve quality of life. In instances where conservative measures fail, early-stage surgical management can be beneficial for select patients, though does carry risk of recurrence and operative morbidity. Optimal treatment strategies are formed with an invested multidisciplinary team over years of follow-up.

REFERENCES

1. Greene AK, Grant FD, Slavin SA. Lower-extremity lymphedema and elevated body-mass index. N Engl J Med. 2012 May 31;366(22):2136–37.
2. Dean SM, Valenti E, Hock K, Leffler J, Compston A, Abraham WT. The clinical characteristics of lower extremity lymphedema in 440 patients. J Vasc Surg Venous Lymphat Disord. 2020 Sep;8(5):851–59.
3. Peters AM, Mortimer PS. "Latent" and "constitutional" lymphedema, useful terms to complement the terms "primary" and "secondary" lymphedema. J Vasc Surg Venous Lymphat Disord. 2021 Sep;9(5):1089–92.
4. Rockson SG. Current concepts and future directions in the diagnosis and management of lymphatic vascular disease. Vasc Med Lond Engl. 2010 Jun;15(3):223–31.
5. Fu MR, Deng J, Armer JM. Putting evidence into practice: Cancer-related lymphedema: Evolving evidence for treatment and management from 2009–2014. Clin J Oncol Nurs. 2014 Dec 1;18(s6):68–79.
6. Cormier JN, Askew RL, Mungovan KS, Xing Y, Ross MI, Armer JM. Lymphedema beyond breast cancer. Cancer. 2010;116(22):5138–49.
7. Executive Committee of the International Society of Lymphology. The diagnosis and treatment of peripheral lymphedema: 2020 Consensus document of the international society of lymphology. Lymphology. 2020;53(1):3–19.
8. Goss JA, Greene AK. Sensitivity and specificity of the stemmer sign for lymphedema: A clinical lymphoscintigraphic study. Plast Reconstr Surg Glob Open. 2019 Jun 25;7(6):e2295.
9. Polomska AK, Proulx ST. Imaging technology of the lymphatic system. Adv Drug Deliv Rev. 2021 Mar;170:294–311.
10. Hassanein AH, Maclellan RA, Grant FD, Greene AK. Diagnostic accuracy of lymphoscintigraphy for lymphedema and analysis of false-negative tests. Plast Reconstr Surg Glob Open. 2017 Jul;5(7):e1396.
11. Rockson SG. Advances in lymphedema. Circ Res. 2021 Jun 11;128(12):2003–16.
12. Pappalardo M, Cheng MH. Lymphoscintigraphy for the diagnosis of extremity lymphedema: Current controversies regarding protocol, interpretation, and clinical application. J Surg Oncol. 2020 Jan;121(1):37–47.

13. Vaqueiro M, Gloviczki P, Fisher J, Hollier LH, Schirger A, Wahner HW. Lymphoscintigraphy in lymphedema: An aid to microsurgery. J Nucl Med Off Publ Soc Nucl Med. 1986 Jul;27(7):1125–30.
14. Iimura T, Fukushima Y, Kumita S, Ogawa R, Hyakusoku H. Estimating lymphodynamic conditions and lymphovenous anastomosis efficacy using 99mTc-phytate lymphoscintigraphy with SPECT-CT in patients with lower-limb lymphedema. Plast Reconstr Surg Glob Open. 2015 Jun 5;3(5):e404.
15. Unno N, Inuzuka K, Suzuki M, Yamamoto N, Sagara D, Nishiyama M, et al. Preliminary experience with a novel fluorescence lymphography using indocyanine green in patients with secondary lymphedema. J Vasc Surg. 2007 May;45(5):1016–21.
16. Akita S, Unno N, Maegawa J, Kimata Y, Fukamizu H, Yabuki Y, et al. HAMAMATSU-ICG study: Protocol for a phase III, multicentre, single-arm study to assess the usefulness of indocyanine green fluorescent lymphography in assessing secondary lymphoedema. Contemp Clin Trials Commun. 2020 Jun 16;19:100595.
17. Granoff MD, Johnson AR, Lee BT, Padera TP, Bouta EM, Singhal D. A Novel approach to quantifying lymphatic contractility during indocyanine green lymphangiography. Plast Reconstr Surg. 2019 Nov;144(5):1197–201.
18. Akita S, Nakamura R, Yamamoto N, Tokumoto H, Ishigaki T, Yamaji Y, et al. Early detection of lymphatic disorder and treatment for lymphedema following breast cancer. Plast Reconstr Surg. 2016 Aug;138(2):192e–202e.
19. Narushima M, Yamamoto T, Ogata F, Yoshimatsu H, Mihara M, Koshima I. Indocyanine green lymphography findings in limb lymphedema. J Reconstr Microsurg. 2016 Jan;32(1):72–9.
20. Yamamoto T, Yamamoto N, Doi K, Oshima A, Yoshimatsu H, Todokoro T, et al. Indocyanine green-enhanced lymphography for upper extremity lymphedema: A novel severity staging system using dermal backflow patterns. Plast Reconstr Surg. 2011 Oct;128(4):941–47.
21. Koelmeyer LA, Thompson BM, Mackie H, Blackwell R, Heydon-White A, Moloney E, et al. Personalizing conservative lymphedema management using indocyanine green-guided manual lymphatic drainage. Lymphat Res Biol. 2021 Feb;19(1):56–65.
22. Hara H, Mihara M. Multi-area lymphaticovenous anastomosis with multi-lymphosome injection in indocyanine green lymphography: A prospective study. Microsurgery. 2019 Feb;39(2):167–73.
23. Cellina M, Oliva G, Menozzi A, Soresina M, Martinenghi C, Gibelli D. Non-contrast magnetic resonance lymphangiography: An emerging technique for the study of lymphedema. Clin Imaging. 2019 Feb;53:126–33.
24. Arrivé L, Derhy S, El Mouhadi S, Monnier-Cholley L, Menu Y, Becker C. Noncontrast magnetic resonance lymphography. J Reconstr Microsurg. 2016 Jan;32(1):80–86.
25. Mitsumori LM, McDonald ES, Neligan PC, Maki JH. Peripheral magnetic resonance lymphangiography: Techniques and applications. Tech Vasc Interv Radiol. 2016 Dec;19(4):262–72.
26. Mazzei MA, Gentili F, Mazzei FG, Gennaro P, Guerrieri D, Nigri A, et al. High-resolution MR lymphangiography for planning lymphaticovenous anastomosis treatment: A single-centre experience. Radiol Med (Torino). 2017 Dec;122(12):918–27.
27. Neligan PC, Kung TA, Maki JH. MR lymphangiography in the treatment of lymphedema. J Surg Oncol. 2017 Jan;115(1):18–22.
28. Zeltzer AA, Brussaard C, Koning M, De Baerdemaeker R, Hendrickx B, Hamdi M, et al. MR lymphography in patients with upper limb lymphedema: The GPS for feasibility and surgical planning for lympho-venous bypass. J Surg Oncol. 2018 Sep;118(3):407–15.
29. International Society of Lymphology. The diagnosis and treatment of peripheral lymphedema: 2013 consensus document of the international society of lymphology. Lymphology. 2013 Mar;46(1):1–11.
30. Rockson SG. Diagnosis and management of lymphatic vascular disease. J Am Coll Cardiol. 2008 Sep 2;52(10):799–806.
31. Mayrovitz HN. The standard of care for lymphedema: Current concepts and physiological considerations. Lymphat Res Biol. 2009;7(2):101–8.
32. Ko DS, Lerner R, Klose G, Cosimi AB. Effective treatment of lymphedema of the extremities. Arch Surg Chic Ill 1960. 1998 Apr;133(4):452–58.

33. Bobrek K, Nabavizadeh R, Nabavizadeh B, Master V. How to Care and Minimize the sequelae of lower extremity lymphedema. Semin Oncol Nurs. 2022 Jun;38(3):151270.
34. Ezzo J, Manheimer E, McNeely ML, Howell DM, Weiss R, Johansson KI, et al. Manual lymphatic drainage for lymphedema following breast cancer treatment. Cochrane Database Syst Rev. 2015 May 21;(5):CD003475.
35. Cheville AL. Current and future trends in lymphedema management: Implications for women's health. Phys Med Rehabil Clin N Am. 2007 Aug;18(3):539–53.
36. Shao Y, Qi K, Zhou QH, Zhong DS. Intermittent pneumatic compression pump for breast cancer-related lymphedema: A systematic review and meta-analysis of randomized controlled trials. Oncol Res Treat. 2014;37(4):170–74.
37. Kerchner K, Fleischer A, Yosipovitch G. Lower extremity lymphedema update: Pathophysiology, diagnosis, and treatment guidelines. J Am Acad Dermatol. 2008 Aug;59(2):324–31.
38. Brown JC, Chu CS, Cheville AL, Schmitz KH. The prevalence of lymphedema symptoms among survivors of long-term cancer with or at risk for lower limb lymphedema. Am J Phys Med Rehabil. 2013 Mar;92(3):223–31.
39. Bakar Y, Tuğral A. Lower extremity lymphedema management after gynecologic cancer surgery: A review of current management strategies. Ann Vasc Surg. 2017 Oct;44:442–50.
40. Ki EY, Park JS, Lee KH, Hur SY. Incidence and risk factors of lower extremity lymphedema after gynecologic surgery in ovarian cancer. Int J Gynecol Cancer Off J Int Gynecol Cancer Soc. 2016 Sep;26(7):1327–32.
41. Fife CE, Carter MJ. Lymphedema in the morbidly obese patient: Unique challenges in a unique population. Ostomy Wound Manage. 2008 Jan;54(1):44–56.
42. Savetsky IL, Torrisi JS, Cuzzone DA, Ghanta S, Albano NJ, Gardenier JC, et al. Obesity increases inflammation and impairs lymphatic function in a mouse model of lymphedema. Am J Physiol Heart Circ Physiol. 2014 Jul 15;307(2):H165–172.
43. Weitman ES, Aschen SZ, Farias-Eisner G, Albano N, Cuzzone DA, Ghanta S, et al. Obesity impairs lymphatic fluid transport and dendritic cell migration to lymph nodes. PLoS One. 2013;8(8):e70703.
44. Blum KS, Karaman S, Proulx ST, Ochsenbein AM, Luciani P, Leroux JC, et al. Chronic high-fat diet impairs collecting lymphatic vessel function in mice. PLoS One. 2014;9(4):e94713.
45. García Nores GD, Cuzzone DA, Albano NJ, Hespe GE, Kataru RP, Torrisi JS, et al. Obesity but not high-fat diet impairs lymphatic function. Int J Obes 2005. 2016 Oct;40(10):1582–90.
46. Khan N, Huayllani MT, Lu X, Boczar D, Cinotto G, Avila FR, et al. Effects of diet-induced obesity in the development of lymphedema in the animal model: A literature review. Obes Res Clin Pract. 2022 Jun;16(3):197–205.
47. Markes M, Brockow T, Resch KL. Exercise for women receiving adjuvant therapy for breast cancer. Cochrane Database Syst Rev. 2006 Oct 18;(4):CD005001.
48. Ahmed RL, Thomas W, Yee D, Schmitz KH. Randomized controlled trial of weight training and lymphedema in breast cancer survivors. J Clin Oncol Off J Am Soc Clin Oncol. 2006 Jun 20;24(18):2765–72.
49. Schmitz KH, Ahmed RL, Troxel A, Cheville A, Smith R, Lewis-Grant L, et al. Weight lifting in women with breast-cancer-related lymphedema. N Engl J Med. 2009 Aug 13;361(7):664–73.
50. Rockson SG, Keeley V, Kilbreath S, Szuba A, Towers A. Cancer-associated secondary lymphoedema. Nat Rev Dis Primer. 2019 Mar 28;5(1):22.
51. Rockson SG, Tian W, Jiang X, Kuznetsova T, Haddad F, Zampell J, et al. Pilot studies demonstrate the potential benefits of antiinflammatory therapy in human lymphedema. JCI Insight. 2018 Oct 18;3(20):123775.
52. Cacchio A, Prencipe R, Bertone M, De Benedictis L, Taglieri L, D'Elia E, et al. Effectiveness and safety of a product containing diosmin, coumarin, and arbutin (Linfadren®) in addition to complex decongestive therapy on management of breast cancer-related lymphedema. Support Care Cancer Off J Multinatl Assoc Support Care Cancer. 2019 Apr;27(4):1471–80.
53. Lessiani G, Iodice P, Nicolucci E, Gentili M. Lymphatic edema of the lower limbs after orthopedic surgery: Results of a randomized, open-label clinical trial with a new extended-release preparation. J Biol Regul Homeost Agents. 2015 Dec;29(4):805–12.

54. Olszewski WL, Zaleska MT. Long-Term benzathine penicillin prophylaxis lasting for years effectively prevents recurrence of dermato-lymphangio-adenitis (cellulitis) in limb lymphedema. Lymphat Res Biol. 2021 Dec;19(6):545–52.
55. Oh CC, Ko HCH, Lee HY, Safdar N, Maki DG, Chlebicki MP. Antibiotic prophylaxis for preventing recurrent cellulitis: A systematic review and meta-analysis. J Infect. 2014 Jul;69(1):26–34.
56. de Sire A, Losco L, Lippi L, Spadoni D, Kaciulyte J, Sert G, et al. Surgical treatment and rehabilitation strategies for upper and lower extremity lymphedema: A comprehensive review. Med Kaunas Lith. 2022 Jul 19;58(7):954.
57. Notohamiprodjo M, Weiss M, Baumeister RG, Sommer WH, Helck A, Crispin A, et al. MR lymphangiography at 3.0 T: Correlation with lymphoscintigraphy. Radiology. 2012 Jul;264(1):78–87.
58. Becker C, Vasile JV, Levine JL, Batista BN, Studinger RM, Chen CM, et al. Microlymphatic surgery for the treatment of iatrogenic lymphedema. Clin Plast Surg. 2012 Oct;39(4):385–98.
59. Schaverien MV, Badash I, Patel KM, Selber JC, Cheng MH. Vascularized lymph node transfer for lymphedema. Semin Plast Surg. 2018 Feb;32(1):28–35.
60. Basta MN, Gao LL, Wu LC. Operative treatment of peripheral lymphedema: A systematic meta-analysis of the efficacy and safety of lymphovenous microsurgery and tissue transplantation. Plast Reconstr Surg. 2014 Apr;133(4):905–13.
61. Dayan JH, Dayan E, Smith ML. Reverse lymphatic mapping: A new technique for maximizing safety in vascularized lymph node transfer. Plast Reconstr Surg. 2015 Jan;135(1):277–85.
62. Park JKH, Seo J, Yang EJ, Kang Y, Heo CY, Myung Y. Association of lymphatic flow velocity with surgical outcomes in patients undergoing lymphovenous anastomosis for breast cancer-related lymphedema. Breast Cancer Tokyo Jpn. 2022 Sep;29(5):835–43.
63. Cha HG, Oh TM, Cho MJ, Pak CSJ, Suh HP, Jeon JY, et al. Changing the paradigm: Lymphovenous anastomosis in advanced stage lower extremity lymphedema. Plast Reconstr Surg. 2021 Jan 1;147(1):199–207.
64. Campisi C, Boccardo F, Zilli A, Macciò A, Napoli F. Long-term results after lymphatic-venous anastomoses for the treatment of obstructive lymphedema. Microsurgery. 2001;21(4):135–39.
65. Gupta N, Verhey EM, Torres-Guzman RA, Avila FR, Jorge Forte A, Rebecca AM, et al. Outcomes of lymphovenous anastomosis for upper extremity lymphedema: A systematic review. Plast Reconstr Surg Glob Open. 2021 Aug 25;9(8):e3770.
66. Brorson H. Liposuction in arm lymphedema treatment. Scand J Surg SJS Off Organ Finn Surg Soc Scand Surg Soc. 2003;92(4):287–95.
67. Schaverien MV, Munnoch DA, Brorson H. Liposuction treatment of lymphedema. Semin Plast Surg. 2018 Feb;32(1):42–47.
68. Miller TA, Wyatt LE, Rudkin GH. Staged skin and subcutaneous excision for lymphedema: A favorable report of long-term results. Plast Reconstr Surg. 1998 Oct;102(5):1486–98; discussion 1499–1501.
69. Bolletta A, di Taranto G, Losco L, Elia R, Sert G, Ribuffo D, et al. Combined lymph node transfer and suction-assisted lipectomy in lymphedema treatment: A prospective study. Microsurgery. 2022 Jul;42(5):433–40.
70. Granzow JW, Soderberg JM, Dauphine C. A novel two-stage surgical approach to treat chronic lymphedema. Breast J. 2014 Aug;20(4):420–22.
71. Sapountzis S, Ciudad P, Lim SY, Chilgar RM, Kiranantawat K, Nicoli F, et al. Modified charles procedure and lymph node flap transfer for advanced lower extremity lymphedema. Microsurgery. 2014 Sep;34(6):439–47.

Section 3

Management of Symptomatic Central Venous Disease

Chapter 14

Contemporary Management of Non-Thrombotic and Thrombotic Iliocaval Compression Syndrome

Ariela Zenilman and Brian Derubertis

INTRODUCTION

Iliocaval compression syndrome is a well-described pathophysiologic entity that has taken over 150 years of investigation to define. As first described by Virchow, iliofemoral DVTs were five times more likely to occur on the left lower extremity rather than the right. May and Thurner then described iliocaval compression due to the chronic pulsation and mechanical obstruction by the right iliac artery as a cause of left lower extremity venous hypertension. The association of this with or without iliofemoral DVT became known as May-Thurner syndrome (MTS). As the pathophysiology of the disease became more widely studied and understood, MTS became recognized as the major contributing factor in lower extremity edema, iliofemoral DVT, and the associated long-term sequela of post-thrombotic syndrome chronic venous insufficiency.[1, 2] Management of iliocaval compression syndromes has changed considerably in the last decade. While symptomatic patients went undiagnosed or untreated for several years, the progression of imaging and endovascular treatment modalities has offered options for management. The focus of this chapter will be on management and treatment algorithms of thrombotic and non-thrombotic iliocaval compression.

PATHOPHYSIOLOGY

Although there are several variants of iliac compression syndrome, MTS is described as compression of the left common iliac vein against the fifth lumbar vertebral body by the right common iliac artery as the artery crosses anterior to the vein. The exact point of compression differs from individual to individual, and compression of the caval confluence has also been described as well. Left iliac vein compression is a prevalent finding in the general population, but only a small percentage of individuals with this radiographically recognized phenomenon are symptomatic, so the true prevalence of iliac vein compression consistent with the clinical diagnosis of MTS is unknown. Kibbe et al identified a 24% prevalence of iliac vein compression in an asymptomatic population and concluded that this is a normal anatomic variant.[3] In the setting of DVT, however, iliac vein compression can be present in 18–49% of cases.[3, 4]

When the right common iliac artery crosses over the left common iliac vein it induces a partial obstruction in two ways: (1) mechanical obstruction caused by compression of the vein between the artery and vertebral body and (2) intimal hypertrophy of the vein from repeated pulsation of overlying artery causing shear stress between the anterior and posterior vein walls.[5, 6] Generally, patients remain asymptomatic until exposed to a stressor that predisposes them to thrombosis such as surgery, initiation of oral contraceptives, prolonged immobility, malignancy, or a hypercoagulable state. The most common risk factors in patients who progress to thrombosis are history of recent surgery or cancer (11.2%), hypercoagulable

DOI: 10.1201/9781003316626-17

disorder (9.6%), immobilization (9%), hormone replacement therapy (6%), trauma (4.6%), and pregnancy (3.2%).[4] The pathophysiology of disease in patients is important to understand as it will guide management and categorize patients as candidates for intervention.

CLINICAL PRESENTATION

When a patient with venous disease is encountered, a careful history can help differentiate between an acute DVT, chronic sequelae of DVT or post-thrombotic syndrome, or chronic venous disease unrelated to venous thrombosis, including primary venous insufficiency. Left-sided clinical findings are presumed to be more likely associated with an obstructive iliac vein lesion, but lesions are also reported near the confluence of the internal and external veins, so right-sided findings can also indicate a pelvic source of obstruction.[7] A literature review in 2009 concluded that the disease predominantly affects female patients, and those with symptoms of acute iliofemoral venous thrombosis tended to be young women in the second to fourth decades of life.[8, 9] As recognition of the disease process was investigated further, studies found that while women tended to have a higher degree of stenosis, anatomic compression is commonly present in both sexes.[7]

Patients with occlusive or stenotic lesions of the iliocaval venous system tend to present as two distinct scenarios: 1) May-Thurner compression of left common iliac vein with or without acute thrombosis or 2) post-thrombotic venous occlusion because of a prior deep venous thrombosis from the iliac venous obstruction.[10] The degree of disability these presentations cause is variable. On the milder end of the spectrum of symptoms of venous occlusive disease, symptoms vary from mild swelling to unilateral leg heaviness, aching, and vague discomfort. In the acute presentation, patients typically present with sudden onset of leg pain and swelling, and the diagnosis of deep venous thrombosis is confirmed with duplex ultrasound. While the thrombus may be isolated to the iliac system, in those with thrombotic MTS, involvement of the deep venous system is more extensive and symptoms are more severe in comparison to those with DVT in the absence of compression syndromes.[3, 11] Furthermore, patients with chronic venous occlusive disease and post thrombotic syndrome with symptoms of valvular incompetence, varicosities, lower leg discoloration, and venous ulcerations can oftentimes be attributed to underlying undiagnosed compression syndrome. With advancement in imaging leading to changes in diagnosis, treatment of obstructive vein lesions has expanded as well.

DIAGNOSTIC EVALUATION

Initial evaluation of patients involves duplex sonography followed by computed tomography venography (CTV) or magnetic resonance venography (MRV). Even with negative findings, however, in patients with high suspicion of MTS, catheter-based venography with use of intravascular ultrasound (IVUS) is still warranted. These measures are both diagnostic and therapeutic.

MANAGEMENT

The current treatment of choice for venous compression syndrome is venography with IVUS and consideration of endovascular iliac venous stenting. Before any treatment is undertaken, a thorough history and physical exam that guides imaging is necessary. In those with acute thrombosis, this includes hypercoagulable workup and investigation of underlying reasons for thrombosis and the initiation of anticoagulation. In those with non-thrombotic compression syndrome, this includes compression therapy, exercise advancement, and weight loss as conservative means. If compression therapy has failed, venography with IVUS would be offered to assess the venous system with possible intervention as well.[3, 6, 11]

Technique

Catheter-Based Venography

Catheter-based venography is the gold standard for diagnosis of venous compression syndrome and allows for treatment in the same setting. Venous access is via the ipsilateral popliteal or femoral veins. Imaging is obtained in two orthogonal views as single-plane venography provides a sensitivity of only 45% in diagnosing a venous stenosis of >70%.[12] The iliac vein may appear "pancaked" in the anterior-posterior plane: it can have a normal to slightly widened diameter with a central translucency at the site of compression.[4, 7] Venography will also show thrombus if present or venous collaterals in non-thrombotic or chronic lesions (Figure 14.1). Without these more obvious findings though, pressure gradients and use of IVUS are necessary to determine the presence of hemodynamically significant lesions.

Intravascular Ultrasound

IVUS is invaluable when it comes to investigation, confirmation, and intervention in venous compression syndrome. It will provide intraluminal measurement of diameter in order to guide stent sizing and will also localize the site of maximal compression. The examination of intraluminal characteristics ensures no lesions are missed particularly by illustrating lesions near the iliac vein confluence that may be missed on standard venography. Up to one-third of venous compressions detected on IVUS can be missed on initial CTV.[14] Studies have also shown that standard venography underestimates the degree of stenosis by 30% compared to IVUS. The full 360-degree field offered by IVUS better appreciates a stenotic lumen and intravascular webs[15] (Figure 14.2, Figure 14.3).

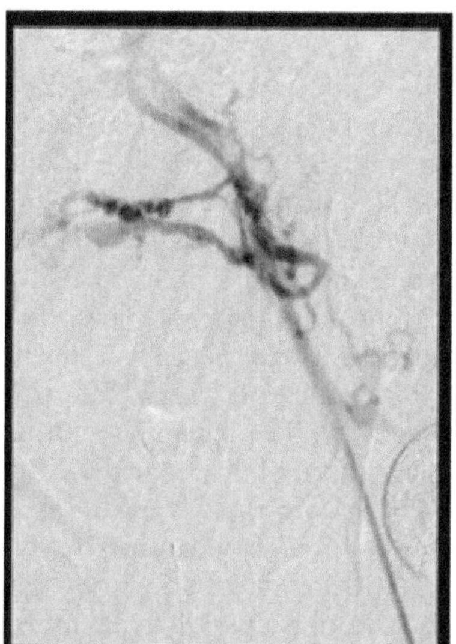

Figure 14.1 Venography showing occlusion of iliac vein with collateral formation.[13]

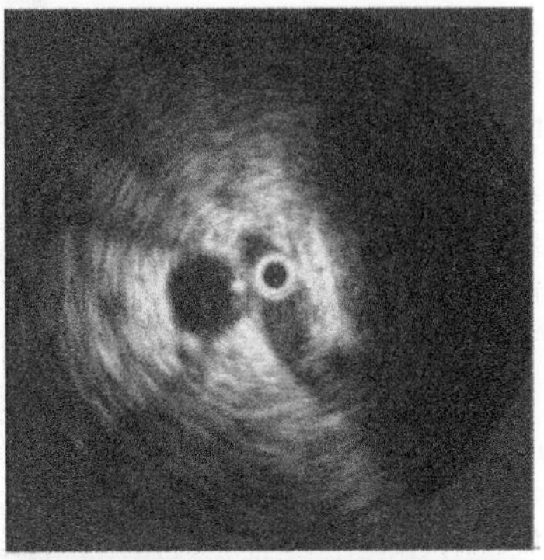

Figure 14.2 IVUS demonstrating stenotic lesion. Left iliac vein is externally compressed by crossing of right iliac artery.[4]

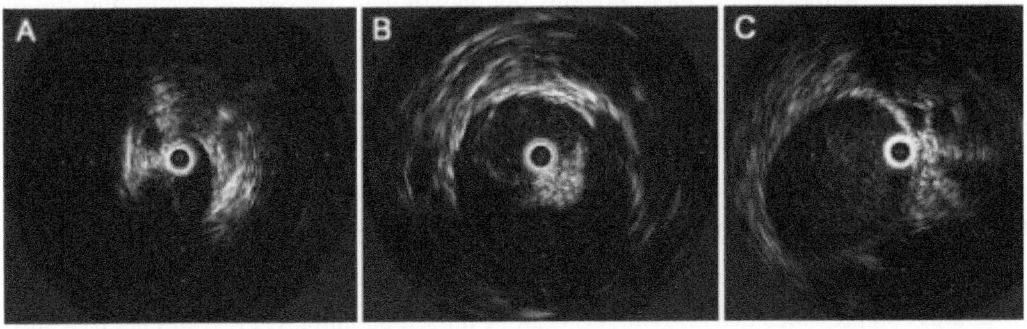

Figure 14.3 IVUS demonstrating non-stenotic venous lesions: (A) a network of echogenic intraluminal trabeculae; (B) a chronic web with associated thrombus; or (C) an eccentric increase in vein wall echogenicity with otherwise preserved vein wall and lumen.[7]

Non-Thrombotic Syndrome

As mentioned earlier, first-line therapy for non-thrombotic compression syndrome in patients with symptoms of unilateral left leg swelling is a trial of compression, exercise, and weight loss. If conservative management fails, patients with life-limiting symptoms are then considered for venography with IVUS. Findings concerning for hemodynamically significant vein compression include contrast stagnation within the left iliac venous system, reversal of flow into the internal iliac system and drainage into the right iliac vein, and extensive collateralization pelvic collateralization. In the non-thrombotic presentation, access is typically via the common femoral vein. In anticipation of stent placement, the puncture should be done below all diseased segments to allow for stenting of all diseased segments of vein, although this is generally a consideration reserved for MTS patients presenting with signs and symptoms of chronic venous disease from a prior thrombotic episode. Crossing of the lesion is generally straightforward, and a wire is placed into the IVC. IVUS is used to assess the iliac system and identify the point of maximal compression of the left common iliac vein. If the degree of stenosis requires intervention (>50% reduction in cross-sectional areal relative to normal vein by IVUS measurements), the sheath is upsized to an appropriately size for stent delivery (generally 10Fr), the patient is anticoagulated to a therapeutic level.[10, 16]

Stent sizing based on IVUS includes diameters of the compressed vein and the proximal vein. Oversizing of 20% is appropriate given the concern in the venous system for stent

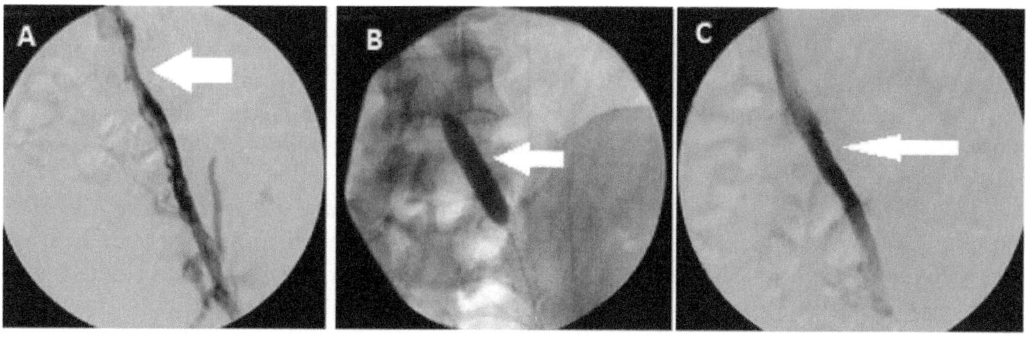

Figure 14.4 Venography (A) point of compression of left iliac vein, (B) balloon dilation, (C) following stent placement.[16]

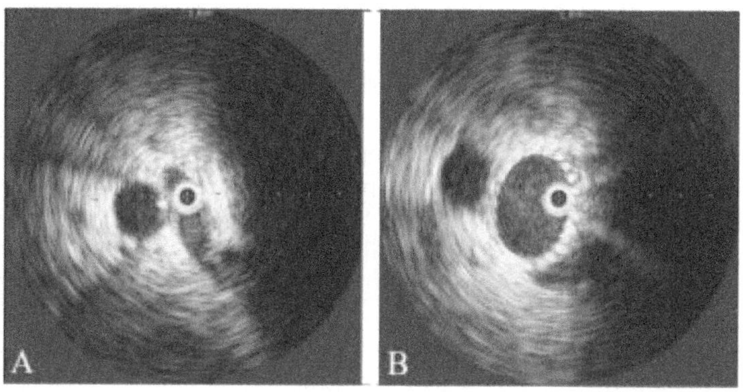

Figure 14.5 IVUS. (A) Left iliac vein is externally compressed by crossing of right iliac artery, (B) luminal gain achieved after stent placement.[4]

migration. Stents are extended about 5 mm beyond the point of maximal compression, even if this requires extension into the IVC. Balloon angioplasty follows stent deployment for wall apposition. Completion venography and repeat IVUS should be performed to confirm adequate luminal gain and stent apposition (Figures 14.4 and 14.5).

Patients with non-thrombotic vein lesions have been shown to have better long-term patency rates than patients presenting with thrombotic MTS. In one study, 98% primary stent patency was observed with four years of follow-up.[17] In another, primary and secondary patency rates were 79% and 100% for non-thrombotic lesions and 57% and 86% in those with a DVT history at 72 months.[18] For this reason, most patients with non-thrombotic lesions do not require anticoagulation. There are no specific guidelines for postoperative antiplatelet, and it is generally at the discretion of the physician. Generally, dual antiplatelet is recommended for a period of 6 weeks to 3 months, after which aspirin can be continued as single therapy.[4, 17]

Thrombotic Syndrome

Acute DVT Associated with Iliac Vein Obstructive Lesion

Although the mainstay of treatment for an acute DVT is anticoagulation, severely symptomatic patients generally require thromboreductive therapy. In thrombotic MTS patients presenting with acute iliofemoral DVT (<2 weeks duration), the need for intervention is based on symptom severity and extent of thrombosis, but most venous specialists believe that iliofemoral DVT with presumed or documented iliac vein compression warrant an aggressive strategy of thrombus removal with catheter-directed thrombolysis or mechanical thrombectomy. When intervention is planned, clearance of clot burden is generally performed to allow for identification and treatment of underlying venous compression pathology.[4] The goal of intervention is to reduce the long-term sequelae of post thrombotic syndrome. The ATTRACT trial, which randomized patients with acute proximal DVT to catheter-directed thrombolysis or anticoagulation arms, did not find any difference in the development of post-thrombotic syndrome. However, subset analysis of the ATTRACT trial demonstrated a decreased incidence of severe post-thrombotic symptoms in those treated with aggressive thrombus removal strategies, especially in those with extensive iliofemoral DVT.[19] The decision to intervene is therefore individually based with consideration given to these factors, as well as the age and functional status of the patient.

Given the iliofemoral location, access is obtained via the popliteal vein as the common femoral vein is commonly involved. A wire is crossed into the IVC, which in the chronic phase can be more challenging and require a stiffer wire with a support catheter. Once crossed, the decision of to perform catheter-directed thrombolysis overnight or in a single session thrombectomy is then made, generally based on the chronicity and ease of wire crossing. For patients with less than 1–2 weeks duration, an attempt at a single-session clearance of the thrombus with pharmacomechanical thrombectomy is reasonable. The AngioJet system (Boston Scientific, Minneapolis, MN) in the "power pulse" mode will lace the thrombus with alteplase which can dwell for 10–20 minute. The system can then be switched to aspiration mode to aspirate the lysed thrombus.[16, 20] Newer devices, such as the ClotTriever (Inari Medical, Irvine CA) and Lightning 12 (Penumbra Inc, Alameda, CA) provide clot clearance in a single session, but their comparison to catheter-directed thrombolysis in terms of outcomes is not known in the setting of iliac compression syndromes.[4] Both modalities, catheter-directed and pharmomechanical thrombectomy, however have shown similar rates of thrombus removal overall (70% in catheter-directed and 75% in pharmomechanical).[21] Patients with a longer interval between initial symptom onset and treatment, overnight catheter-directed thrombolysis, typically at tissue plasminogen activator drip rates of 0.5–1.0 mg/hr is recommended.

Following thrombus removal, venographic and IVUS evaluation for May-Thurner compression of the left common iliac vein is nearly identical to that discussed for non-thrombotic May-Thurner patients. These patients, however, are more likely to have additional post-thrombotic occlusive lesion. These residual occlusive lesions generally extend from the common femoral vein to the caval confluence and should be stented as angioplasty alone may not be durable.[22] Studies have shown that leaving these lesions unstented lead to a higher rate of postoperative early thrombosis.[23, 24]

In patients that present with stent thrombosis and recurrent symptoms, undersizing of the stent and inadequate extension should be considered as etiologies for these complications. Reintervention can be difficult as these lesions are now more chronic, yet the same principles of catheter-directed thrombolysis and pharmocomechanical thrombectomy still apply for those with recent symptoms presumed to be due to acute stent thrombosis. Once recanalization is achieved, assessment and correction of the underlying pathology is required.[4, 17]

Post-Thrombotic Syndrome with Iliac Vein Stenosis or Occlusion

The diagnosis of PTS is based on clinical signs and symptoms the patient experiences in the affected leg after a DVT. IVUS remains the most sensitive examination to detect the extent of

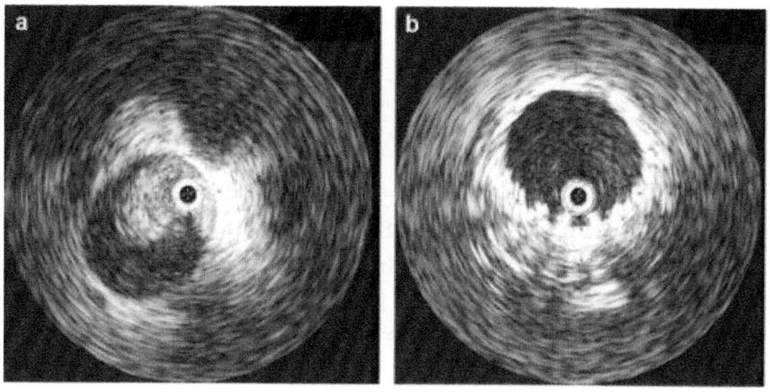

Figure 14.6 (a) IVUS with trabeculations of the vein in a patient with PTS, (b) patent vein following stenting.[13]

the lesion and typically will show trabeculations, thickness of the vein wall, external compression, and thrombus formation. Studies have shown that iliac vein stenting alone is sufficient to control symptoms in a patient with outflow obstruction and deep reflux in the setting of a chronic venous obstruction.

A similar technique of venography and intervention is performed. After confirming the obstruction and the existence of collaterals, a stiff hydrophilic wire and supporting catheter is usually needed to pass these obstructions. Pre-dilation of the obstructed venous tract is performed next. After balloon dilation without stenting, immediate recoil occurs in most cases and stenting is mandatory. Stenting with a self-expanding stent should be carried out throughout the complete diseased post-thrombotic vein segment, from healthy segment to healthy segment. To achieve the best possible alignment of the stent, the balloon used for predilation should have at least the same diameter as the stent. In patients with long-segment post-thrombotic iliofemoral obstructions who need more than one stent, stent placement should have 1–2 cm of overlap with stenting of the common iliac first to the common femoral vein. Post-dilation must always be performed, and completion venography obtained in two views to exclude recoil and complications. IVUS upon completion is preferred as well (Figure 14.6).

Venous Stents

Veins have greater diameters than the corresponding arteries, therefore stenting of the iliofemoral venous system require stents of larger diameter. These typically include self-expandable, longitudinally flexible stents of diameters from 12 mm to 18 mm.[7] Additionally, post thrombotic veins are typically fibrotic and compressed and need stents with more radial force. There are venous stents that exhibit these characteristics, but the literature about their outcomes is limited. Rollo et al, on the other hand, describes using braided stainless steel stents, typically in diameters of 16–20 mm, for iliac vein stenting with good results prior to the advent of dedicated venous stents.[20] The largest study investigating stenting for reconstruction of the femoroiliocaval venous system was published in 2017 by van Vuuren et al. In 221 patients operated on (196 for PTS), outcomes at 60 months, including primary patency, assisted primary patency, and secondary patency rates were 64%, 81%, and 89%. Thirty-six patients had a thrombotic stent occlusion, requiring thrombolysis and secondary stenting in 19 patients. All stents implanted in this study were dedicated venous stents [(sinus-XL), sinus-XL Flex, sinus-Venous, and sinus-Obliquus (OptiMed); Vici Venous Stent (Veniti Inc); Zilver

Vena (Cook Medical); and Venovo (Bard)]. Mortality was 0%, and significant improvement of Villalta score was noticed.[25]

CONCLUSIONS

Iliocaval compression syndromes are increasingly diagnosed due to increased awareness and improved recognition of symptoms in the acute and chronic phases. Improved technology of both imaging and intervention have improved patient outcomes and quality of life. Anatomic anomalies are amenable to endovascular surgical techniques and stenting of these lesions, while the literature is still ongoing, do show favorable short and long-term outcomes and patency rates.

REFERENCES

1. Cockett, F.B., M.L. Thomas, and D. Negus, *Iliac vein compression.–its relation to iliofemoral thrombosis and the post-thrombotic syndrome.* Br Med J, 1967. **2**(5543): pp. 14–19.
2. Cockett, F.B., and M.L. Thomas, *The iliac compression syndrome.* Br J Surg, 1965. **52**(10): pp. 816–821.
3. Cheng, L., H. Zhao, and F.X. Zhang, *Iliac vein compression syndrome in an asymptomatic patient population: a prospective study.* Chin Med J (Engl), 2017. **130**(11): pp. 1269–1275.
4. Fereydooni, A., and J.R. Stern, *Contemporary treatment of May-Thurner Syndrome.* J Cardiovasc Surg (Torino), 2021. **62**(5): pp. 447–455.
5. Taheri, S.A., et al., *Iliocaval compression syndrome.* Am J Surg, 1987. **154**(2): pp. 169–172.
6. Heniford, B.T., et al., *May-Thurner Syndrome: Management by endovascular surgical techniques.* Ann Vasc Surg, 1998. **12**(5): pp. 482–486.
7. Birn, J., and S. Vedantham, *May-Thurner Syndrome and other obstructive iliac vein lesions: Meaning, myth, and mystery.* Vasc Med, 2015. **20**(1): pp. 74–83.
8. Foit, N.A., et al., *Iliofemoral deep vein thrombosis after tibial plateau fracture fixation related to undiagnosed May-Thurner Syndrome: A case report.* Patient Saf Surg, 2013. **7**(1): p. 12.
9. Boyd, D.A., *Unilateral lower extremity edema in May-Thurner Syndrome.* Mil Med, 2004. **169**(12): pp. 968–971.
10. DeRubertis, B.G., et al., *Endovascular management of nonmalignant iliocaval venous lesions.* Ann Vasc Surg, 2013. **27**(5): pp. 577–586.
11. Radaideh, Q., N.M. Patel, and N.W. Shammas, *Iliac vein compression: Epidemiology, diagnosis and treatment.* Vasc Health Risk Manag, 2019. **15**: pp. 115–122.
12. Derubertis, B.G., and R. Patel, May-Thurner Syndrome: Diagnosis and management. In *Current Management of Venous Diseases* (p. 463–477). Springer International Publishing, 2018.
13. Schleimer, K., et al., *Update on diagnosis and treatment strategies in patients with post-thrombotic syndrome due to chronic venous obstruction and role of endovenous recanalization.* J Vasc Surg Venous Lymphat Disord, 2019. **7**(4): pp. 592–600.
14. Gagne, P.J., et al., *Venography versus intravascular ultrasound for diagnosing and treating iliofemoral vein obstruction.* J Vasc Surg Venous Lymphat Disord, 2017. **5**(5): pp. 678–687.
15. Neglen, P., and S. Raju, *Intravascular ultrasound scan evaluation of the obstructed vein.* J Vasc Surg, 2002. **35**(4): pp. 694–700.
16. Waheed, K.B., et al., *Left lower limb deep venous thrombosis, May-Thurner Syndrome and endovascular management.* Saudi Med J, 2022. **43**(1): pp. 108–112.
17. Ye, K., et al., *Long-term outcomes of stent placement for symptomatic nonthrombotic iliac vein compression lesions in chronic venous disease.* J Vasc Interv Radiol, 2012. **23**(4): pp. 497–502.

18. Neglen, P., et al., *Stenting of the venous outflow in chronic venous disease: Long-term stent-related outcome, clinical, and hemodynamic result.* J Vasc Surg, 2007. **46**(5): pp. 979–990.
19. Vedantham, S., et al., *Pharmacomechanical catheter-directed thrombolysis for deep-vein thrombosis.* N Engl J Med, 2017. **377**(23): pp. 2240–2252.
20. Rollo, J.C., et al., *Contemporary outcomes after venography-guided treatment of patients with May-Thurner Syndrome.* J Vasc Surg Venous Lymphat Disord, 2017. **5**(5): pp. 667–676 e1.
21. Lin, P.H., et al., *Catheter-direct thrombolysis versus pharmacomechanical thrombectomy for treatment of symptomatic lower extremity deep venous thrombosis.* Am J Surg, 2006. **192**(6): pp. 782–788.
22. Neglen, P., T.P. Tackett, Jr., and S. Raju, *Venous stenting across the inguinal ligament.* J Vasc Surg, 2008. **48**(5): pp. 1255–1261.
23. Mickley, V., et al., *Left iliac venous thrombosis caused by venous spur: Treatment with thrombectomy and stent implantation.* J Vasc Surg, 1998. **28**(3): pp. 492–497.
24. Hartung, O., et al., *Late results of surgical venous thrombectomy with iliocaval stenting.* J Vasc Surg, 2008. **47**(2): pp. 381–387.
25. van Vuuren, T., et al., *Editor's choice – reconstruction of the femoro-ilio-caval outflow by percutaneous and hybrid interventions in symptomatic deep venous obstruction.* Eur J Vasc Endovasc Surg, 2017. **54**(4): pp. 495–503.

Chapter 15

Evidence-Based Diagnosis and Management of Pelvic Congestion Syndrome

Neeraj Rastogi, Nii-Kabu Kabutey, and Ducksoo Kim

INTRODUCTION

Pelvic congestion syndrome (PCS) as a clinical entity was first described in 1949 by Taylor, suggesting pelvic venous insufficiency/incompetence (PVI) as an etiologic factor contributing to pelvic pain pathology.[1–3] PVI can present with a plethora of abdominal symptoms and can be a diagnostic challenge for physicians. PCS usually occurs in premenopausal and multiparous women.[1, 2] Fifteen percent of women experience PCS between the ages of 20 and 50, but not all patient with PVI will experience abdominal or pelvic symptoms.[4]

Pain secondary to PCS or PVI is defined as non-cyclical pelvic pain that has been present for at least a 6-month duration. Patients will have dilated ovarian, periuterine, or vaginal veins. The pain is often associated with prolonged standing and sexual intercourse. Clinically, the term PVI is preferred over PCS, female varicocele, or pelvic vascular congestion (PVC) because it defines the etio-pathology associated with pelvic congestion and venous engorgement.

Overall, there is overlapping of the clinical presentations that may be seen with PVI, May-Thurner syndrome, and Nutcracker syndrome (NCS). Recently, an international panel at the American Vein and Lymphatic Society developed a descriptive and instrumental classification for 'Pelvic Venous Disease' (PeVD). The Symptoms-Varices-Pathophysiology ('SVP') classification for PeVD, includes three domains: symptoms (S), varices (V), and pathophysiology (P), with the pathophysiology domain encompassing the anatomic (A), hemodynamic (H), and etiologic (E) features of the patient's disease.[5] An individual patient's classification is designated as SVPA,H,E (Table 15.1).

Preliminary diagnostic laboratory tests are obtained to rule out common pelvic pathologies that can cause pelvic pain. Testing should include a pregnancy test and Pap smear to ensure pregnancy or cervical cancer is not the cause for pain. Pelvic duplex ultrasounds (US) and/or computed tomography (CT) scans are usually the first imaging modalities in the evaluation of patients with chronic pelvic pain. Cross-sectional imaging studies in the form of CT and magnetic resonance imaging (MRI) with 3-dimensional reconstructions maximum intensity projection (MIP) and volume rendered (VR) images are useful to determine whether there may be an anatomical issue that is causing the symptoms. Non-invasive imaging techniques such as CT, MRI, and pelvic venous duplex ultrasound are increasingly gaining favor as helpful diagnostic tools. Selective ovarian venography[1, 2, 6] remains the most effective method for both identification of pelvic venous pathology, including reno-caval pressure gradient and its ability to provide treatment options. Pelvic varices are treatable using ovarian suppression, ligation of the pelvic veins, or endovascular embolization therapy with utilization of sclerosant agent or coils. Procedural interventions, including coil embolization of ovarian vein, can be performed for females with PCS that do not respond to medical treatment.[7–11] In this chapter we define primary and secondary PCS, highlight the role of ovarian venography, and

DOI: 10.1201/9781003316626-18

The Symptoms-Varices-Pathophysiology (SVP) Classification of Pelvic Venous Disorders

A Report of the American Vein & Lymphatic Society International Working Group on Pelvic Venous Disorders

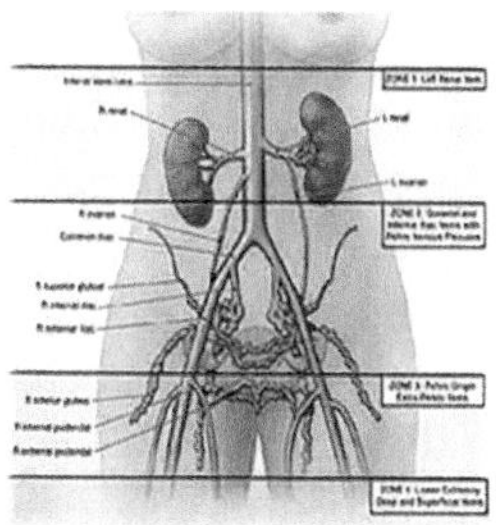

	(S) SYMPTOMS		(V) VARICES		(P) PATHOPHYSIOLOGY
S_0	No symptoms	V_0	No abdominal, pelvic, or pelvic origin extra-pelvic varices	Anatomy	IVC Left renal vein Gonadal vein Common iliac vein External iliac vein Internal iliac vein Pelvic escape vein
S_1	Renal symptoms of venous origin				
S_2	Chronic pelvic pain of venous origin	V_1	Renal hilar varices		
S_3	Extra-pelvic symptoms of venous origin	V_2	Pelvic varices		
		V_3	Pelvic origin extra-pelvic varices		
a	Localized symptoms associated with veins of the external genitalia	a	Genital varices (vulvar varices and varicocele)	Hemo dynamics	Obstruction (O) Reflux (R)
b	Localized symptoms associated with pelvic origin non-saphenous leg veins	b	Pelvic origin lower extremity varicose veins arising from pelvic escape points, extending into the thigh.	Etiology	Thrombotic (T) Non-thrombotic (NT) Congenital (C)
c	Venous claudication				

JVS-VL Journal of Vascular Surgery Venous and Lymphatic Disorders

Meissner et al, *J Vasc Surg Venous Lymphat Disord. May 2021*

LinkedIn @TheJVascSurg @JVascSurg

Table 15.1 The Symptoms-Varices-Pathophysiology (SVP) Classification of Pelvic Venous Disorders.

describe the role of sclerotherapy and endovascular coil embolization as a safe and effective treatment modality in the management of PCS. Additionally, this chapter will provide a literature review of various treatment modalities that have been adopted for pelvic congestion syndrome.

PATHOPHYSIOLOGY

The etiology of pelvic pain can be very difficult to discern. Referred pain from the abdominal viscera and neurogenic and psychogenic factors can all contribute to pelvic pain pathology. Pain within the pelvis can occur due to several pelvic conditions such as endometriosis, fibroids, pelvic inflammatory disease, uterine prolapse/malposition, and ovarian cysts[1–3] Therefore, it can be very challenging for physicians that deal with pelvic pain including primary care doctors, general surgeons, vascular surgeons, gynecologists, gastroenterologists, pain specialist/anesthesiologist, urological surgeons, and interventional radiologists to confirm a diagnosis of PCS. No definitive diagnosis is usually made in 60% of patients with pelvic pain.[4, 12] The presence of varices of the pelvic veins has been shown to be the underlying etiology in most patients with PCS.[1, 12–16] Primary PCS including congenital or acquired ovarian vein incompetence from non-obstructive causes is considered a diagnosis of exclusion. Patients with secondary PCS develop ovarian and/or pelvic vein collateral pathways to circumvent an obstructive process.

Development of symptomatic ovarian/pelvic varices is caused by a combination of pelvic venous valvular insufficiency and endocrine and mechanical factors. Obstructing anatomic anomalies such as NCS, May-Thurner syndrome, uterine malposition and pelvic tumors may lead to secondary PCS, where the ovarian and/or pelvic veins contribute to the development of the collateral pathways to relieve antegrade obstruction. In some cases, a left retroaortic renal vein may obstruct the drainage from the left ovarian vein leading to symptomatic pelvic varices. Ovarian veins in premenopausal women are exposed to high concentrations of estradiol and estrone compared to the peripheral circulation.[17] Estrogen overstimulation may be responsible in greater than 50% of women diagnosed with PCS. Of note, most patients with PCS do not have amenorrhea or demonstrate hirsutism. Estrogen stimulation leads to venodilatation, which results in pelvic venous engorgement and thereby weakening of the venous walls, leading to enlargement of the pelvic veins/varicosities. Frequently, ovarian and pelvic varicosities are seen after pregnancy. The capacity of pelvic veins may increase by 60-fold over the non-pregnant state due to increased blood volume during pregnancy, which contributes to venous dilatation and valvular insufficiency. The venous distension may also cause pelvic pain in some woman.

Other contributing factors to PCS include mechanical factors such as damaged or absent venous valves that lead to retrograde flow. Weight gain and anatomic changes in the pelvic structures during pregnancy, external vascular compression such as renal NCS, and iliac vein compression/May-Thurner syndrome may all lead to PCS. NCS is described as left renal vein compression by the superior mesenteric artery. May-Thurner syndrome can occur due to left common iliac vein compression from the right common iliac artery against the pelvic brim, which may cause iliofemoral stenosis or deep venous thrombosis with or without the pelvic varices of PCS. Additionally, a few rare cases of combined PCS secondary to both May-Thurner syndrome and NCS have been reported.[11, 12, 14, 15] Mechanical factors result in pooling and delayed clearance of blood in the pelvic and ovarian veins may be a predisposing factor for venous thrombosis and pelvic pain secondary to mass effect on the lumbosacral plexus.

CLINICAL PICTURE

Clinical symptoms of pelvic congestion are likely the result of the presence of ovarian and pelvic varicosities secondary to PCS, renal NCS, or iliac vein compression/May-Thurner syndrome. The spectrum of pelvic pain symptoms is comparable to lower extremity varicose vein symptomatology, where leg pain and discomfort arises during ambulation resulting from lower extremity chronic venous hypertension secondary to superficial veins valvular incompetence.

PCS is associated with constant dull pain in the pelvis, vulvar region, and upper thighs. Heaviness just before the onset of menses with or without dyspareunia and/or post-coital pain may also occur. A pelvic exam may demonstrate cervical motion and ovarian point tenderness. Exacerbations of symptoms often occur after prolonged walking/standing or activities that typically increase intra-abdominal pressure. Diurnal variations are frequently reported; the patients are asymptomatic in the morning and pain typically worsens with time during the day, in the premenstrual period, and/or during pregnancy. The symptoms usually continue to worsen after each subsequent pregnancy and, therefore, multiparous women are predisposed to develop PCS due to a significant increase in intravascular volume and increased venous capacity with each term of gestation.[18, 19]

Pelvic varices develop during pregnancy and continue to progress in size during each term of gestation. Continued venous engorgement predisposes to venous valvular insufficiency. As a result, venous varicosities may be seen internally around the pelvis and sometimes externally at the buttocks, varices extending onto the legs, or in the vulvar area under soft tissue resulting in labial asymmetry.[4] Vulvar or perineal varicosities are reported in greater than 10% of the patients with lower extremity superficial venous insufficiency and may accompany and reflect ovarian vein insufficiency. These varices can extend over the buttock and posteromedial thigh and communicate with both greater and small saphenous veins. They most commonly manifest during pregnancy and regress in the postpartum period. Missed diagnosis of PVI may explain treatment failure in patients treated solely for lower extremity superficial venous insufficiency.[20]

APPLIED CLINICAL ANATOMY

Normal ovarian veins are usually less than 5 mm in diameter and have functional valves.[6, 13, 14] The left ovarian plexus drains into the left ovarian vein, which empties into the left renal vein at an angle of 90 degrees. The right ovarian plexus drains into the right ovarian vein, which usually empties directly into the IVC antero-laterally at a 45-degree angle just below the right renal vein. Rarely, the right ovarian vein may drain into the right renal vein. It is important to understand that veins draining the bladder, vagina, uterus, and rectum are interconnected and highly variable. The uterus and vagina drain into the uterine veins and ovarian plexus via utero-ovarian and salpingo-ovarian veins and then into branches of the internal iliac veins. Vulvar and perineal veins drain into the internal pudendal vein and then into the inferior gluteal vein, then the external pudendal vein, which drains into the great saphenous vein, or into the circumflex femoral vein, and then into the femoral vein.[21]

The main trunks of ovarian veins have valves particularly at the terminus of the ovarian vein to maintain antegrade flow. Most other pelvic venous plexuses and the internal iliac veins are relatively devoid of valves.[19, 21] This is an additional contributing factor involved in venous dilation of the pelvic venous anatomy in some patients even without pregnancy. Congenital absence of venous valves in ovarian veins has been demonstrated in 15% of the PCS patients on the left and 6% on the right.[22] Moreover, valvular incompetency has been recorded in more than one-third of patients both in the right and left ovarian veins.

The development of ovarian/pelvic varices is caused by a combination of factors: (i) valvular incompetence leading to reversal of flow, (ii) mechanical venous obstruction, and (iii) endocrine/hormonal factors. Of note, all three may play a role in the delayed clearance of pelvic venous flow in the utero-ovarian and salpingo-ovarian veins resulting in pelvic venous congestion.

The diagnosis of PCS is defined by the presence of (i) ovarian vein reflux and (ii) pelvic varicosities. Ovarian vein reflux can also be present in healthy asymptomatic parous women. During pregnancy, pelvic venous capacity increases by 60% due to mechanical compression of the gravid uterus and the vasodilator action of progesterone. Mechanical obstruction caused by the gravid uterus is a main contributing factor in the development of pelvic varicosities. Ovarian vein valvular incompetence leads to reversal of venous flow in the ovarian vein with dilation of veins in the pelvis and development of ovarian and internal iliac varices. This explains why successive pregnancies may cause venous valves to break down and allow varices to extend to the adjoining pelvic venous plexus, e.g., around uterus (uterovaginalis), bladder (vesicalis), vulva (vulvaris), rectum (rectalis), and finally the right ovarian vein.[15, 23, 24]

DIAGNOSTIC IMAGING

CT scan has greater sensitivity for showing pelvic varicosities, however, duplex ultrasound, retrograde venography, and intravascular ultrasound (IVUS) are increasingly gaining favor as imaging modalities to diagnosis PCS as they can provide dynamic information about visualized venous blood flow and therefore can be used to evaluate pelvic varicosities, detect venous reflux, and diagnose compression syndromes (e.g., NCS and May-Thurner syndrome). Diagnostic criteria for pelvic duplex sonography include (i) visualization of enlarged ovarian veins, measuring >6 mm in diameter; (ii) presence of pelvic varicocele (>5 mm) and dilated and tortuous myometrial arcuate veins (>5 mm) communicating with pelvic varicose veins/varicocele, bilaterally; and (iii) reversed and slow flow (less than 3 cm/s) particularly in the left ovarian vein.[25] Pelvic ultrasonography is a good screening tool, but it can lead to false-negative studies due to slow blood flow in pelvic varicosities.[26] Likewise, advanced imaging techniques such as CT and magnetic resonance venography (MRV) can be used to detect dilated pelvic varicosities and areas of venous compression to demonstrate renal NCS and iliac vein compression/May-Thurner syndrome and to rule out other potential etiologies for pelvic pain including underlying malignancies.

Pelvic MRI typically demonstrates dilated, tortuous, enhancing tubular structures (enlarged pelvic veins) near the uterus and ovary extending to the broad ligament and pelvic sidewall (dilated utero-ovarian and salpingo-ovarian veins). Contrast enhancement with gadolinium not only improves visualization but increases sensitivity if MR sequences are obtained while patients perform a Valsalva maneuver. Of note, CT or duplex ultrasound of the pelvis has a relatively lower sensitivity 13 and 20%, respectively for PCS compared with MRI/MRV (59%) or diagnostic venogram. Diagnostic laparoscopy is sometimes used in patients with chronic pelvic pain to rule out other etiologies, especially pelvic endometriosis. Examinations performed in the supine position may not recognize PCS in 80–90% of patients.[21, 27, 28]

PCS can be a difficult diagnosis to make and often one or more imaging modalities may already have been used by the time PCS patients are referred to venous specialist. The diagnosis of PCS is best made with ovarian venography.[4, 6, 7] For compete evaluation left renal, bilateral ovarian, and iliac, including internal iliac venography, is performed. Intravascular pressure gradients across the renal (reno-caval) and left common iliac vein are obtained whenever an abnormality like NCS is visualized on diagnostic imaging. A gradient of less than 1 mmHg is normal. The pressure gradient between the left renal vein and IVC should be less than 2 mmHg. A pressure gradient greater than 3 mmHg at the level of compression can confirm the diagnosis of NCS. Even though regarded as the most informative method, renal, ovarian, and iliac venography should not be used as first-line diagnostic tests but rather as means to confirm the findings of non-invasive testing and should not routinely be performed in patients who do not have severe symptoms of primary or secondary PCS.

MRI/MRV is a preferred primary imaging modality as it helps to rule out other potential etiologies for pelvic pain, detect venous reflux, diagnose compression syndromes (e.g., NCS and May-Thurner syndrome), analyze the severity of the PCS, and assess if the patient is a candidate for endovascular treatment. Additionally, venographic demonstration of ovarian vein incompetency and pelvic varicosities are the most common clinical signs that should raise suspicion for the diagnosis of PCS.

In order to perform catheter-based venography, the common femoral vein is accessed using a 21-gauge micropuncture needle. A catheter is then advanced into the inferior vena cava via a sheath to select and image the ovarian and/or pelvic veins following contrast injection under fluoroscopic guidance. Diagnostic criteria on the selective ovarian and pelvic venography are (i) ovarian vein measuring >6 mm in diameter, upper limit of normal is considered to be 5 mm; (ii) retrograde ovarian or pelvic venous flow; (iii) presence of pelvic varicosities and multiple tortuous cross pelvic venous collaterals from left-to-right/contralateral reflux; (iv) stagnation and delayed clearance of contrast in the pelvic veins; and (v) visualization of vulvoperineal or posteromedial thigh varices.[27] De Schepper explained this phenomenon by the so-called 'left-to-right' theory of PCS and graded the pelvic varicosities as follows: Grade I = dilated left ovarian vein/plexus, Grade II = + dilated left utero-vaginal vein plexus, and Grade III = + dilated right utero-vaginal plexus and right ovarian vein.[24]

The direct relationship between varices and chronic pelvic pain remains difficult to ascertain, indicating that other causes of pelvic pain may coexist with pelvic varicosities.[4, 6] Moreover, ovarian veins (left more commonly than right) can show reflux in healthy asymptomatic parous women, and no definitive diagnosis is usually made in 60% of patients.[15]

TREATMENT OPTIONS FOR PELVIC CONGESTION SYNDROME

Treatment of PCS may consist of medical management, open surgical techniques, and endovascular therapy. Currently, many minimally invasive therapeutic choices with excellent results are available for these patients. Pain caused by PCS can be managed by analgesics alone or in combination with drug producing ovarian suppression (medroxyprogesterone acetate [MPA: 30 mg per day, PO for 6 months] or gonadotropins receptor agonists [GnRH; goserelin to be given parenterally 3.6 mg, monthly × 6 doses]). Chemical ovarian suppression with MPA or GnRH blocks the direct vasodilator effect of estrogen and thereby provides relief in pelvic congestion and patients symptoms by reducing venous distention.[28] Failed medical treatment or recurrence of symptoms is an indication for open or laparoscopic surgery. Open procedures that have been utilized to alleviate PCS include ligation of ovarian veins and hysterectomy with or without bilateral salpingo-oophorectomy. Endovascular interventions such as ovarian vein coil embolization or embolization therapy using detachable balloons, sclerosing agents such as 3% sodium tetradecyl sulfate (STS) foam, or glue such as Enbucrilate (Butyl cyanoacrylate) have all been utilized with high success rates for the treatment of PCS. The goal of the interventional treatment is elimination of ovarian vein reflux with or without direct sclerosis of enlarged pelvic varicosities. Endovascular therapy has been validated with standardized pain assessment surveys before and after embolization therapy and during follow-up using a visual analog scale. Currently, embolization therapy of ovarian veins with and without internal iliac vein embolization is an effective endovascular treatment for PCS. This should always be performed prior to varicose vein treatment of lower limb. Ovarian and internal iliac veins are in close communication, and therefore, in some cases, embolization of the iliac veins may also be required. The internal iliac vein embolization is performed after treatment of the ovarian vein.

Case Example 1

Thirty-six-year-old female presented with chronic pelvic pain of moderate severity without dyspareunia. Associated symptoms included right lower extremity swelling and varicose veins over pubic area for over 10 years. She complained of continuous discomfort requiring daily analgesics to get relief and denied abdominal or urogynecological pain. The patient's past medical history is significant for normal menstrual cycle, two pregnancies via C-section, right hip fracture 12 years ago, and deep vein thrombosis (DVT) in the right lower extremity (RLE). Peripheral vascular exam showed normal distal pulses, with gross varicosities over the pubic area extending to the right labia majora, diffuse swelling of RLE. Initial venous duplex US of the RLE were consistent with normal phasic flow and good augmentation at all levels, incompetent deep venous system with severe reflux involving the popliteal

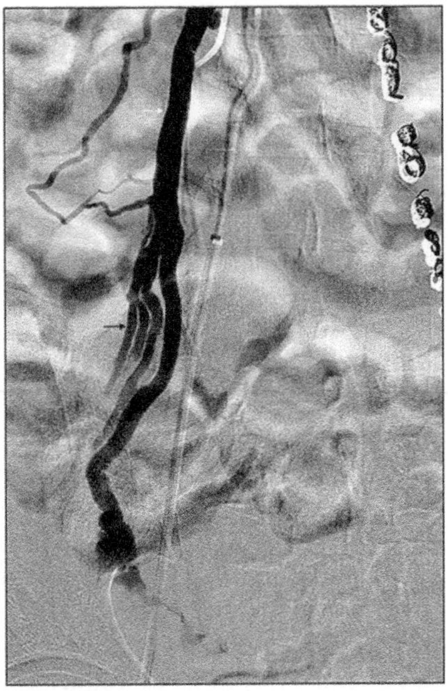

Figure 15.1 A 36-year-old female patient with PCS confirmed on ovarian venography. DSA image shows dilated Rt. ovarian vein (white arrow) with reverse blood flow and multiple collaterals (black arrow).

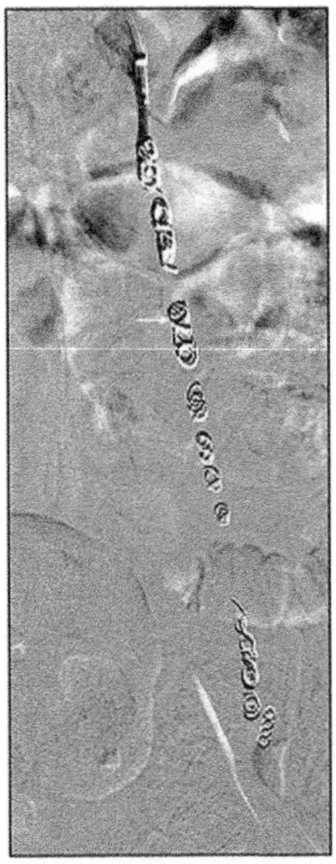

Figure 15.2 A 36-year-old female patient with PCS confirmed on ovarian venography. DSA image shows complete coil embolization of Lt. ovarian vein (white arrow) without any reflux.

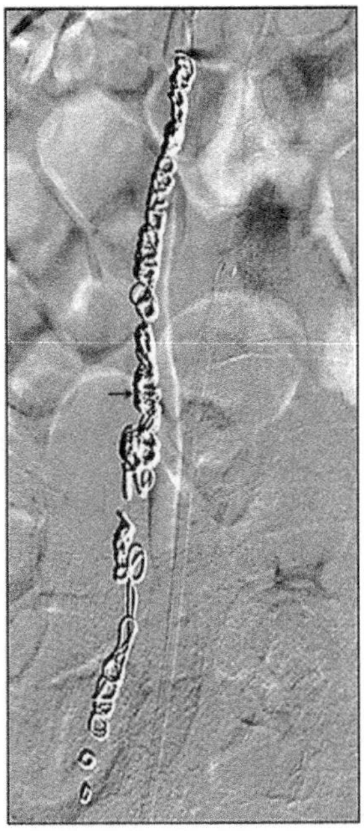

Figure 15.3 A 36-year-old female patient with PCS confirmed on ovarian venography. DSA image shows complete coil embolization of Rt. ovarian vein (black arrow) without any reflux.

vein, and an incompetent superficial venous system with severe reflux involving the greater saphenous vein.

Based on patient's history of chronic pelvic pain, multiparous status, and gross varicosities over the pubic area/vulval varices a diagnosis of PCS was considered.

The patient was scheduled for bilateral ovarian venography under monitored anesthesia care in reverse Trendelenburg position. Venography demonstrated bilateral enlarged ovarian veins measuring greater than 6 mm in diameter. Both veins were individually cannulated and coil embolized (Figures 15.1, 15.2, and 15.3). Postoperative follow-up pelvic duplex imaging of the adnexal vasculature 6 weeks after the procedure demonstrated no significant change in size of the pelvic vasculature with Valsalva. Likewise, during the follow-up office visit her pain was resolved and remained asymptomatic as of 2-year post-procedural follow-up.

Case Example 2

A 32-year-old female was referred to us for the evaluation of recurrent post-phlebitic pelvic and groin pain of moderate severity and dyspareunia requiring narcotic analgesics for over 5 years. On complete evaluation she was diagnosed with May-Thurner syndrome, which was managed with left common iliac vein stenting. Due to persistent pelvic pain and swelling in the left thigh, repeat venography was performed that demonstrated a moderate stenosis of the left external iliac vein below the previously placed left common iliac stent. This was treated with percutaneous transluminal angioplasty and stent placement in the left external iliac vein.

The patient continued to have persistent mild swelling in the left thigh, left leg pain and dyspareunia requiring narcotic analgesics. A left renal venogram was performed, which demonstrated retrograde filling of left ovarian and pelvic veins via collaterals. A left ovarian vein coil embolization was performed at the same outside hospital. The patient's leg swelling and pain were improved, but pelvic pain and dyspareunia continued.

Due to persistent venous disability with previously stented May-Thurner syndrome and left ovarian vein coil embolization, a pre-procedural diagnosis of incompletely resolved PCS was considered. She was then scheduled for ilio-caval and ovarian venography. Complete procedural steps were recorded as follows: Anterior-posterior spot fluoroscopic imaging of the abdomen was taken in supine position (Figure 15.4). Preliminary iliocaval venography demonstrated patent iliac veins and patent IVC. Next, left renal venogram showed a patent left renal vein without hilar dilatation and occluded left ovarian vein from previous embolization without any evidence of collaterals (Figure 15.5 and Figure 15.6). Subsequent right ovarian venogram revealed a patent but grossly dilated right ovarian vein (diameter above the iliac crest: 10.4 mm, at iliac crest: 8.9 mm, and below the iliac crest: 10.1 mm; mean: 9.8 mm) with retrograde flow and cross pelvic collaterals confirming grade-III PCS (Figure 15.7). Tornado coils were successfully deployed in the right ovarian vein starting from lower border of right iliac crest toward the level of entry of right ovarian vein into the IVC. Post coil embolization selective right ovarian venogram demonstrated occlusion of the right ovarian vein (Figure 15.8). Follow-up pelvic duplex images of the adnexal vasculature after 2 months of the procedure demonstrated no significant change in size of the pelvic vasculature with Valsalva. During the follow-up office visit her pain was resolved and remained asymptomatic until 2-year post-procedural follow-up. Persistent PCS despite left ovarian vein embolization and iliac venous stentings in the index case was likely due to unrecognized co-existing right ovarian vein incompetency.

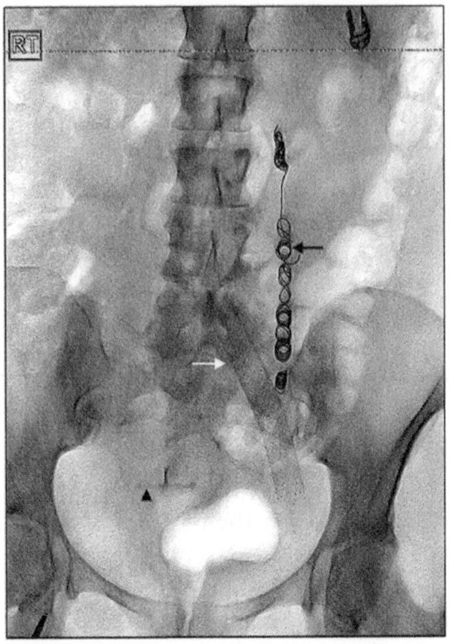

Figure 15.4 A 32-year-old multiparous woman with unresolved incapacitating PCS and history of previous successfully stented May-Thurner syndrome and left ovarian vein embolization. Plain X-ray abdomen shows iliac stenting on the left side (white arrow), multiple embolization coils blocking the left ovarian vein (black arrow), and an intrauterine contraceptive device in the pelvis (arrowhead).

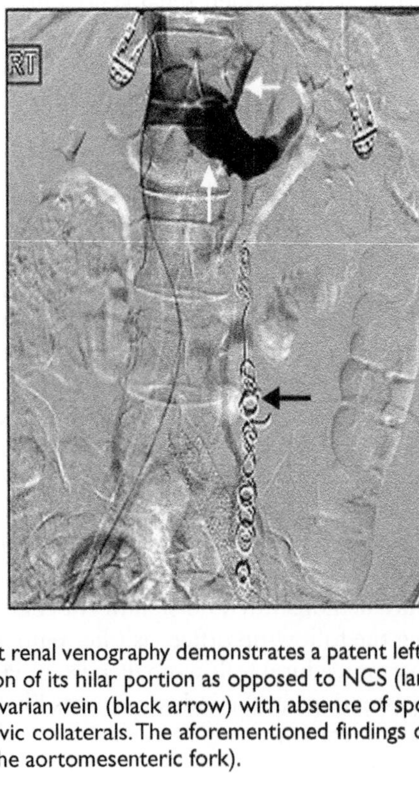

Figure 15.5 DSA image from left renal venography demonstrates a patent left adrenal vein (small white arrow) and renal vein without distension of its hilar portion as opposed to NCS (large white arrow). Multiple embolization coils blocking the left ovarian vein (black arrow) with absence of spontaneous retrograde flow in the left ovarian vein or any parapelvic collaterals. The aforementioned findings did not represent NCS (extrinsic left renal vein compression at the aortomesenteric fork).

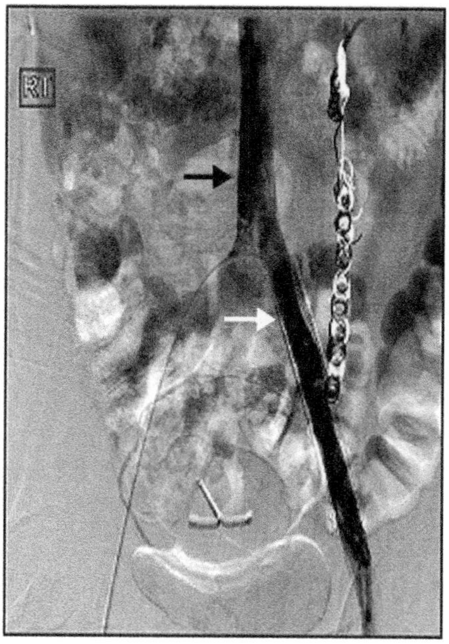

Figure 15.6 DSA image from inferior venacavogram and iliac venogram demonstrates patent IVC (black arrow) and iliac stents on the left side (white arrow) with multiple embolization coils blocking the left ovarian vein.

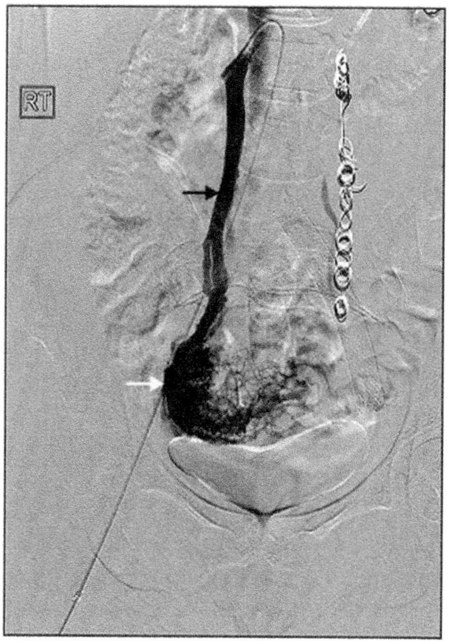

Figure 15.7 DSA image during right selective ovarian venography demonstrates the catheter in the patient's right ovarian vein with contrast traversing down into the dilated right ovarian vein (black arrow). Note the reversed/caudal flow in ovarian vein and retrograde filling of varicose veins in the pelvis lying around the ovaries, uterus, bladder and bowel (white arrow).

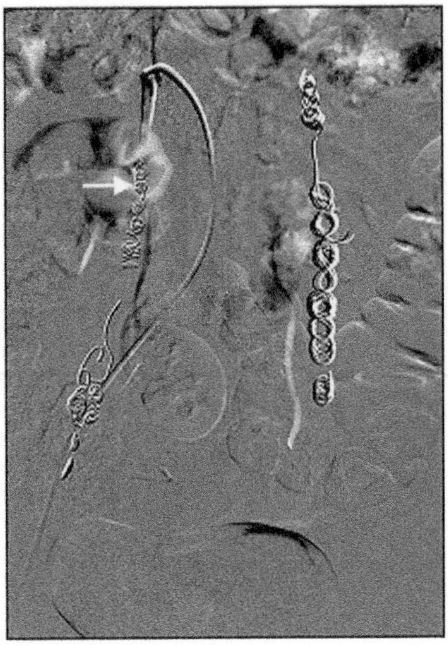

Figure 15.8 A 32-year-old female patient with unresolved PCS confirmed on right ovarian venography. Post coil embolization final DSA image during Valsalva demonstrates sets of embolization coils – all completely blocking the right ovarian vein (white arrow) without any reflux.

TREATMENT RESULTS PCS

Medical treatment suppresses the ovarian function and/or increases venous contraction; several studies have reported both MPA and goserelin to be equally effective with 71% of the women reported ≥ 50% reduction in pain score at less than 1 year follow-up.[29] Chemical ovarian ligation is not without adverse effects; estrogen replacement therapy is often required. It is unclear if the benefits of chemical ligation for pelvic varices are long lasting.

Hysterectomy with removal of one or both ovaries was performed with a response rate of 75%. However, studies reported residual pain in 33% of patients after hysterectomy. This led to the advent of less invasive procedures such as extra-peritoneal surgical ligation or resection of ovarian veins as described by Rundqvist E et al.[30] Laparoscopic ligation of bilateral ovarian veins gained popularity with a response rate of 75%.[31] However, the carbon dioxide insufflations into the peritoneal cavity during laparoscopy cause venous decompression, thus not allowing accurate estimation of pelvic varices, decreasing procedural efficacy.

Successful bilateral ovarian vein embolization using steel endovascular coils was first reported by Edwards RD et al, in 1993.[32] The procedure is usually performed at the time of diagnostic venography. Laborda et al., in 2013 analyzed the clinical outcome and satisfaction surveys for PCS coil embolization in patients with chronic pelvic pain that initially consulted for lower limb venous insufficiency (n = 202; mean age: 43.5 years; range: 27–57; follow-up at 1, 3, and 6 months and every year for 5 years). Patients with lower limb varices and chronic pelvic pain (>6 months), >6 mm pelvic venous caliber in ultrasonography, and venous reflux or presence of communicating veins/collaterals were recruited prospectively.[20] They used coil occlusion and targeted all refluxing veins including both ovarian and refluxing branches of both internal iliac veins. Pain level was assessed before and after embolization therapy and during follow-up using a visual analog scale (VAS). Technical and clinical success and recurrence of leg varices were recorded as 100%, 93.85 % (n = 168), and 12.5% (n = 24), respectively. VAS was 7.34 ± 0.7 pre-procedurally versus 0.78 ± 1.2 at the end of follow-up (P < 0.0001). Complications were reported as follows: groin hematoma (n = 6), coil migration (n = 4), reaction to contrast media (n = 1), and post-procedural pain (n = 23).

In 2008, Gandini R et al. reported the use of 3% STS as a sclerosant without using endovascular coils in patients with PVI (n = 38; 2 mL of STS mixed with 8 mL of air). Total injection volumes used were 30 and 20 mL on the left and right, respectively. Of note, the right-sided incompetency was treated only when varices did not cross the midline from left to right. Clinical success rate was reported in 100% of their cases. Less procedural cost and less radiation time are the benefits with a sclerosant-only approach over coil embolization.[33]

Kim et al., in 2006 evaluated the long-term clinical outcome of transcatheter embolization therapy in women with PCS caused by ovarian and pelvic varices (n = 131; mean age, 34.0 years+/−12.5). Basal female hormonal levels were obtained before and after treatment and compared. Percutaneous transfemoral venography confirmed the presence of ovarian varices in 127/131 (97.0%), and all were treated with embolization therapy. In summary, 108/127 (85%) underwent internal iliac embolization. In 97/127 at long-term clinical follow-up (mean 45 months+/−18) the mean pelvic pain level improved significantly from 7.6+/−1.8 before treatment to 2.9+/−2.8 after embolization therapy (P < .0001). Overall, 83% of the patients exhibited clinical improvement at long-term follow-up, Thirteen percent had no significant change, and 4% exhibited worsened condition. No significant change was noted in hormone levels after treatment, and successful pregnancies were noted in two patients after ovarian and pelvic vein embolization.

Maleux et al., in 2000 reported their results of ovarian vein embolization for the treatment of PCS.[34] In their study all cases (n = 41; mean age, 37.8 years) had pelvic pain and varicosities detected on ovarian venography. Of 41 cases, 32 patients underwent unilateral embolization, and nine patients underwent bilateral embolization. Embolizing material used were the mixture of Enbucrilate + lipiodized oil (n = 40) and Enbucrilate + minicoils (n = 1). They reported technical success rate of 98% with pain relief in 58.5% of their cases (mean clinical follow-up: 19.9 months). Later, Kwon et al., in 2007 evaluated the therapeutic effectiveness of ovarian vein embolization using coils for PCS.[22] They enrolled 67 patients, all confirmed on ovarian venography and underwent left ovarian vein embolization (n = 64), right ovarian vein embolization (n = 1), and bilateral ovarian vein embolization (n = 2) using 0.035–0.038-inch coils (5–15 mm; average: 5.8 coils; range: 3–8; COOK, US). 55 of 67 patients (82%) experienced pain reduction with coil embolization alone; all were satisfied and did not pursue any further treatment (mean follow-up: 44.8+/− 21 months). Immediate complications of coil migration were recorded in 3% (n = 2) of the cases (pulmonary circulation = 1 [retrieved with snare], and left renal vein = 1 [retrieved with snare]).

Rastogi et al., in 2011 reported a case of PCS managed by bilateral ovarian vein coil embolization, complicated with migration of a small coil to the right ventricle.[35] Coil migration occurred partly because of disparity in the size of coils and dilated ovarian veins, which can change in their diameters depending on pelvic venous hemodynamics. Authors preferred Tornado coils because of their tornadolike configuration and various coil lengths in deployed state maximizes coil exposure to cross-sectional lumen to obstruct blood flow and promote thrombogenicity. Unlike the Kwon et al., approach of retrieving the coil from the pulmonary circulation, authors opted not to attempt retrieval of the unintended migrated coil from the right ventricle, considering its smaller size (3 mm 2 cm) and position adjacent to the tricuspid annulus. Retrieving the coil would have increased the procedure time and may have subjected the patient to additional radiation exposure and cardiac complications such as arrhythmia. Authors concluded that in the setting of unintended coil migration into the Rt. ventricle without hemodynamic or electrocardiographic changes, it can be safe to leave the coil in situ.

Results from aforementioned studies have demonstrated that PCS patients who underwent ovarian vein embolization have an acceptable result in reduction of their pelvic pain. Both ovarian veins usually have multiple branches; of note, multiple main trunks off the ovarian vein exist in as many as 40% and 25% on the left and right, respectively; and furthermore, most communicating pelvic venous plexus are devoid of valves.[21, 28] Therefore, incomplete embolization of the tributaries often leads to recurrence and clinical failure of the procedure for both endovascular embolization and laparoscopic ligation.

COMPLICATIONS

Complications that have been reported during or following ovarian vein coil embolization are as follows: bleeding, post-embolization syndrome (up to 80% of cases), ovarian vein thrombophlebitis, coil migration (3–4%), and recurrence of varices (5%).[10–12, 14] Kwon et al., in their study reported coil migration occurred 3% (n = 2) of the cases (pulmonary circulation = 1 [retrieved with snare] and left renal vein = 1 [retrieved with snare]). Coil migration in rare circumstances can occur partly because of disparity in size of coils and dilated ovarian veins, which can change in their diameters depending on pelvic venous hemodynamics. A guide catheter can be used to provide additional stability and support for coil delivery. However, in the setting of incompetent veins assessing the true diameter of the dilated vein can be a difficult task.

CONCLUSIONS

Most pelvic vein insufficiency patients are asymptomatic. Diagnosis of PCS is made by clinical history, physical examination findings, and imaging that demonstrates ovarian and pelvic varicosities.

Patients with severe venous disability symptoms may benefit from an endovascular intervention after failed conservative medical treatment. In addition to being less expensive than surgery, endovascular ovarian vein embolization offers a safe, effective, minimally invasive treatment option that restores patient's quality of life. The procedure is highly successful in blocking the retrograde blood flow with a success rate of 95–100%. Overall, 85–95% of women have demonstrated improvement in their pain symptoms after embolization therapy.

REFERENCES

1. Taylor HC. Vascular congestion and hyperemia: Their effect on function and structure in the female reproductive organs. Part I. Physiological basis and history of the concept. Am J Obstet Gynecol. 1949;57:211–230.
2. Taylor HC. Vascular congestion and hyperemia: Their effect on function and structure in the female reproductive organs. Part II. Clinical concepts of the congestion-fibrosis syndrome. Am J Obstet Gynecol. 1949;57:637–653.
3. Taylor HC. Vascular congestion and hyperemia: Their effect on function and structure in the female reproductive organs. Part III. Etiology and therapy. Am J Obstet Gynecol. 1949;57:654–668.

4. Mathias SD, Kuppermann M, Liberman RF, Lipschutz RC, Steege JF. Chronic pelvic pain: Prevalence, health-related quality of life, and economic correlates. Obstet Gynecol. 1996;87(3):321–327.
5. Meissner MH, Khilnani NM, Labropoulos N, et al. The Symptoms-Varices-Pathophysiology classification of pelvic venous disorders: A report of the American vein & lymphatic society international working group on pelvic venous disorders. J Vasc Surg Venous Lymphat Disord. 2021;9(3):568–584.
6. Rudloff U, Holmes RJ, Prem JT, Faust GR, Moldwin R, Siegel D. Mesoaortic compression of the left renal vein (nutcracker syndrome): Case reports and review of the literature. Ann Vasc Surg. 2006;20(1):120–129.
7. Barsoum MK, Shepherd RF, Welch TJ. Patient with both wilkie syndrome and nutcracker syndrome. Vasc Med. 2008;13(3):247–250.
8. Fu WJ, Hong BF, Xiao YY, et al. Diagnosis of the nutcracker phenomenon by multislice helical computed tomography angiography. Chin Med J (Engl). 2004;117(12):1873–1875.
9. Scultetus AH, Villavicencio JL, Gillespie DL. The nutcracker syndrome: Its role in the pelvic venous disorders. J Vasc Surg. 2001;34(5):812–819.
10. Rogers A, Beech A, Braithwaite B. Transperitoneal laparoscopic left gonadal vein ligation can be the right treatment option for pelvic congestion symptoms secondary to nutcracker syndrome. Vascular. 2007;15(4):238–240.
11. Hartung O, Grisoli D, Boufi M, et al. Endovascular stenting in the treatment of pelvic vein congestion caused by nutcracker syndrome: Lessons learned from the first five cases. J Vasc Surg. 2005;42(2):275–280.
12. Farquhar CM, Rogers V, Franks S, Pearce S, Wadsworth J, Beard RW. A randomized controlled trial of medroxyprogesterone acetate and psychotherapy for the treatment of pelvic congestion. Br J Obstet Gynaecol. 1989;96(10):1153–1162.
13. Park SJ, Lim JW, Ko YT, et al. Diagnosis of pelvic congestion syndrome using transabdominal and transvaginal sonography. AJR Am J Roentgenol. 2004;182(3):683–688.
14. Park YB, Lim SH, Ahn JH, et al. Nutcracker syndrome: Intravascular stenting approach. Nephrol Dial Transplant. 2000;15(1):99–101.
15. Rozenblit AM, Ricci ZJ, Tuvia J, Amis ES Jr. Incompetent and dilated ovarian veins: A common CT finding in asymptomatic parous women. AJR Am J Roentgenol. 2001;176(1):119–122.
16. Kurklinsky AK, Rooke TW. Nutcracker phenomenon and nutcracker syndrome. Mayo Clin Proc. 2010;85(6):552–559.
17. Stones RW. Pelvic vascular congestion-half a century later. Clin Obstet Gynecol. 2003;46(4):831–836.
18. Hodgkinson CP. Physiology of the ovarian veins during pregnancy. Obstet Gynecol. 1953;1(1):26–37.
19. Viala JL, Flandre O, Girardot B, Maamer M. [Histology of the pelvic vein. Initial approach]. Phlebologie. 1991;44(2):369–372; discussion 373.
20. Laborda A, Medrano J, de Blas I, Urtiaga I, Carnevale FC, de Gregorio MA. Endovascular treatment of pelvic congestion syndrome: Visual analog scale (VAS) long-term follow-up clinical evaluation in 202 patients. Cardiovasc Intervent Radiol. 2013;36(4):1006–1014.
21. Durham JD, Machan L. Pelvic congestion syndrome. Semin Intervent Radiol. 2013;30(4):372–380. doi: 10.1055/s-0033-1359731.
22. Belenky A, Bartal G, Atar E, Cohen M, Bachar GN. Ovarian varices in healthy female kidney donors: Incidence, morbidity, and clinical outcome. AJR Am J Roentgenol. 2002;179(3):625–627.
23. Kwon SH, Oh JH, Ko KR, Park HC, Huh JY. Transcatheter ovarian vein embolization using coils for the treatment of pelvic congestion syndrome. Cardiovasc Intervent Radiol. 2007;30(4):655–661.
24. d'Archambeau O, Maes M, De Schepper AM. The pelvic congestion syndrome: Role of the "nutcracker phenomenon" and results of endovascular treatment. JBR-BTR. 2004;87(1):1–8.
25. Park SJ, Lim JW, Ko YT, et al. Diagnosis of pelvic congestion syndrome using transabdominal and transvaginal sonography. AJR Am J Roentgenol. 2004;182(3):683–688.

26. Kim HS, Malhotra AD, Rowe PC, Lee JM, Venbrux AC. Embolotherapy for pelvic congestion syndrome: Long-term results. J Vasc Interv Radiol. 2006;17(2, Pt 1):289–297.
27. Beard RW, Highman JH, Pearce S, Reginald PW. Diagnosis of pelvic varicosities in women with chronic pelvic pain. Lancet. 1984;2(8409):946–949.
28. Venbrux AC, Sharma GK, Jackson ET, et al. Pelvic varices embolization. In Women's Health in Interventional Radiology (pp. 37–59). 2012, XVI.
29. Soysal ME, Soysal S, Vicdan K, et al. A randomized controlled trial of goserelin and medroxyprogesterone acetate in the treatment of pelvic congestion. Hum Reprod. 2004;19(1):160–167.
30. Rundqvist E, Sandholm LE, Larsson G. Treatment of pelvic varicosities causing lower abdominal pain with extraperitoneal resection of the left ovarian vein. Ann Chir Gynaecol. 1984;73(6):339–341.
31. Carter JE. Surgical treatment for chronic pelvic pain. JSLS. 1998;2(2):129–139.
32. Edwards RD, Robertson IR, MacLean AB, Hemingway AP. Case report: Pelvic pain syndrome – successful treatment of a case by ovarian vein embolization. Clin Radiol. 1993;47(6):429–431.
33. Gandini R, Chiocchi M, Konda D, et al. Transcatheter foam sclerotherapy of symptomatic female varicocele with sodium-tetradecyl-sulfate foam. Cardiovasc Intervent Radiol. 2008;31(4):778–784. doi: 10.1007/s00270-007-9264-6.
34. Maleux G, Stockx L, Wilms G, et al. Ovarian vein embolization for the treatment of pelvic congestion syndrome: Long-term technical and clinical results. JVIR. 2000;11:859–864.
35. Rastogi N, Kabutey NK, Kim D. Unintended coil migration into the right ventricle during the right ovarian vein coil embolization. Vasc Endovascular Surg. 2011;45(7):660–664. doi: 10.1177/1538574411414924.

Chapter 16

Nutcracker Syndrome

Diagnosis and Endovascular Management

Ana Fuentes, Roberta Lozano Gonzalez, and Young Erben

INTRODUCTION

Nutcracker syndrome (NS), also known as left renal vein entrapment syndrome, is a rare vascular disorder that occurs when the left renal vein (LRV) is compressed between the aorta and the superior mesenteric artery (SMA). This phenomenon was first described by Grant in 1937[1] and can cause a range of symptoms, such as abdominal, flank, or pelvic pain; varicocele; hematuria; and proteinuria.[2, 3] The diagnosis of NS can be challenging due to the variety of symptoms that patients may present with; however, a contributing factor is the lack of awareness among healthcare providers of this disease entity.[3] Fortunately, advances in imaging modalities, such as computed tomography (CT), magnetic resonance imaging (MRI), and duplex ultrasonography (DUS), have improved the diagnosis of NS.[4] Endovascular treatments, including stenting and balloon angioplasty, have emerged as minimally invasive options for managing NS with high rates of technical success and symptom improvement.[2, 4–6] This chapter will review the current state of knowledge on NS, with an emphasis on its diagnosis and the endovascular management approach. By the end of this chapter, readers will have a better understanding of NS, its diagnosis, and the available treatment options.

CLINICAL PRESENTATION

The nutcracker phenomenon refers specifically to the compression of the LRV between the aorta and the SMA, leading to increased pressure in the LRV and symptoms of pelvic congestion (**Figure 16.1**).[3, 7] There are variations of this condition, such as posterior NS, where the LRV is compressed between the aorta and the vertebral body (**Figure 16.2**).[5, 8] This disease entity is more common in women, with the most frequent age of presentation around the third decade of life.[7, 9] Low body mass index has also been correlated with the phenomenon.[7, 9]

Patients with NS can present with a variety of clinical symptoms, which include abdominal or flank pain, hematuria (micro or macro), proteinuria, varicocele, or in the case of female patients' symptoms of pelvic congestion.[2, 3] There are two subtypes of clinical presentation: the typical or renal presentation, which is characterized by hematuria and orthostatic proteinuria with or without flank pain, and the atypical or urologic presentation, which includes abdominal pain, dyspareunia, dysmenorrhea, varicocele, fatigue, and orthostatic intolerance.[9] Due to the non-specific nature of NS symptoms, it is important to maintain a high index of suspicion and perform appropriate diagnostic testing to confirm the diagnosis. Differential diagnosis includes renal calculi, glomerulonephritis, endometriosis, vascular malformation of the renal pelvis, primary varicocele, and other pathologies associated with pelvic congestion.[2, 3, 6]

DOI: 10.1201/9781003316626-19

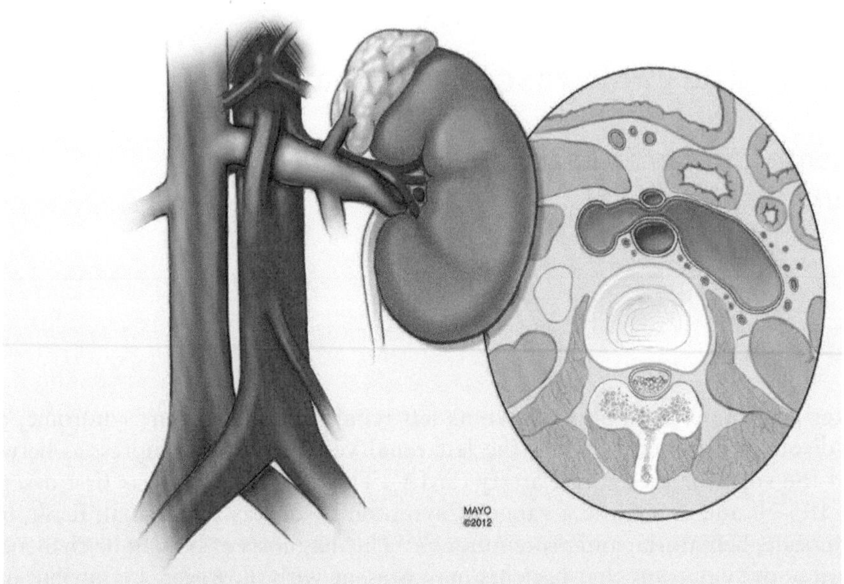

Figure 16.1 Anterior nutcracker syndrome.

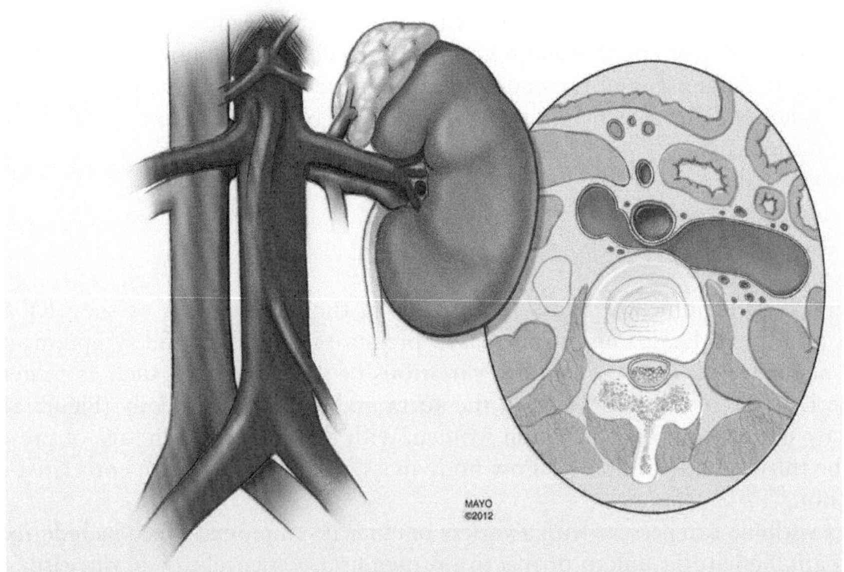

Figure 16.2 Posterior nutcracker syndrome.

DIAGNOSTIC EVALUATION

The diagnosis of NS is challenging for healthcare providers, as it requires a high suspicion index and is often a diagnosis of exclusion.[5] When NS is suspected, several diagnostic tools may be used. DUS is the first recommended approach, as it allows for anatomical assessment as well as hemodynamic evaluation. One of the diagnostic criteria for this syndrome is a ratio of peak systolic velocity of the aortomesenteric segment to the hilar portion of >4.2 to 5.0. While DUS has a high sensitivity and specificity, its limitations must not be overlooked. These include the required 6 to 8 hours of fasting, positional changes (upright or supine), interobserver variability, and difficulties faced by the operator due to limited space for the study performance, which might interfere with its accuracy.[3, 5]

Additional diagnostic tools that may be used to confirm the diagnosis of NS include CT and MRI. CT angiography and MRI can provide detailed anatomical information and can help differentiate NS from other conditions that present with similar symptoms. However, these imaging modalities may not be as sensitive for detecting hemodynamic changes in the renal vasculature as DUS. In some cases, venography may be necessary to confirm the diagnosis of NS. Indeed, vein diameters, an aorta-to-SMA angle <35, a hilar-to-aortomesenteric diameter ratio ≥4.9 and "beak sign" may be evaluated with CT and MRI and are part of the radiological features of NS. Meanwhile, venography with direct pressure measurements with or without intravascular ultrasound (IVUS) is considered the diagnostic gold standard. Additionally, a pressure gradient between the LRV and the IVC ≥ 3 mmHg is considered diagnostic for venous hypertension. However, it is noteworthy to clarify during venography that many patients may have developed collateral circulation and thus, do not present with venous hypertension.[5]

TREATMENT

The available treatment options for NS depend on the severity of symptoms and the patient's individual factors. Currently there are no guidelines for the management of NS. In younger patients, conservative management should be considered initially, with the goal of delaying or avoiding surgical intervention.[3, 10] Conservative management includes surveillance and lifestyle modifications, especially focusing on weight gain to increase retroperitoneal fat.[10] Medical management can also be utilized, with a focus on pain management, and may involve pharmacotherapy with angiotensin converting enzyme inhibitors and aspirin to manage orthostatic hypotension and increase renal perfusion.[3, 5] Studies have shown that approximately 30–68.7% of patients respond to conservative management, making it a reasonable option to try before considering surgical intervention.[5, 10, 11]

Open Revascularization

Current surgical intervention can be done either open, laparoscopically, endovascular, or robotically assisted. Transposition of the LRV from the inferior vena cava has been shown to be an effective open surgical procedure, in which through a midline transperitoneal approach, the LRV is transected and anastomosed to the left lateral aspect of the IVC more distally to ensure less compression and assuring minimal tension.[10–12] However, there are other surgical approaches that have been described. Among them, Mejia et al. described 29 patients with NS and noted that through a robotic-assisted kidney auto-transplantation, there was complete resolution of symptoms in 63% of patients.[13] Shaper et al. performed initially venolysis and concomitant LRV transposition with a reported resolution of hematuria in 80% of patients.[14] Scultetus et al. described a cohort of three patients in whom gonadocaval bypass was performed preceded by embolization of the internal iliac vein tributaries connecting with varicose veins in the lower extremities. This cohort demonstrated resolution of hematuria in 100% of patients during follow-up.[15]

An emerging alternative technique is laparoscopic extravascular stenting, where through pneumoperitoneal access and without clamping of vessels, the fibrous tissue in the aortomesenteric angle is excised and a synthetic graft is opened and placed longitudinally around the LRV.[6, 16–19] Wang et al., described 13 patients that underwent this procedure with symptom resolution in 77% and partial resolution in 15%. Migration of the synthetic graft occurred in one patient.[18] In the same fashion, Zang et al. described three patients that had either complete or partial symptom resolution.

Endovascular Revascularization

The first case reported of endovascular treatment for NS was in 1996 by Nestle et al. Since then, this approach has become a valuable tool.[20] Endovascular treatment options for NS include balloon angioplasty and stenting.[21–23] Concomitant gonadal vein embolization can also be done periprocedurally at the time of stenting. Venous access under ultrasound guidance can be achieved via the transfemoral, jugular, or basilic vein routes, with studies showing similar outcomes for each approach.[6, 23–25] Procedures can be performed under general anesthesia or with conscious sedation, which may be preferable for patients who cannot tolerate general anesthesia. Typically sheaths used for LRV access are 9F–10F with 4F–5F angled catheters.[6, 24, 25] Venous pressures should be documented, and it is also useful to implement intravascular ultrasound to accurately measure the vessels' diameter. Advantageously under fluoroscopy, collateral vessels can be evaluated before stent placement and balloon angioplasty.[22–24] Generally, percutaneous access of the vein is obtained, and the LRV is selectively catheterized, venography is useful for confirmation with visualization of contrast washout or with reno-caval pressure gradient measurement.[24] The sheath is placed through the area of stenosis and by repositioning the wire, a stent is deployed across the lesion.[24] A systematic review of studies that describe patients treated with endovascular therapy determined symptom resolution in 86% of patients with a reintervention rate of 4.9%.[6] A retrospective series with a median follow-up of 66 months that included 61 patients, who underwent stenting reported symptom relief in 59 of them within 6 months. They also reported one stent migration.[22] Endovascular treatment is not without possible complications, including restenosis, symptom recurrence, stent migration, and stent thrombosis.[22, 24, 26–28] The main contributors to preventing stent migration include correct sizing, avoidance of balloon dilatation, and operator experience.[24] Table 16.1 summarizes all the studies with more than five patients that underwent endovascular treatment for NS up to January 2023.

A hybrid procedure has also been described, which on one hand decreases the rate of restenosis and on the other hand decreases the risk of stent migration. It entails transposition of the LRV with immediate deployment of a stent, that is sutured to the LRV to avoid migration. This procedure allows for placement of a vein patch in cases where the vein might be too small to allow the deployment of a 12–14 mm stent. This procedure may require oral anticoagulation for at least 3 months after the index procedure.[10, 26, 28, 29]

CONCLUSIONS

Overall, treatment for NS is individualized based on the patient's clinical presentation and specific circumstances and requires a multidisciplinary approach involving urologists, interventional radiologists, and vascular surgeons. Minimally invasive procedures, endovascular, laparoscopic, and robotically assisted have demonstrated high technical success rates and

Table 16.1 Studies of Endovascular Management for Nutcracker Syndrome

Author	*Country*	*Study Design*	*Number of Patients*	*Female Sex % (n/total)*	*Outcomes at Follow-Up*	*Reintervention % (n/total)*	*Follow-Up (months)*
Cronan et al.	USA	RCS	10	40 (4/10)	Symptom resolution, 70 (7/10); hematuria resolution, 80 (8/10), flank and pelvic pain resolution, 90 (9/10)	3 (3/30)	Median, 8 (3–37)
Chen et al.	China	RCS	61	26 (16/61)	Symptom resolution, 73.7 (45/61); partial symptom resolution, 22.9 (14/61); symptoms unchanged, 3.27 (2/61); flank pain resolution, 81.2 (13/16); partial flank pain resolution, 18.7 (3/16); hematuria resolution, 77.2 (44/57); partial hematuria resolution, 19.2 (11/57); unchanged hematuria, 35 (2/57); proteinuria resolution, 72.7 (24/33); partial proteinuria resolution, 24.2 (8/33); proteinuria unchanged, 3 (1/33)	1.6 (1/61)	Median, 66 (12–144)
Avgerinos et al.	USA	RC	18	94 (17/18)	Symptom resolution, 50 (9/18); partial symptom resolution, 22.2, (4/18); hematuria resolution, 60 (6/10); atypical GI pain, resolution, 62.5 (5/8)	16.7 (3/18)	Median ± SD 41.4 ± 26.6
Leal Monedero et al.	France	RSC	40	90 (36/40)	Symptom resolution at 12 months, 83.9 (26/31); hematuria resolution at 12 months, 100 (31/31)	3.6 (2/55)	Range 12–60
Li et al.	China	RCS	6	0 (0/6)	Hematuria resolution, 83.3 (5/6); flank pain resolution, 50 (3/6)	0 (0/6)	Median ± SD 25.5 ± 15
Wang et al.	China	RCS	30	7 (2/30)	Flank and abdominal pain resolution, 100 (30/30); left varicocele, resolution at 1 month, 69.2 (18/26); at 3 months, 92.3 (24/26); hematuria relief at 1 month, 92.8 (26/28); at 3 months, 100 (28/28)	0 (0/30)	Median (range) 36 (12–18)
Hartung et al.	France	RCS	5	100 (5/5)	Symptom resolution, 60 (3/5)	0 (0/5)	Mean, 14.3 (4.2–26.5)
Total			170	47 (80/170)		4.9 (9/185)	

Abbreviations: RCS: Retrospective case series, RC: Retrospective cohort, SD: Standard deviation.

symptom improvement. However, there is a risk of complications such as stent migration, restenosis, or thrombosis. Long-term outcomes are still being studied, and there is not enough evidence to provide clear recommendations regarding the newer techniques.

REFERENCES

1. Boileau Grant JC. A method of anatomy: Descriptive and deductive. Baltimore: The Williams and Wilkins Co., 1944.
2. Erben Y, Gloviczki P, Kalra M, Bjarnason H, Reed NR, Duncan AA, et al. Treatment of nutcracker syndrome with open and endovascular interventions. J Vasc Surg Venous Lymphat Disord. 2015;3(4):389–96.
3. Kolber MK, Cui Z, Chen CK, Habibollahi P, Kalva SP. Nutcracker syndrome: Diagnosis and therapy. Cardiovasc Diagn Ther. 2021;11(5):1140–49.
4. Ahmed K, Sampath R, Khan MS. Current trends in the diagnosis and management of renal nutcracker syndrome: A review. Eur J Vasc Endovasc Surg. 2006;31(4):410–16.
5. Velasquez CA, Saeyeldin A, Zafar MA, Brownstein AJ, Erben Y. A systematic review on management of nutcracker syndrome. J Vasc Surg Venous Lymphat Disord. 2018;6(2):271–78.
6. Fuentes-Perez A, Bush RL, Kalra M, Shortell C, Gloviczki P, Brigham TJ, et al. Systematic review of endovascular versus laparoscopic extravascular stenting for treatment of nutcracker syndrome. J Vasc Surg Venous Lymphat Disord. 2023;11(2):433–41.
7. Orczyk K, Łabetowicz P, Lodziński S, Stefańczyk L, Topol M, Polguj M. The nutcracker syndrome. Morphology and clinical aspects of the important vascular variations: A systematic study of 112 cases. Int Angiol. 2016;35(1):71–77.
8. Skeik N, Gloviczki P, Macedo TA. Posterior nutcracker syndrome. Vasc Endovascular Surg. 2011;45(8):749–55.
9. Gulleroglu K, Gulleroglu B, Baskin E. Nutcracker syndrome. World J Nephrol. 2014;3(4):277–81.
10. Erben Y, Gloviczki P. The management of nutcracker Syndrome. In: Gloviczki P (Ed.), Handbook of Venous and Lymphatic Disorders: Guidelines of the American Venous Forum (4th ed.). London and New York: CRC Press.
11. Reed NR, Kalra M, Bower TC, Vrtiska TJ, Ricotta JJ, Gloviczki P. Left renal vein transposition for nutcracker syndrome. J Vasc Surg. 2009;49(2):386–93; discussion 93–94.
12. Dieleman F, Hamming JF, Erben Y, van der Vorst JR. Nutcracker syndrome: Challenges in diagnosis and surgical treatment. Ann Vasc Surg. 2023;94:178–185. doi:10.1016/j.avsg.2023.03.030
13. Mejia A, Barrera Gutierrez JC, Vivian E, Shah J, Dickerman R. Robotic assisted kidney autotransplantation as a safe alternative for treatment of nutcracker syndrome and loin pain haematuria syndrome: A case series report. Int J Med Robot. 2023;19(3):e2508.
14. Shaper KR, Jackson JE, Williams G. The nutcracker syndrome: An uncommon cause of haematuria. Br J Urol. 1994;74(2):144–46.
15. Scultetus AH, Villavicencio JL, Gillespie DL. The nutcracker syndrome: Its role in the pelvic venous disorders. J Vasc Surg. 2001;34(5):812–19.
16. He D, Liang J, Wang H, Jiao Y, Wu B, Cui D, et al. 3D-printed peek extravascular stent in the treatment of nutcracker syndrome: Imaging evaluation and short-term clinical outcome. Front Bioeng Biotechnol. 2020;8:732.
17. Wang H, Guo YT, Jiao Y, He DL, Wu B, Yuan LJ, et al. A minimally invasive alternative for the treatment of nutcracker syndrome using individualized three-dimensional printed extravascular titanium stents. Chin Med J (Engl). 2019;132(12):1454–60.
18. Wang SZ, Zhang WX, Meng QJ, Zhang XP, Wei JX, Qiao BP. Laparoscopic extravascular stent placement for nutcracker syndrome: A report of 13 cases. J Endourol. 2015;29(9):1025–29.
19. Chen FM, Chen XL, Jiang XN, Tang S, Shi JQ, Li DB, et al. A new technique: Laparoscopic resection of fibrous ring and placing extravascular stent in patients with nutcracker syndrome: A report of 5 cases. Urology. 2019;126:110–15.

20. Neste MG, Narasimham DL, Belcher KK. Endovascular stent placement as a treatment for renal venous hypertension. J Vasc Interv Radiol. 1996;7(6):859–61.
21. Cronan JC, Hawkins CM, Kennedy SS, Marshall KW, Rostad BS, Gill AE. Endovascular management of nutcracker syndrome in an adolescent patient population. Pediatr Radiol. 2021;51(8):1487–96.
22. Chen S, Zhang H, Shi H, Tian L, Jin W, Li M. Endovascular stenting for treatment of Nutcracker syndrome: Report of 61 cases with long-term followup. J Urol. 2011;186(2):570–75.
23. Li H, Sun X, Liu G, Zhang Y, Chu J, Deng C, et al. Endovascular stent placement for nutcracker phenomenon. J Xray Sci Technol. 2013;21(1):95–102.
24. Avgerinos ED, McEnaney R, Chaer RA. Surgical and endovascular interventions for nutcracker syndrome. Semin Vasc Surg. 2013;26(4):170–77.
25. Avgerinos ED, Saadeddin Z, Humar R, Salem K, Singh M, Hager E, et al. Outcomes of left renal vein stenting in patients with nutcracker syndrome. J Vasc Surg Venous Lymphat Disord. 2019;7(6):853–9.
26. Chen Y, Mou Y, Cheng Y, Wang H, Zheng Z. Late stent migration into the right ventricle in a patient with nutcracker syndrome. Ann Vasc Surg. 2015;29(4):839.e1–4.
27. Tabiei A, Cifuentes S, DeMartino RR. Spiral saphenous vein graft for left renal vein reconstruction after endovascular failure in the treatment of nutcracker syndrome. J Vasc Surg Cases Innov Tech. 2023;9(1):101085.
28. Rana MA, Oderich GS, Bjarnason H. Endovenous removal of dislodged left renal vein stent in a patient with nutcracker syndrome. Semin Vasc Surg. 2013;26(1):43–47.
29. Chen S, Zhang H, Tian L, Li M, Zhou M, Wang Z. A stranger in the heart: LRV stent migration. Int Urol Nephrol. 2009;41(2):427–30.

Chapter 17

Endovascular and Open Management of Benign Disease of the Deep Venous System

Indrani Sen and Manju Kalra

INTRODUCTION

Benign disease of the deep venous system occurs most commonly due to post-thrombotic occlusion or congenital atresia. Superior vena cava (SVC) occlusion is most commonly secondary to metastatic malignant disease but there has been a steady increase in occlusions from benign disease mostly attributable to central lines/pacemakers, which have outpaced mediastinal fibrosis. Rarer etiologies include granulomatous fungal disease, mediastinal radiation, retrosternal goiter, or aortic dissection.(1, 2) Benign inferior vena cava (IVC) occlusion can occur due to central propagation of iliofemoral venous thrombosis, congenital atresia or thrombosis around an IVC filter, the latter gaining prominence in last two decades. The management of non- obstructive iliocaval obstruction and management of IVC occlusion from filters are described in other chapters.

CLINICAL PRESENTATION

Patients with SVC and/or innominate vein obstruction present with clinical manifestations of cerebral venous hypertension: swelling and fullness in the head and neck, upper extremity swelling, orthopnea, dizziness and blurring of vision, which is most severe in the morning after being recumbent overnight, bending over or laying flat. Asymptomatic SVC occlusion may be unmasked by the creation of a hemodialysis arteriovenous access; patients present with rapid arm swelling and neck engorgement. Emergent or life-threatening symptoms like respiratory compromise or altered mentation due to cerebral edema may occur. Exclusion of a malignant etiology by history and clinical examination as well as imaging is essential.

Stenosis or occlusion following an episode of acute lower extremity deep venous thrombosis (DVT) can present with heaviness, pain, swelling, discoloration and cramping as well as advanced chronic venous insufficiency with lower extremity venous claudication, swelling, lipodermatosclerosis and venous ulceration (post thrombotic syndrome). Additional symptoms like non-specific back, abdominal or pelvic pain and genital swelling; history of phlegmasia; pulmonary embolism or renal failure from extension across renal veins may point to the diagnosis of IVC occlusion. Congenital IVC atresia may be underdiagnosed because lower extremity edema may be present without specific signs especially in the presence of well-developed collaterals. Symptom severity in both SVC syndrome and IVC occlusion/atresia may not correlate with the degree of anatomic obstruction if there is extensive venous collateralization.

 DOI: 10.1201/9781003316626-20

IMAGING

Contrast enhanced computed tomography (CTV) and/or magnetic resonance imaging (MRI) have become first-line imaging studies to definitely diagnose and ascertain the extent of the central venous obstruction, for both the SVC and IVC.[3] Conventional venography, previously a gold standard, is now performed in conjunction with endovenous intervention. Although the SVC cannot be directly imaged on duplex ultrasound (DUS), SVC occlusion can be suspected on DUS of the internal jugular, subclavian and innominate veins. Initial imaging with duplex ultrasound (DUS) to detect indirect evidence from loss of femoral venous phasicity or blunting of waveforms is reasonable but may be limited due to obesity or overlying bowel gas.

SVC occlusion was classified into four venographic patterns by Stanford and Doty,[4] based on the site and extent of SVC obstruction as well as the collateral network pattern. Type I is partial SVC obstruction. Type II is complete or near-complete SVC stenosis, with antegrade azygos vein flow. Type III is 90% to 100% SVC stenosis with reversed azygos vein flow and type IV is extensive mediastinal/central venous occlusion with occlusion of the azygos veins as well and venous return through the IVC (Figure 17.1). IVC occlusion is classified as

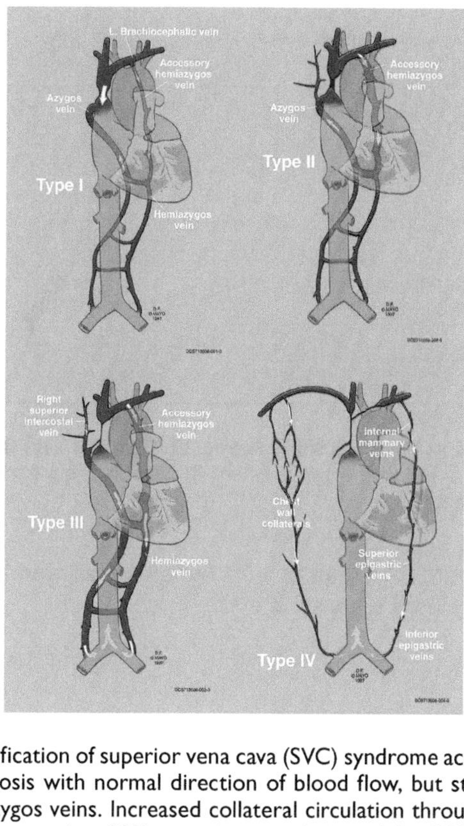

Figure 17.1 Venographic classification of superior vena cava (SVC) syndrome according to Stanford and Doty. Type I: High-grade SVC stenosis with normal direction of blood flow, but still normal direction of blood flow through the SVC and azygos veins. Increased collateral circulation through hemiazygos and accessory hemiazygos veins. Type II: Greater than 90% stenosis or occlusion of the SVC, but patent azygos vein with normal direction of blood flow. Type III: Occlusion of the SVC with retrograde flow in both the azygos and hemiazygos veins. Type IV: Extensive occlusion of the SVC and innominate and azygos veins with chest wall and epigastric venous collaterals. (From Alimi YS, Gloviczki P, Vrtiska TJ, et al: Reconstruction of the superior vena cava: The benefits of postoperative surveillance and secondary endovascular interventions. J Vasc Surg 27:298–99, 1998.)

Clasafication type	*Disease characteristics*	*Examples*
Type I	Single-segment stenosis	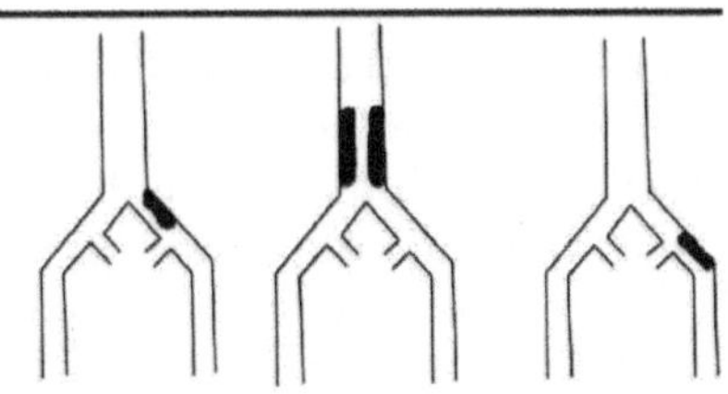
Type II	Multiple-segment stenosis	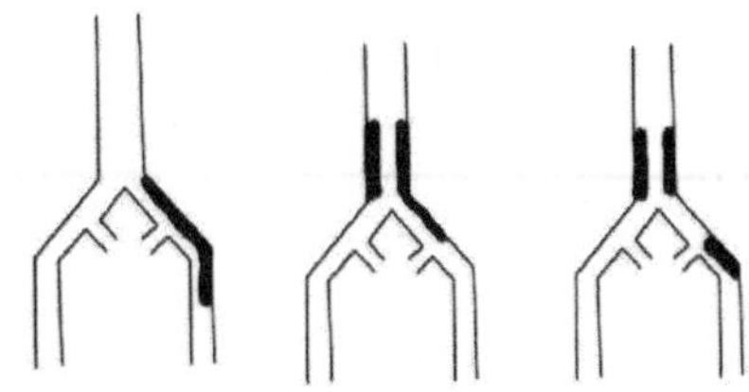
Type III	Single-segment occlusion	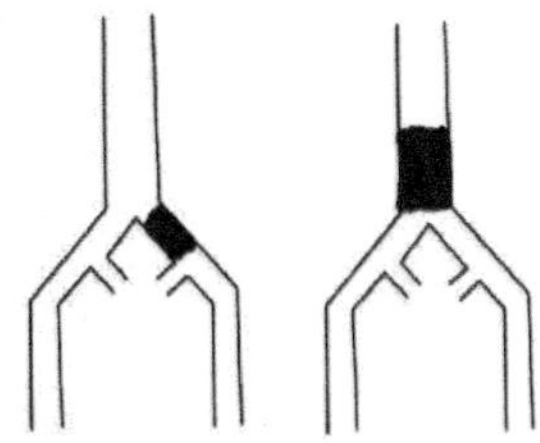
Type IV	Multiple-segment occlusion	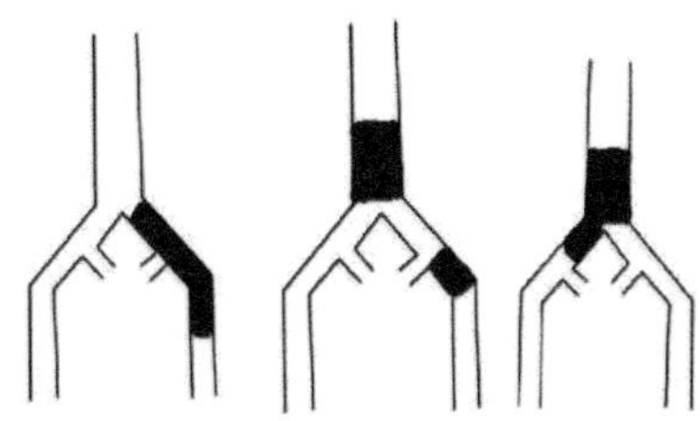

Figure 17.2 Crowner classification: Type I is a single segment IVC or iliac vein stenosis. Type II is multiple segment IVC or iliac vein stenosis. Type III is single segment IVC or iliac vein occlusion, and Type IV is multiple segment IVC or iliac vein occlusion.

infrarenal, suprarenal or both. Crowner et al. proposed an additional classification of iliocaval thrombosis into four types (Figure 17.2).[5]

MANAGEMENT

Patients with mild symptoms are advised conservative management. Those with SVC syndrome are advised to make lifestyle changes such as elevation of the head during the night on pillows, avoiding bending over and wearing constricting garments or a tight collar) and diuretic therapy. Those with IVC occlusion are advised to use compression stockings or garments and make lifestyle changes like avoiding long periods of standing and lower extremity elevation. Patients may benefit from therapeutic anticoagulation to treat acute/subacute thrombsois and preserve collaterals.

INTERVENTION

In symptomatic patients, interventional treatment, surgical or endovascular, is offerred to patients with incapacitating symptoms not responding to conservative therapy. Endovascular therapy is the first-line therapy for benign SVC and IVC occlusion. Open surgical treatment for SVC syndrome is indicated in patients with extensive chronic venous thrombosis not anatomically suitable for endovascular treatment or those who have failed prior endovascular treatment (even if pattern of occlusion is less extensive). Intervention for IVC occlusion is indicated in severely symptomatic patients (C4–6 or lifestyle limiting venous claudication). Endovenous treatment for both SVC and IVC pathology includes percutaneous transluminal balloon angioplasty (PTA), stenting and thrombolysis performed alone or in combination.(4, 6) Life-threatening symptoms from SVC syndrome or phlegmasia may warrant emergent endovenous intervention. In the next sections, technical details of intervention are discussed separately for SVC and IVC pathology.

SVC Occlusion: Endovenous Treatment

Endovascular intervention is performed under monitored local anesthesia or under general anesthesia in a severely symptomatic patient, requiring aggressive balloon dilatation or if treating a complex lesion. Vascular access is established under ultrasound guidance via the right internal jugular or arm vein (basilic/brachial) and/or the right common femoral with placement of 6–12Fr sheaths. A diagnostic venogram is obtained to identify the stenosis/occlusion and the central reformation.

Lesions can be crossed with a hydrophilic guidewire and standard catheter for short stenosis; more complex lesions may require using stiffer wires as well as establishing femoral through-and-through wire access. Primary PTA using standard 10–16 mm high-pressure angioplasty balloons is performed, (eg. Mustang, Atlas) with concomitant stenting for residual stenosis with persistent collateral flow or perforation. A variety of balloon-expandable and self-expanding stents have been used over the last few decades. The risk of fatal complications is 1–2%, with a total complication rate around 9%. SVC rupture leading to pericardial tamponade can be fatal, most often when treating recurrent stenosis. Rapid diagnosis, prolonged balloon inflation, placement of a covered stent and immediate ultrasound-guided pericardial drainage is essential. Endovascular therapy reports high technical success (establishment of patency of the SVC, resolution of collateral flow) and clinical success (alleviation of symptoms) of around 90–98%, with rapid symptoms relief.(7) The overall restenosis and recurrence rate reported is 10%.(4, 6, 8–17)

Benign SVC syndrome is rare, and three recent meta-analysis did not compare the patency between stent types in benign pathology alone.(18) Overall, the highest primary patency is reported with stent grafts (96%, Viabahn, iCast) as compared to Wallstents (83%, the latter has been the most commonly used self-expanding stent due to the larger sizes available). The secondary patency of Wallstents in one metanalysssssis on malignant disease was 93%.(19) Other available stent options include steel stents (Gianturco and Palmaz; balloon expandable, precise deployment and good radial force, limited stent flexibility) and nitinol stents (E-Luminexx [Bard], Sinus-XL [Optimed], Zilver Vena [Cook Medical], Symphony [Boston Scientific], Smart stents [Cordis Endovascular], Protégé stents [ev3] and Memotherm [Bard]), which offer differing flexibility and are ss in a range of sizes and lengths.(4, 6, 9, 19–27) Experience is being accrued with the use of dedicated venous stents (Venovo, Vena) since their introduction a few years ago. Comparison between dedicated venous- and non-venous-dedicated stents, as well as use of Paclitaxel coated balloons has not been specifically studied in SVC syndrome.[28] Pacemaker wire/line induced SVC syndrome requires pre-procedure planning and discussion with other specialities for removal of the offending central line or pacemaker wires. If pacemaker wire removal is not feasible, it may require the procedure to be performed with electrophysiologic monitoring and replacement of the lead wires through the new stent.[6] Newer leadless pacing devices can also be considered.

Catheter-directed thrombolysis prior to PTA with a short infusion length side-hole catheter is helpful to resolve the thrombosis and reveal the underlying stenotic lesion in patients with acute/subacute central venous thrombosis (usually line related).[6, 29–32] Laser-assisted venous thrombectomy for recurrent in-stent stenosis[33] and use of aspiration or pharmacomechanical thrombectomy (AngioJet/INARI clotreiver) can also be considered.[34, 35] Use of bilateral stents in a kissing/Y configuration is described but not always necessary, as reestablishment of flow through a unilateral innominate/SVC stent is usually sufficient for symptom resolution.[7, 12, 36]

Post-procedure anticoagulation/antiplatelet use varies depending on the etiology, type and length of stents and surgeon preference. Oral anticoagulation is continued for 3–6 months in those with acute/subacute thrombosis until the stent is lined with pseudointima and the risk of re-thrombosis decreases. Antiplatelet therapy alone (aspirin/clopidogrel) may be used in those with mediastinal fibrosis.

IVC Occlusion: Endovenous Treatment

IVC, venoplasty ± stenting should be considered in severely symptomatic patients (C4–6 or lifestyle limiting venous claudication), this offers symptom relief and helps in healing venous ulcers. Recanalization, balloon venoplasty and self-expandable stenting is reported to have patency rates >85% at 36 months.[37] The technique is not different from that described for iliac vein stenting for May-Thurner syndrome or if performed after IVC filter removal (see Chapter 16 and Chapter 2623). Similar to SVC stenosis, through-and-through femoral-right jugular access to facilitate crossing of highly fibrotic iliocaval segments may be required. Self-expandable stents such as Wallstents and Gianturco stents are preferred for endofibrosis. In addition to radial force and flexibility, the main stent characteristic to be considered during IVC stenting is the degree of foreshortening, which is maximum for the Wallstent as compared to the Cook Z stent or the Cook Vena. The majority of IVC stenoses involve the iliocaval segment, and most studies of dedicated venous stents are in this patient group. Intravascular ultrasound (IVUS) is essential to identify fibrotic webs and ensure adequate coverage and stent expansion. Although many configurations have been described for recreating the iliocaval confluence (double barrel, side butting, side piercing) it is best recreated by a single stent in the IVC and iliac veins with a bare triangle at the confluence.[37]

Self-expandable stents are placed without leaving uncovered diseased veins behind between the stents, with a few millimeters overlap. The IVC is stented using a single-barrel technique with a large-diameter stent, such as the Wallstent (20 × 40 mm and 22 × 45 mm; Boston Scientific), in combination with the Gianturco (20 mm; Cook Medical, Bloomington, Ind) stent. At the bifurcation, we simultaneously bring stents across the common iliac veins (CIVs); the inferior edges of the CIV stents just touch at the bifurcation, without bringing the stents higher/parallel into the IVC. The Gianturco stents add radial force to the distal and weakest part of the Wallstent. These also extend past the Wallstent and thus allow inflow from the hepatic or renal veins proximally and from the CIVs distally,

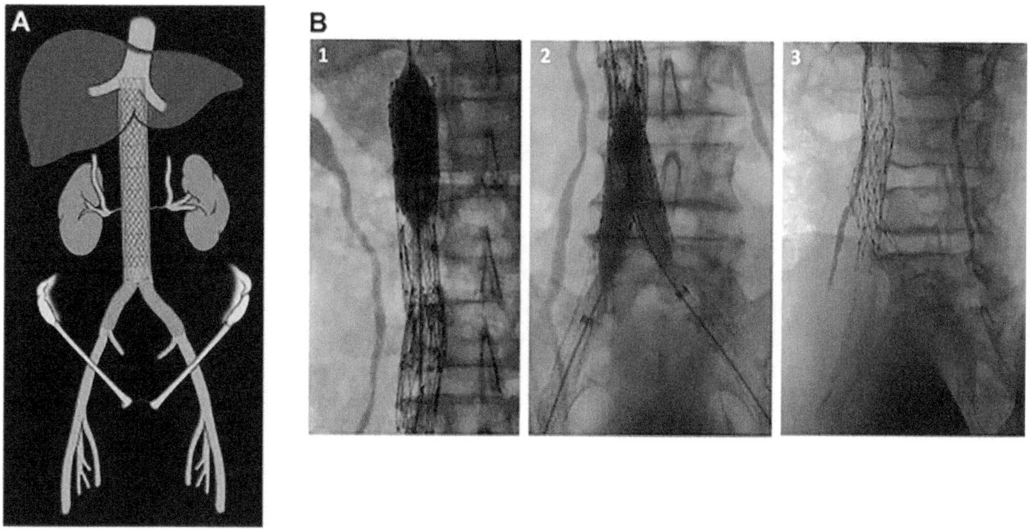

Figure 17.3 (A) Diagrammatic representation of a recanalized inferior vena cava (IVC). (B) Important tips in the process of IVC recanalization: stent overlap (1), recreation of the iliac bifurcation using kissing balloon technique (2), and stenting of the iliac bifurcation (3). The Gianturco stents are used to offer radial strength at the level of the *hepatic veins* without compromising inflow from them.

helping recreate the IVC confluence. This is followed by balloon dilatation with XXL balloons (Figure 17.3).[37]

Technical success for IVC recanalization is 85–90%; the primary patency drops from 78% to 52% between 3 and 5 years respectively.[37,38] Nevertheless, secondary patency is excellent at 93% even for complex endovenous reconstruction. Most studies reported improvement in clinical symptoms.[39] Hypercoagulable states are a risk factor for reocclusion.[37]

SVC Occlusion: Open Surgical Treatment

The patient is under general anesthesia, positioned supine with the neck, chest, abdomen and lower limbs prepped and draped. Central venous access is established via the common femoral vein. Redo sternotomy and any operation for extensive SVC obstruction often requires participation of a cardiac or thoracic surgeon as control of hemorrhage from large venous collaterals during median sternotomy can be challenging. The upper end of the incision is extended into the neck on the side of the internal jugular vein being used for inflow.

Dissection proceeds with dividing or excising the thymus or an occluded left innominate vein in the anterior mediastinum to create room for the new bypass. The innominate veins are dissected and the pericardium opened to expose the SVC. The right atrial appendage or a patent SVC central to the occlusion is the most frequent site for the central anastomosis.

After therapeutic heparinization, the peripheral anastomosis is performed first to the internal jugular or innominate vein in an end-to-side or, preferably, an end-to-end fashion. We recommed a partial or total interrupted technique for this anastomosis. Next, a side-biting Satinsky clamp on the right atrial appendage, which is opened longitudinally for about 2 cm, and the trabecular muscle in the appendage is excised. This optimizes inflow inflow into the heart. An oblique end-to-side anastomosis is performed with running 5–0 monofilament suture.[36, 40] Before declamping the appendage, the graft is allowed to fill with blood, the patient is placed in the Trendelenburg position and a Valsalva maneuvers is perfomed to prevent air embolization. The graft is de-aired with a needle before unclamping the atrial appendage. In rare cases the central anastomosis may be performed first, filling the graft with salin before unclamping. Especially if the conduit is very short or very long; it is much easier to perform the peripheral anastomosis first to distend the graft, avoid kinking and determine appropriate length for the central anastomois.

Specific attention to closure is critical to not compress the low pressure venous graft at the thoracic inlet. The posterior portion manabrium and/or the sternoclavicular joint should be shaved or partially excised for during sternal closure. Excision of soft tissues and portions of the strap muscles may also be required (Figure 17.4).

Both biologic (great saphenous vein graft, SSVG or femoral vein) and prosthetic (PTFE) conduits can be used for bypass. SSVG is the choice of conduit for short segment occlusion. To calculate the final length of the spiral vein graft (L) that will be generated, the formula

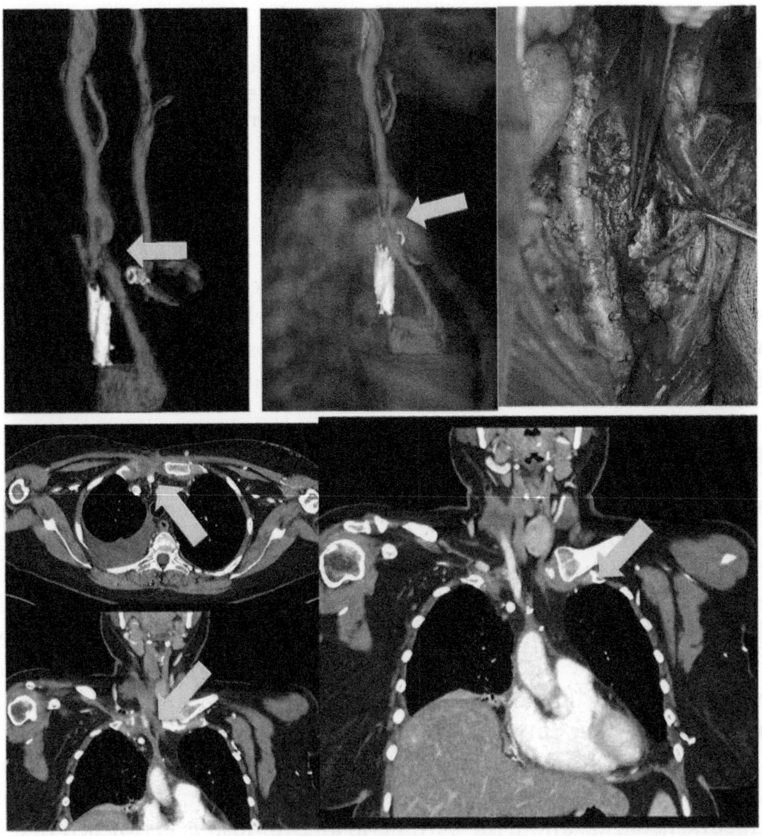

Figure 17.4 Compression on a SVC bypass at the thoracic outlet on imaging (yellow arrows) causing graft thrombosis; excision of the medial head of the clavicle and part of manubrium demonstrated in the intraoperative picture, with postop imaging demonstrating no compression, excision of clavicle (yellow arrows) resolved venous compression at the thoracic outlet with a patent graft.

(RL = rl) is used, where R is the planned diameter of the spiral graft, l is the length and r is the diameter of the available GSV.[41] To create the spiral graft, the GSV is harvested, distended with papaverine-saline solution, opened longitudinally and the valves excised. The vein is then wrapped around a 32- or 36-F polyethylene chest tube as a mandril. The edges of the vein are sutured together with running 6–0 or 7–0 monofilament nonabsorbable sutures, interrupting the suture line at every three-quarter turn. Femoral vein is preferred for longer lesions (>15 cm) because long length (>60 cm) of GSV is rarely available.

Short length, large-diameter (10–14 mm) intrathoracic ePTFE grafts fare well in patients with mediastinal fibrosis as these can resist external compression better and high innominate vein flow (more than 1000 mL/min). In our experience these short, intramediastinal synthetic grafts yielded excellent patency, while longer grafts with inflow from the neck veins did not. Unilateral reconstruction is sufficient to relieve symptoms unless the collateral circulation is inadequate. In the latter scenario, two separate bypasses are preferred to a bifurctaed graft.[42] Anticoagulation on postoperative day 1 is with low or very low-dose heaprin; this is increased to therapeutic levels by postoperative day 3 or 4. Graft patency is confirmed in the first few postoperative days with CT venography. Patients are discharged on an oral anticoagulation; lifelong anticoagualtion is considered for those with PTFE grafts or an abnormal thrombophilia profile. Patients with SSVGs or femoral vein without a known hypercoagulable state are maintained on warfarin (Coumadin) or NOAC (new oral anticoagulants) for 3–6 months only.

Technical and clincial success of open SVC reconstruciton are between 93–100%.[36, 40, 43–51] The primary, assisted primary and secondary patency rates of surgical bypass grafts in a large series form the Mayo Clinic are reported to be 45%, 68% and 75% at 3 and 5 years, respectively. Assisted primary patency is higher for vein grafts than for ePTFE grafts. Clinical and radiological surveillance is recommended with duplex ultrasound, CTV or MRV at 6 monthly intervals during the first 2 years. This is followed by annually surveillance or follow-up whenever symptoms recur as recurrent stenoses are invariably associated with recurrent symptoms.[36, 40, 52] Reintervention for restenosis is mostly endovenous; secondary interventions are required to maintain patency following both endovascular and open repair (Figure 17.5). The need for reintervention remains persistent for those treated with an initial endovascular procedure as compared to patients undergoing surgical repair, where the need for reinterventions mostly subsides after 24–36 months (Figure 17.6).

IVC Occlusion: Open Surgical Treatment

Open surgical reconstruction for benign IVC occlusion with femorocaval or iliocaval bypass is extremely challenging and rare. Patency in these long bypass grafts is low due to low venous pressure, poor inflow secondary to infrainguinal chronic post-thrombotic venous changes and underlying prothrombotic conditions. Ringed ePTFE is the preferred as this is the only graft with the appropriate length and size to bypass these long, occlusive lesions. Successful bypass around an IVC occlusion provides excellent relief of venous stasis symptoms and does promote ulcer healing.[53] Secondary patency of femorocaval bypasses at 1 and 5 years is 76% and 67%, respectively.[54] These invasive procedures should therefore only be considered for patients with severe disability from chronic venous insufficiency after multiple failed attempts at endovenous reconstruction. Postoperative management and follow-up are similar to patients undergoing SVC reconstruction, but in this situation most patients are continued on therapeutic anticoagulation.

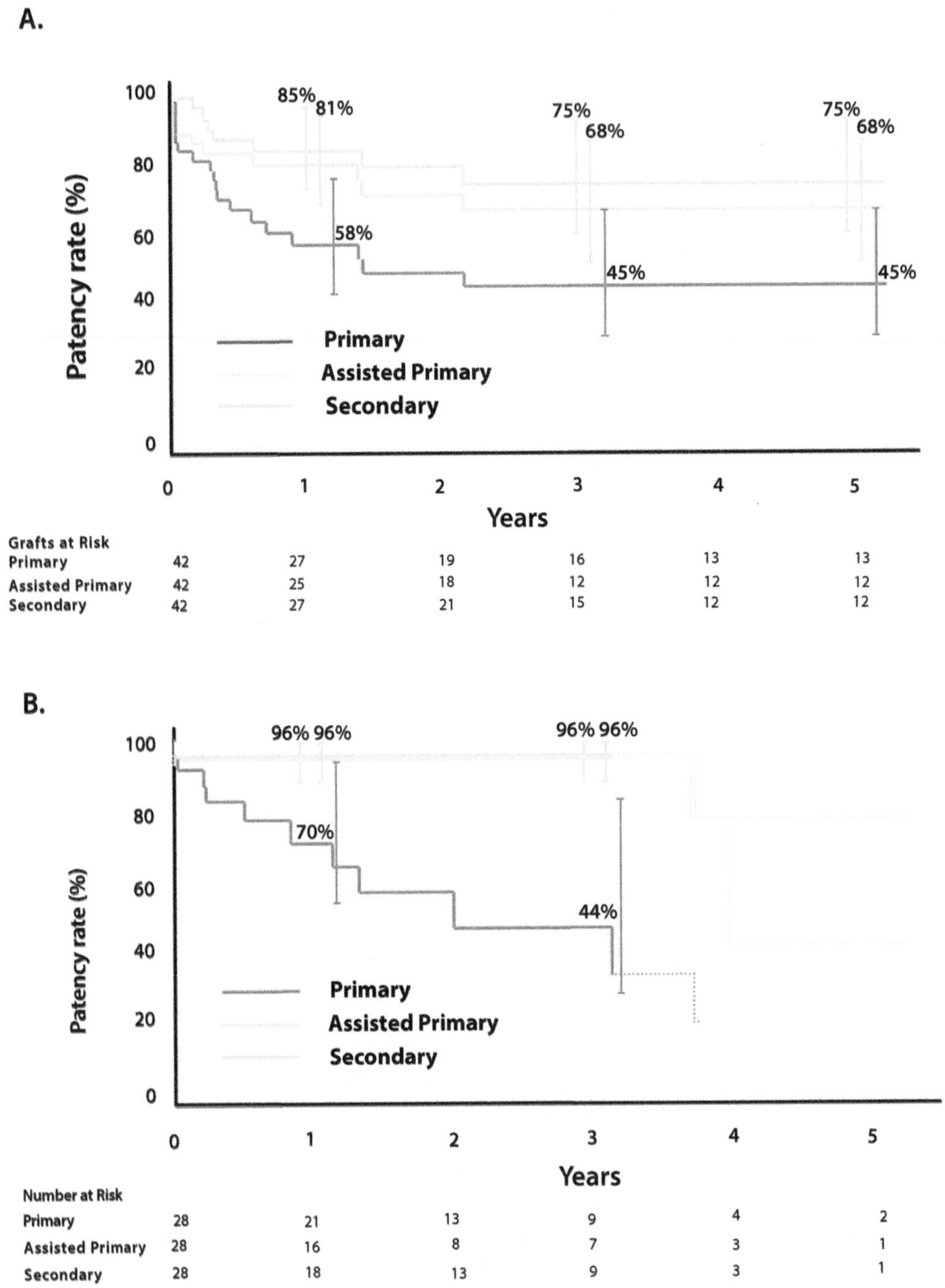

Figure 17.5 (A) Cumulative primary, assisted primary and secondary patency rates at 1, 3 and 5 years of open surgical reconstruction (n = 42). Solid bars represent SEM <10%. (B) Cumulative primary, assisted primary and secondary patency rates at 1 and 3 years of endovascular repair (n = 28). Solid bars represent SEM <10%. (From Rizvi, AZ, et al. Benign superior vena cava syndrome: stenting is now the first line of treatment. J Vasc Surg 47(2): 372–380, 2008.)

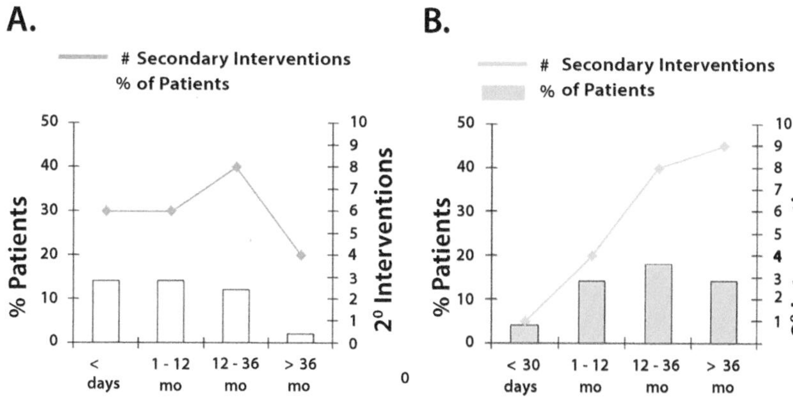

Figure 17.6 Treatment of benign superior vena cava syndrome. Secondary interventions are required to maintain patency in (A) the open surgical group (n = 42) and (B) the endovascular group (n = 28). The bars represent the percentage of patients in each group, and the line graphs represent the total number of interventions. (From Rizvi, AZ, et al. Benign superior vena cava syndrome: stenting is now the first line of treatment. J Vasc Surg 47(2): 372–380, 2008.)

REFERENCES

1. Wilson LD, Detterbeck FC, Yahalom J. Superior vena cava syndrome with malignant causes. New England Journal of Medicine. 2007;356(18):1862–9.
2. Rice TW, Rodriguez RM, Light RW. The superior vena cava syndrome: Clinical characteristics and evolving etiology. Medicine (Baltimore). 2006;85(1):37–42.
3. Stanford W, Doty DB. The role of venography and surgery in the management of patients with superior vena cava obstruction. Annals of Thoracic Surgery. 1986;41(2):158–63.
4. Gwon DI, Ko GY, Kim JH, Shin JH, Yoon HK, Sung KB. Malignant superior vena cava syndrome: A comparative cohort study of treatment with covered stents versus uncovered stents. Radiology. 2013;266(3):979–87.
5. Crowner J, Marston W, Almeida J, McLafferty R, Passman M. Classification of anatomic involvement of the iliocaval venous outflow tract and its relationship to outcomes after iliocaval venous stenting. Journal of Vascular Surgery: Venous and Lymphatic Disorders. 2014;2(3):241–5.
6. Haddad MM, Thompson SM, McPhail IR, Bendel EC, Kalra M, Stockland AH, et al. Is long-term anticoagulation required after stent placement for benign superior vena cava syndrome? Journal of Vascular and Interventional Radiology. 2018;29(12):1741–7.
7. Azizi AH, Shafi I, Zhao M, Chatterjee S, Roth SC, Singh M, et al. Endovascular therapy for superior vena cava syndrome: A systematic review and meta-analysis. EClinicalMedicine. 2021;37:100970.
8. Maleux G, Gillardin P, Fieuws S, Heye S, Vaninbroukx J, Nackaerts K. Large-bore nitinol stents for malignant superior vena cava syndrome: Factors influencing outcome. American Journal of Roentgenology. 2013;201(3):667–74.
9. Haddad MM, Simmons B, McPhail IR, Kalra M, Neisen MJ, Johnson MP, et al. comparison of covered versus uncovered stents for benign superior vena cava (svc) obstruction. Cardiovascular and Interventional Radiology. 2018;41(5):712–7.
10. Fagedet D, Thony F, Timsit J-F, Rodiere M, Monnin-Bares V, Ferretti G, et al. Endovascular treatment of malignant superior vena cava syndrome: Results and predictive factors of clinical efficacy. Cardiovascular and Interventional Radiology. 2013;36(1):140–9.

11. Fagedet D, Thony F, Timsit JF, Rodiere M, Monnin-Bares V, Ferretti GR, et al. Endovascular treatment of malignant superior vena cava syndrome: Results and predictive factors of clinical efficacy. Cardiovascular and Interventional Radiology. 2013;36(1):140–9.
12. Dinkel HP, Mettke B, Schmid F, Baumgartner I, Triller J, Do DD. Endovascular treatment of malignant superior vena cava syndrome: Is bilateral wallstent placement superior to unilateral placement? Journal of Endovascular Therapy. 2003;10(4):788–97.
13. Dartevelle PG, Chapelier AR, Pastorino U, Corbi P, Lenot B, Cerrina J, et al. Long-term follow-up after prosthetic replacement of the superior vena cava combined with resection of mediastinal-pulmonary malignant tumors. Journal of Thoracic and Cardiovascular Surgery. 1991;102(2):259–65.
14. Da Ines D, Chabrot P, Cassagnes L, Merle P, Filaire M, Ravel A, et al. [Endovascular treatment of SVC syndrome from neoplastic origin: A review of 34 cases]. Journal de Radiologie. 2008;89(7–8 Pt 1):881–90.
15. Borsato GW, Rajan DK, Simons ME, Sniderman KW, Tan KT. Central venous stenosis associated with pacemaker leads: Short-term results of endovascular interventions. Journal of Vascular and Interventional Radiology. 2012;23(3):363–7.
16. Barshes NR, Annambhotla S, El Sayed HF, Huynh TT, Kougias P, Dardik A, et al. Percutaneous stenting of superior vena cava syndrome: Treatment outcome in patients with benign and malignant etiology. Vascular. 2007;15(5):314–21.
17. Anton S, Oechtering T, Stahlberg E, Jacob F, Kleemann M, Barkhausen J, et al. Endovascular stent-based revascularization of malignant superior vena cava syndrome with concomitant implantation of a port device using a dual venous approach. Supportive Care in Cancer: Official Journal of the Multinational Association of Supportive Care in Cancer. 2018;26(6):1881–8.
18. Sen I, Kalra M, Gloviczki P. Interventions for superior vena cava syndrome. Journal of Cardiovascular Surgery (Torino). 2022;63(6):674–81.
19. Léon D, Rao S, Huang S, Sheth R, Yevich S, Ahrar K, et al. Literature review of percutaneous stenting for palliative treatment of malignant superior vena cava syndrome (SVCS). Academic Radiology. 2022;29 (Suppl 4):S110–S20.
20. Anaya-Ayala JE, Smolock CJ, Colvard BD, Naoum JJ, Bismuth J, Lumsden AB, et al. Efficacy of covered stent placement for central venous occlusive disease in hemodialysis patients. Journal of Vascular Surgery. 2011;54(3):754–9.
21. Smayra T, Otal P, Chabbert V, Chemla P, Romero M, Joffre F, et al. Long-term results of endovascular stent placement in the superior caval venous system. Cardio Vascular and Interventional Radiology. 2001;24(6):388–94.
22. García Mónaco R, Bertoni H, Pallota G, Lastiri R, Varela M, Beveraggi EM, et al. Use of self-expanding vascular endoprostheses in superior vena cava syndrome. European Journal of Cardio-Thoracic Surgery: Official Journal of the European Association for Cardio-Thoracic Surgery. 2003;24(2):208–11.
23. Breault S, Doenz F, Jouannic AM, Qanadli SD. Percutaneous endovascular management of chronic superior vena cava syndrome of benign causes: Long-term follow-up. European Radiology. 2017;27(1):97–104.
24. Karakhanian WK, Karakhanian WZ, Belczak SQ. Superior vena cava syndrome: Endovascular management. Journal Vascular Brasileiro. 2019;18:e20180062.
25. McDevitt JL, Goldman DT, Bundy JJ, Hage AN, Jairath NK, Gemmete JJ, et al. Gianturco Z-stent placement for the treatment of chronic central venous occlusive disease: Implantation of 208 stents in 137 symptomatic patients. Diagnostic and Interventional Radiology (Ankara, Turkey). 2021;27(1):72–8.
26. Aung EY, Khan M, Williams N, Raja U, Hamady M. Endovascular stenting in superior vena cava syndrome: A systematic review and meta-analysis. Cardiovascular and Interventional Radiology. 2022;45(9):1236–54.
27. Kordzadeh A, Askari A, Hanif MA, Gadhvi V. Superior vena cava syndrome and wallstent: A systematic review. Annals of Vascular Diseases. 2022;15(2):87–93.

28. Kitrou PM, Steinke T, El Hage R, Ponce P, Lucatelli P, Katsanos K, et al. Paclitaxel-coated balloons for the treatment of symptomatic central venous stenosis in vascular access: Results From a European, multicenter, single-arm retrospective analysis. Journal of Endovascular Therapy. 2021;28(3):442–51.
29. Kee ST, Kinoshita L, Razavi MK, Nyman UR, Semba CP, Dake MD. Superior vena cava syndrome: Treatment with catheter-directed thrombolysis and endovascular stent placement. Radiology. 1998;206(1):187–93.
30. Danışman N, Çeneli D, Kültürsay B, Yılmaz C, Alizade E. Endovascular treatment of vena cava superior syndrome using angiojet thrombectomy due to COVID-19 infection. Kardiologia Polska. 2022.
31. Ramjit A, Chen J, Konner M, Landau E, Ahmad N. Treatment of superior vena cava syndrome using angiojet™ thrombectomy system. Cardiovascular and Interventional Radiology Endovascular. 2019;2(1):28.
32. Sessions KL, Anderson JH, Johnson JN, Taggart NW. AngioJet(™) thrombolysis of SVC thrombosis after orthotopic heart transplantation: A case report. Pediatric Transplantation. 2016;20(5):723–6.
33. Ahmed O, Kuo WT. Laser-assisted venous thrombectomy for treatment of recurrent in-stent restenosis and superior vena cava syndrome. Journal of Vascular and Interventional Radiology. 2016;27(4):603–6.
34. Sousou JM, Sherard DM, Edwards JR, Negron-Rubio E. Successful removal of a thrombus in the setting of SVC syndrome using the INARI FlowTriever device. Radiology Case Reports. 2022;17(3):744–7.
35. Hanser A, Sieverding L, Hauser TK, Wiegand G, Hofbeck M. Stent-retriever thrombectomy in the treatment of infants with acute thrombosis of the superior vena cava and innominate vein. Catheterization and Cardiovascular Interventions: Official Journal of the Society for Cardiac Angiography & Interventions. 2019;93(6):E357–E61.
36. Rizvi AZ, Kalra M, Bjarnason H, Bower TC, Schleck C, Gloviczki P. Benign superior vena cava syndrome: Stenting is now the first line of treatment. Journal of Vascular Surgery. 2008;47(2):372–80.
37. Erben Y, Bjarnason H, Oladottir GL, McBane RD, Gloviczki P. Endovascular recanalization for nonmalignant obstruction of the inferior vena cava. Journal of Vascular Surgery: Venous and Lymphatic Disorders. 2018;6(2):173–82.
38. Murphy EH, Johns B, Varney E, Raju S. Endovascular management of chronic total occlusions of the inferior vena cava and iliac veins. Journal of Vascular Surgery: Venous and Lymphatic Disorders. 2017;5(1):47–59.
39. Morris RI, Jackson N, Smith A, Black SA. A systematic review of the safety and efficacy of inferior vena cava stenting. European Journal of Vascular and Endovascular Surgery. 2023;65(2):298–308.
40. Kalra M, Gloviczki P, Andrews JC, Cherry KJ, Bower TC, Panneton JM, et al. Open surgical and endovascular treatment of superior vena cava syndrome caused by nonmalignant disease. Journal of Vascular Surgery. 2003;38(2):215–23.
41. Chiu CJ, Terzis J, MacRae ML. Replacement of superior vena cava with the spiral composite vein graft. A versatile technique. The Annals of Thoracic Surgery. 1974;17(6):555–60.
42. Manju Kalra IS, Bjarnason H, Gloviczki P. Superior vena cava occlusion and management. Rutherford's Vascular Surgery and Endovascular Therapy. 2023, Chapter 162, 2148–2162.e2.
43. Mistirian AA, Balmforth DC, Oo A, Lawrence D. Open repair of superior vena cava syndrome with high intracranial pressures using a 'Y' graft. Annals of Thoracic Surgery. 2022;113(4):e283–e6.
44. Uceda PV, Feldtman RW, Ahn SS. Long term results of bypass graft to the right atrium in the management of superior vena cava syndrome in dialysis patients. Annals of Vascular Surgery. 2021;74:321–9.
45. Colombier S, Girod G, Niclauss L, Danzer D, Eeckhout E, Qanadli SD, et al. Total endovascular repair of post-trauma ascending aortic pseudoaneurysm and secondary superior vena cava syndrome. Annals of Vascular Surgery. 2019;61:468.e13–e17.

46. Fichelle JM, Baissas V, Salvi S, Fabiani JN. [Superior vena cava thrombosis or stricture secondary to implanted central venous access: Six cases of endovascular and direct surgical treatment in cancer patients]. Journal de medecine vasculaire. 2018;43(1):20–8.
47. Li H, Jiang X, Sun T. Open surgery repair for superior vena cava syndrome after failed endovascular stenting. Annals of Thoracic Surgery. 2014;97(4):1445–7.
48. Firstenberg MS, Blais D, Abel E, Go MR. Superior vena cava bypass with cryopreserved ascending aorta allograft. Annals of Thoracic Surgery. 2011;91(3):905–7.
49. Kennedy DP, Palit TK. Reconstruction of superior vena cava syndrome due to benign disease using superficial femoral vein. Annals of Vascular Surgery. 2010;24(4):555.e7–e12.
50. Dedeilias P, Nenekidis I, Hountis P, Prokakis C, Dolou P, Apostolakis E, et al. Superior vena cava syndrome in a patient with previous cardiac surgery: What else should we suspect? Diagnostic Pathology. 2010;5:43.
51. Doty JR, Flores JH, Doty DB. Superior vena cava obstruction: Bypass using spiral vein graft. Annals of Thoracic Surgery. 1999;67(4):1111–6.
52. Alimi YS, Gloviczki P, Vrtiska TJ, Pairolero PC, Canton LG, Bower TC, et al. Reconstruction of the superior vena cava: Benefits of postoperative surveillance and secondary endovascular interventions. Journal of Vascular Surgery. 1998;27(2):287–301.
53. AbuRahma AF, Robinson PA, Boland JP. Clinical, hemodynamic, and anatomic predictors of long-term outcome of lower extremity venovenous bypasses. Journal of Vascular Surgery. 1991;14(5):635–44.
54. Garg N, Gloviczki P, Karimi KM, Duncan AA, Bjarnason H, Kalra M, et al. Factors affecting outcome of open and hybrid reconstructions for nonmalignant obstruction of iliofemoral veins and inferior vena cava. Journal of Vascular Surgery. 2011;53(2):383–93.

Chapter 18

Evidence-Based Management of Venous Aneurysms

Reid C. Mahoney, Leo Daab, and Gregory Moneta

INTRODUCTION

Venous aneurysms are rare and were first described by Osler in 1913.[1] They have varying presentations, from asymptomatic, incidentally discovered on imaging or at surgery, to presenting with pain, thrombosis, palpable mass, deep venous thrombosis, pulmonary embolus, or death. There are no management strategies based on level one evidence; management is generally individualized and/or based on case studies and case series.

Venous aneurysms have been reported to involve most major veins.[2] Synonymous terms include aneurysm, varix, and phlebectasia.[3] For the purposes of this chapter, any venous dilatation will be termed "aneurysm." Venous aneurysm can be defined as a solitary area of localized venous dilation that communicates with a main venous structure by a single channel and does not have an association with a surgical arteriovenous communication, pseudoaneurysm, or involve vein proximal to venous stenosis or obstruction.[4]

Herein we present the current understanding of the etiology and pathophysiology of venous aneurysms, including their relation to congenital conditions. This is followed by a discussion of venous aneurysm presentation and management based on anatomic location, size, imaging, and clinical presentation.

ETIOLOGY AND PATHOPHYSIOLOGY

Little is known about the etiology and the pathogenesis of venous aneurysms. Thinning of the venous walls occurs with aging. A combination of congenital and mechanical factors, including potential prior trauma, may also stimulate the formation of venous aneurysms.[5] Venous reflux and venous hypertension are suggested as likely contributors to the etiology of aneurysmal degeneration.[6] Reduced amount and size of smooth muscle cells and elastin fibers in the vein walls are seen histologically; hyalinization of the intima can also occur.[7] An early investigation of the popliteal vein by Lev and Saphir proposed that areas associated with stress were prone to hypertrophy of the vein, while thinning of the venous wall was seen in areas that were in direct apposition with the artery, perhaps indicating external force may be a cause of venous aneurysmal changes.[3] Schatz and Fine, in one of the first series of venous aneurysms, noted two commonly found histologic changes: an increase in fibrous connective tissue with decrease in smooth muscle cells and an increase or decrease in fibrous connective tissue and elastic tissue.[2] Degenerative histologic changes are described for internal jugular venous aneurysms, including increased levels of matrix metalloproteinases.[8] Histology, however, appears to be more variable for popliteal venous aneurysms, perhaps in response to gravitational forces, tending to have thickened and fibrosed intima and regions of increased smooth muscle cells.[7]

DOI: 10.1201/9781003316626-21

Venous aneurysms appear to have equal distribution between sexes and a wide range of age at discovery is noted.[6] Most patients with venous aneurysms will not have an associated genetic mediated pathway or syndrome. However, there are known genetic syndromes that increase a patient's chance of having venous pathology, including malformations and aneurysms. Blue rubber bleb nevus syndrome is a rare syndrome of venous malformations primarily affecting the gastrointestinal tract. It is generally sporadic but can be transmitted in an autosomal dominant manner and has been associated with inferior vena cava (IVC) aneurysm.[9] Klippel-Trenaunay syndrome is a well-known disorder that results in a wide range of lymphatic and venous anomalies including agenesis, hypoplasia, atresia, valvular incompetence, external compression by fibrous bands, and aneurysmal degeneration.[6] These anomalies most frequently involve the lower extremity.

MANAGEMENT

Lower Extremity Venous Aneurysms

Popliteal Venous Aneurysms

The popliteal vein appear to be the most common site of venous aneurysms.[3] Presentation is variable, from asymptomatic to pain, deep venous thrombosis, pulmonary embolism, or death from pulmonary embolism.[7] Popliteal venous aneurysms are the most common venous aneurysm to present with pulmonary embolism (PE), with rates as high as 70% of patients afflicted with popliteal venous aneurysms.[7] Interestingly, size does not appear to impact the risk of pulmonary embolism. Rupture rates are not known but appear to be exceedingly low as there are no reports describing rupture of a primary popliteal venous aneurysm.

Large popliteal venous aneurysms may be palpable to the patient or healthcare provider, but most popliteal venous aneurysms are diagnosed utilizing ultrasound. CT and MRI can also be used for diagnosis and, if elected, operative planning. Size criteria to define a popliteal venous aneurysm has been debated, but most often two to three times the size of a normal popliteal vein is considered aneurysmal. This equates to approximately 1.5 to 2cm in diameter representing an aneurysmal popliteal vein.[7] Once a patient has been diagnosed with a popliteal venous aneurysm, further investigation is warranted to ensure no other venous aneurysms are present, including the contralateral popliteal vein.

Symptoms, aneurysm size, mass effect, and the presence or absence of associated intraluminal thrombus (Figure 18.1) influence management. Medical management with anticoagulation has been the mainstay of treatment for popliteal venous aneurysms. However, anticoagulation alone does not appear to prevent thromboembolic events. Nasr et al demonstrated 43% of patients with popliteal venous aneurysms treated with anticoagulation alone went on to develop thromboembolic complications, including one death from pulmonary embolism.[10] Given their propensity to lead to catastrophic results, including pulmonary embolism and death, intervention for symptomatic aneurysms is widely accepted. Management of asymptomatic popliteal aneurysm is less clear but is likely still best managed surgically in reasonably fit patients to avoid the potential of future complications.

Surgical management of popliteal venous aneurysms is variable between aneurysmectomy and venorrhaphy or resection with venous interposition graft.[1] Posterior approach appears to be the most common. Additional options include the use of PTFE graft and the use of patch venoplasty.[1] Outcomes appear to be similar regardless of surgical approach. This indicates

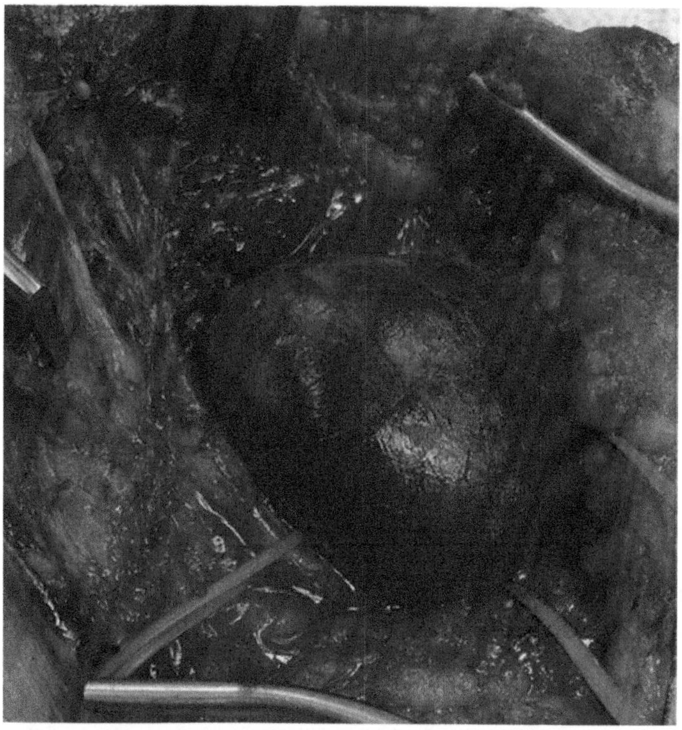

Figure 18.1 Popliteal venous aneurysm with intraluminal thrombus.

individual case planning based on patient presentation, anatomy of the aneurysm, and surgeon preference appears to be a reasonable tactic for treatment. It should be noted that one review does demonstrate higher rates of postoperative thrombosis in venous interposition grafts; this finding has not been replicated in other reviews.[1] The role of anticoagulation pre and postoperatively appears institution dependent, but most surgeons will treat with anticoagulation until the postoperative period, with some surgeons recommending continuing anticoagulation for up to 3 months after surgery.[10]

Iliac and Common Femoral Venous Aneurysms

Iliac venous aneurysms are quite rare, although aneurysms of the common, external, and internal iliac vein have been reported. A recent review reported 50 cases of iliac venous aneurysms, noting a 2:1 male to female ratio.[11] Most cases included in this review were related to trauma or arteriovenous fistula and thus not primary aneurysms. Of those that were primary aneurysms, approximately 70% were found in women, and the majority were found in the left external iliac vein. This is likely due to extrinsic trauma/forces from the right common iliac artery as a variant of May-Thurner syndrome.[12] Abdominal pain, back pain, leg swelling, and pulmonary embolism have been reported in primary iliac venous aneurysm. Most patients are asymptomatic, and rupture has never been reported.[13] Although the data is less compelling than for popliteal venous aneurysms, given the risk of thrombosis and pulmonary embolism, surgical treatment of primary iliac venous aneurysms is reasonable in suitable risk patients. Venorrhaphy, venoplasty, bypass, and ligation are all possible options, although ligation should only be performed if there is adequate collateral drainage.

One report details coil embolization of a common femoral vein aneurysm,[14] but coiling does not seem to eliminate the potential for thromboembolic events, and management akin to popliteal or iliac veins seems more prudent.

Lower Extremity Superficial Venous Aneurysms

Superficial venous aneurysms of the lower extremity are less common than deep aneurysms and likely represent an overall benign process. They may be discovered in an evaluation for symptoms consistent with chronic venous disease (Figure 18.2). The most common presenting symptoms include pain, swelling, and a palpable mass. Cosmesis is the most common reason to intervene. There have been reports of deep venous thrombosis and pulmonary embolism from superficial venous aneurysms of the lower extremity; however, it appears that the risk of thromboembolic events remains quite low.[2] Small saphenous venous aneurysms can compress the sural nerve, causing significant pain within the distribution of the nerve.[4] The most common surgical approaches are aneurysmectomy and venorrhaphy or excision and interposition grafting. Ligation is a viable option if the deep venous system remains patent. Endovascular treatment is likely to leave a large palpable mass if used for superficial venous aneurysms.

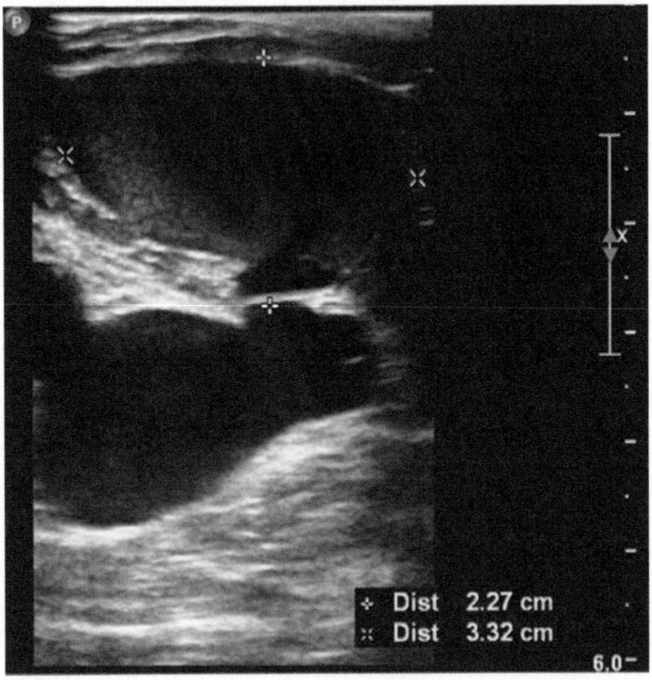

Figure 18.2 Ultrasound of an accessory saphenous vein aneurysm discovered in an evaluation for chronic venous disease.

Upper Extremity, Internal Jugular, and Thoracic Venous Aneurysms

Primary axillary venous aneurysms are distinctly uncommon. Although possible, thromboembolic events are quite rare in upper extremity aneurysms, including in the axillary vein. There is a case report of axillary venous aneurysm and associated pulmonary embolus.[15] However, in a study of 30 patients with venous aneurysms, four axillary venous aneurysms were encountered, and none of these patients had thromboembolic events.[2] Reasons to intervene surgically include symptoms of compression or pain and cosmetic reasons. If there is concern for the possibility of VTE, such as thrombus within the aneurysm, it is reasonable to consider surgical treatment or anticoagulation. Surgical treatment options are similar to those for lower extremity aneurysms, including aneurysmectomy and venorrhaphy, excision with grafting, or ligation.

Cephalic, brachial, and basilic venous aneurysms unrelated to arteriovenous fistula formation are rare, although one case series did include an asymptomatic cephalic vein aneurysm.[4] It is unlikely that they would require intervention unless they are causing significant cosmetic issues or symptoms.

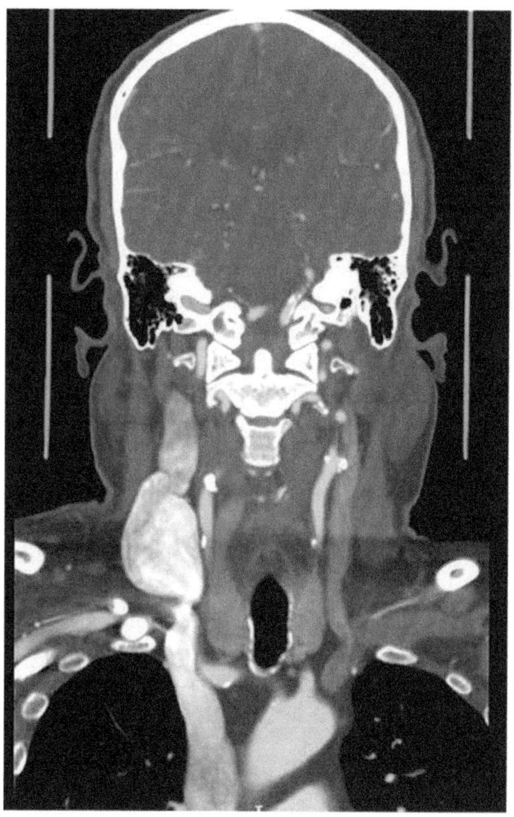

Figure 18.3 Internal jugular venous aneurysm.

Internal jugular (IJ) and external jugular (EJ) aneurysms tend to be benign, fusiform, and most often present as an asymptomatic neck mass.[16] Right-sided IJ aneurysms are more common than left-sided IJ aneurysms (Figure 18.3). EJ aneurysms are equally distributed between left and right sided. Some patients have discomfort from a neck aneurysm, and this is more common in EJ than IJ aneurysms; however, voice changes, cough, and dysphagia are only associated with IJ aneurysms, although the rates of these symptoms are all <5%.[17] Rupture has not been reported. Although thrombosis has been reported in several case studies, the rise of pulmonary embolus appears low.[4]

Neck masses encompass many different pathologies, including neoplasm and cysts, but painless masses that enlarge with Valsalva maneuver should incorporate internal jugular venous aneurysms into the differential diagnosis. IJ venous aneurysms are often diagnosed in the pediatric population, but a wide range of ages at diagnosis have been reported. Pediatric patients tend to have aneurysmal degeneration of the right side, whereas older patients tend to have left-sided aneurysms attributed to calcified arch vessels causing external compression or traumatic forces.[18] Following history and physical, ultrasound is often the only imaging necessary for diagnosis. If there are equivocal findings on ultrasound or an operation is being planned, CT or MRI can be performed. Serial imaging and conservative management are an appropriate treatment strategy for asymptomatic patients once diagnosis is confirmed. Intervention should be considered for growth, pain, localized compression symptoms, and cosmetic reasons. Surgical intervention options include aneurysmectomy and venorrhaphy, bypass, or ligation. Ligation with aneurysm excision is an appropriate option for EJ aneurysms. Patency of the contralateral internal jugular vein should be confirmed if ligation is performed, as there are reports of intracranial hypertension after right side IJ ligation.[17]

Thoracic venous aneurysms include subclavian, innominate, and superior vena cava (SVC) aneurysms. Several case reports and case series have been published encompassing aneurysms in these locations.[1] Most are diagnosed incidentally when imaging is performed for other reasons, frequently by chest X-ray when a widened mediastinum is found.[1] Providers must be aware of the possibility that a thoracic or mediastinal mass may indeed be a venous aneurysm, as biopsy or surgical intervention can be catastrophic.[19] Most thoracic venous aneurysms are managed nonoperatively with low rates of significant complications. Subclavian vein aneurysm patients have been treated nonoperatively, with endovascular surgery, or with open surgery, all of whom recovered without complications in the follow-up period.[1]

Central thoracic venous aneurysms, including the innominate artery and the SVC, tend to have low rates of complications including rupture and pulmonary embolism. It should be noted that fusiform SVC aneurysms portend a more benign course while saccular aneurysms, usually post-infectious or inflammatory, tend to present with more complications.[20] Surgical intervention on any central thoracic venous aneurysm is difficult and should be preceded with appropriate preoperative risk stratification and patient discussion. There are case reports describing intraoperative death including massive pulmonary embolism from manipulation of the aneurysm.[1] Contained ruptures of the SVC have been managed nonoperatively with patient survival, adding to the concept that risks associated with surgical intervention most often outweigh benefit.[3]

Abdominal Venous Aneurysms

Portal Venous System

Superior mesenteric venous aneurysms, as part of the portal venous system, are often described in conjunction with portal venous aneurysms (Figure 18.4). Cirrhosis or malignancy have been associated with PV/SMV aneurysm.[21] Diagnosis can be by ultrasound as an unexpected

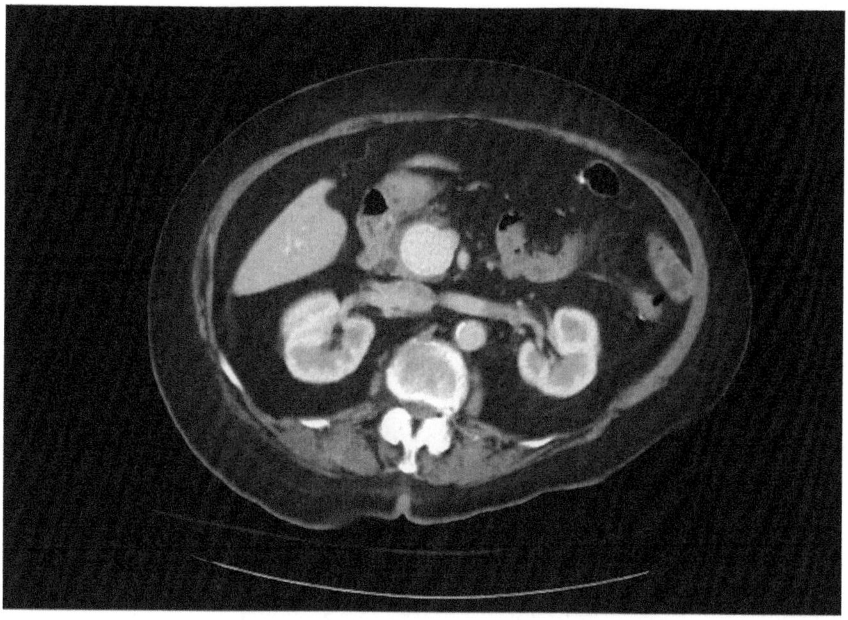

Figure 18.4 Aneurysm of the portal superior mesenteric vein confluence.

finding in a patient being assessed for other pathology, but CT and MRI remain reasonable options for diagnosis in the face of equivocal ultrasound findings. Patients tend to present without symptoms, but vague abdominal pain and GI bleeding can be seen,[1] and there are reports of patients with biliary or duodenal compressive symptoms from aneurysmal degeneration of the portal venous system.[22] Given the preponderance for these aneurysms to be associated with other pathology, it is difficult to determine the true significance of aneurysmal degeneration in these vessels, but case reports describe operative intervention for complications including thrombosis or rupture.[21] A review by Laurenzi et al included 128 patients with aneurysmal degeneration of the portal venous system without known liver disease.[23] Thirty-two of these patients underwent surgical intervention, the majority of which underwent aneurysmectomy with venorrhaphy. Eighty percent, however, were treated nonoperatively, and this appears to be a viable management strategy for asymptomatic or high-risk surgical patients.

Inferior Vena Cava

Inferior vena cava (IVC) aneurysms are also very uncommon. They may be primary, congenital, associated with trauma, arteriovenous fistula, inflammation, or neoplasm. Primary IVC aneurysms may represent a congenital abnormality of persistence, degradation, or fusion of the embryonic cardinal veins from which the IVC is formed (Figure 18.5).[24] Patient presentation ranges from asymptomatic and discovered on incidental imaging finding to acute thrombosis to pulmonary embolism.[9] Ultrasound can be used for diagnosis, but the retrohepatic and suprahepatic IVC is best imaged utilizing CT or MRI.

Gradman and Steinberg described a classification system for IVC aneurysms that has proven useful in describing IVC aneurysms and, as such, can aid in guiding clinical management (Figure 18.6).[25] Wang et al, based on a literature review, summarized IVC aneurysms

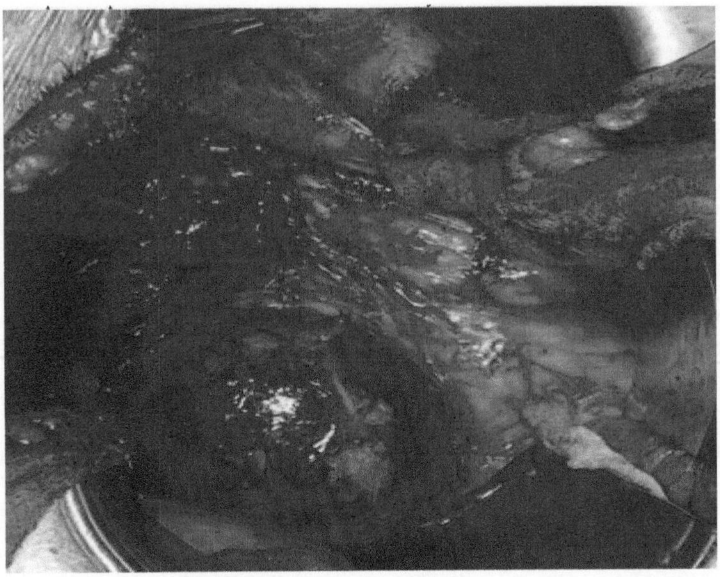

Figure 18.5 Intraoperative photo of infrarenal inferior vena cava aneurysm.

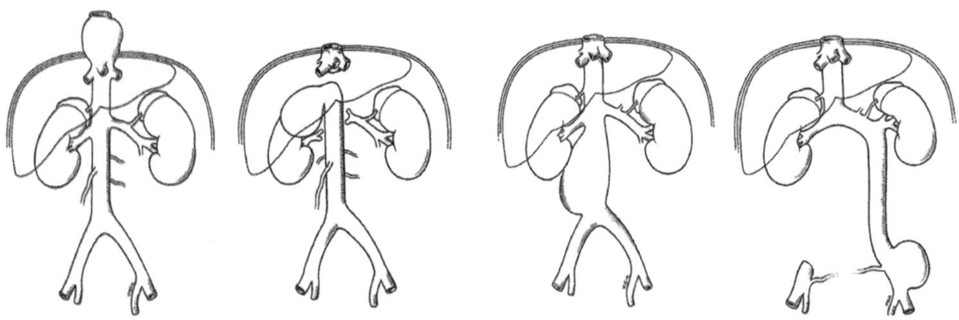

Figure 18.6 Gradman and Steinberg classification of inferior vena cava aneurysms.

according to the Gradman and Steinberg classification system.[9] Type I IVC aneurysms represent 35% of IVC aneurysms, are often fusiform or asymptomatic, and do not appear to be associated thrombosis or VTE complications. Given the complexity of surgical management, type I IVC aneurysms are likely best served with conservative management; successful nonoperative management is reported in over 90% of patients.[9] Type II IVC aneurysms, 18% of IVC aneurysms, appear to be mostly congenital, and more than 90% are saccular. Most patients present with abdominal or back pain as well as limb swelling. IVC thrombosis pulmonary embolism occurs in approximately one-third of these patients. Type III IVC aneurysms appear to be the most common type, accounting for 45% of IVC aneurysms. They tend to present with symptoms including back pain, abdominal pain, leg swelling, IVC thrombosis (42%), DVT (45%), and PE (12%). More than 90% are saccular, and more than 90% are congenital. Type IV IVC aneurysms are rare, accounting for <10% of IVC aneurysms. All reported cases are saccular and congenital. There was one death from rupture in this subgroup.[9] Based on these findings, surgically fit patients that have a type II–IV IVC aneurysm should be intervened on. However, small asymptomatic IVC aneurysms can likely be followed with serial imaging. Montero-Baker et al consider flow dynamics of type II–IV IVC aneurysms to be different than type I and therefore, if surgically accessible, recommend surgical intervention to avoid complications of thrombosis and pulmonary embolism.[26]

CONCLUSIONS

Venous aneurysms may occur in nearly all veins. Their management depends on several important factors including anatomic location, size, and clinical presentation. Decisions regarding management can have significant impact on the patient and should be based on available evidence as discussed in this chapter. Popliteal venous aneurysms are associated with significant clinical problems including pulmonary embolus, are surgically accessible, and therefore should be dealt with promptly. Upper extremity, cervical, and superficial lower extremity venous aneurysms tend to have a more indolent course. Thoracic and abdominal venous aneurysms require an individualized approach with treatment algorithms proposed for IVC aneurysms based on anatomic location.

REFERENCES

1. Teter KA, Maldonado TM, Adelman MA. A systematic review of venous aneurysms by anatomic location. J Vasc Surg Venous Lymphat Disord. 2018;6:408–13.
2. Gillespie DL, Leonel Villavicencio J, Gallagher C, Chang A, Hamelink K, Fiala LA, et al. Presentation and management of venous aneurysms. J Vasc Surg. 1997 Nov;26(5):845–52.
3. Gloviczki P (Eds.). Handbook of Venous and Lymphatic Disorders: Guidelines of the American Venous Forum (4th ed., 675–83). CRC Press, 2017.
4. ElKassaby M, Regal S, Khafagy T, El Alfy K. Surgical management of venous aneurysms. J Vasc Surg Venous Lymphat Disord. 2021 Jan 1;9(1):193–99.
5. Patel R, Hanish S, Baril D, Woo K, Lawrence P. Contemporary management of lower extremity venous aneurysms. J Vasc Surg Venous Lymphat Disord. 2019;860–64.
6. Sivakumaran Y, Duara R, Vasudevan TM. Superficial femoral venous aneurysm in a patient with Klippel-Trenaunay Syndrome: The femoral hernia mimic. Ann Vasc Surg. 2019 May 1;57:274.e15–e18.
7. Johnstone JK, Fleming MD, Gloviczki P, Stone W, Kalra M, Oderich GS, et al. Surgical treatment of popliteal venous aneurysms. Ann Vasc Surg. 2015 Aug 1;29(6):1084–89.
8. Kovacs T, el Haddi S, Lee WA. Internal jugular venous aneurysm – a report of two cases with literature review. J Vasc Surg Cases Innov Tech. 2020;326–30.
9. Wang M, Wang H, Liao B, Peng G, Chang G. Treatment strategies for inferior vena cava aneurysms. J Vasc Surg Venous Lymphat Disord. 2021 Nov 1;9(6):1588–96.
10. Nasr W, Babbitt R, Eslami MH. Popliteal vein aneurysm: A case report and review of literature. Vasc Endovascular Surg. 2008 Dec;41(6):551–55.
11. Zarrintan S, Tadayon N, Kalantar-Motamedi SMR. Iliac vein aneurysms: A comprehensive review. J Cardiovasc Thorac Res. 2019 Feb 19;11(1):1–7.
12. Hurwitz RL, Gelabert H. Thrombosed iliac venous aneurysm: A rare cause of left lower extremity venous obstruction. J Vasc Surg. 1989 Jun;9(6):822–24.
13. Hosaka A, Miyata T, Hoshina K, Okamoto H, Shigematsu K. Surgical management of a primary external iliac venous aneurysm causing pulmonary thromboembolism: Report of a case. Surg Today. 2014;44(9):1771–73.

14. Ross CB, Schumacher PM, Datillo JB, Guzman RJ, Naslund TC. Endovenous stent-assisted coil embolization for a symptomatic femoral vein aneurysm. J Vasc Surg. 2008 Oct;48(4):1032–36.
15. Pierre-Louis WS, Tikhtman R, Bonta A, Meier G. Primary axillary venous aneurysm in a young patient presenting with cardiac arrest. J Vasc Surg Cases Innov Tech. 2019 Sep 1;5(3):375–78.
16. Khashram M, Walker PJ. Internal jugular venous aneurysm. J Vasc Surg Venous Lymphat Disord. 2015 Jan 1;3(1):94.
17. Nucera M, Meuli L, Janka H, Schindewolf M, Schmidli J, Makaloski V. Comprehensive review with pooled analysis on external and internal jugular vein aneurysm. J Vasc Surg Venous Lymphat Disord. 2022;10:778–85.
18. Bartholomew JR, Smolock CJ, Kirksey L, Lyden SP, Badrinathan B, Whitelaw S, et al. Jugular venous aneurysm. Ann Vasc Surg. 2020 Oct 1;68:567.e5–e9.
19. Buehler MA, Ebrahim FS, Popa TO. Left innominate vein aneurysm: Diagnostic imaging and pitfalls. Int J Angiol. 2013 Jun;22(2):127–30.
20. Kapoor H, Gulati V, Pawley B, Lee JT. Massive fusiform superior vena cava aneurysm in a 47-year-old complicated by pulmonary embolism: A case report and review of literature. Clin Imaging. 2022 Jan 1;81:43–45.
21. Sfyroeras GS, Antoniou GA, Drakou AA, Karathanos C, Giannoukas AD. Visceral venous aneurysms: Clinical presentation, natural history and their management: A systematic review. Eur J Vasc Endovasc Surg. 2009;38:498–505.
22. Lerch R, Wolfle KD, Loeprecht H. Superior mesenteric venous aneurysm. Ann Vasc Surg. 1996;10(6):582–88.
23. Laurenzi A, Ettorre GM, Lionetti R, Meniconi RL, Colasanti M, Vennarecci G. Portal vein aneurysm: What to know. Dig Liver Dis. 2015 Nov 1;47(11):918–23.
24. Regoort M, Reekers JA, Kromhout JG. An unusual cause of an inferior vena cava syndrome. Neth J Surg. 1989 Aug;41(4):92–94. PMID: 2779816.
25. Gradman WS, Steinberg F. Aneurysm of the Inferior vena cava: Case report and review of the literature. Phlebology. 2008;23(4):184–88.
26. Montero-Baker MF, Branco BC, Leon LL Jr., Labraopoulos N, Echeverria A, Mills JL Sr. Management of inferior vena cava aneurysm. J Cardiovasc Surg (Torino). 2015 Oct;56(5):769–74.

Chapter 19

Diagnosis and Management of Vascular Malformations

Steven M. Farley

INTRODUCTION

The starting point to the management of vascular malformations is nomenclature. Vascular anomalies are divided into vascular tumors and vascular malformations. Hemangioma is a term commonly misused to describe any vascular anomaly. In reality, a hemangioma is a specific disease – a benign vascular tumor most commonly diagnosed in infants. As a benign tumor, a hemangioma goes through stages of growth and involution. A vascular malformation is not a tumor but an error of embryogenesis.[1]

As such, most malformations do not grow and certainly do not involute. Many parents are told their child's malformation should regress or disappear but see no improvement as the child grows. Another challenge with terminology has been the use of different nomenclature systems over time and a lack of consensus on terminology. The International Society for the Study of Vascular Anomalies (ISSVA) has created a single nomenclature system.[2] Referencing this document is initially challenging due to the high level of detail regarding syndromes and genetic information.

Once identified as a vascular malformation, in clinical practice, a malformation can be best described as low flow or high flow. Low flow malformations are more common, can be purely venous or have a lymphatic component as well. High flow lesions reference a high volume of blood flow through the malformation and denote an arterial component to the lesion. High flow lesions are generally more difficult to manage. They will grow over time with low sheer, high flow characteristics. High flow lesions are more likely to bleed, be painful and cause wounds or tissue loss. Moreover, control of the high flow lesion is more difficult and complex.

LOW FLOW MALFORMATIONS

Presentation

A low flow lesion can present in a variety of ways. Some lesions are superficial and are visible on physical exam with a blueish lesion in the skin. Other lesions cause local tissue swelling, and a visible bump alerts the patient or family. With regard to symptoms, patients can present with venous type complaints – pain, throbbing, local swelling, heaviness, phlebitis – in any location of the body. At times, low flow lesions are asymptomatic and are an incidental finding from cross-sectional imaging. Age at presentation varies, but often lesions are identified by the teenage years.

Imaging

A plain radiograph can be a route to diagnosis. Low flow lesions often demonstrate phleboliths, small calcific spheres (Figure 19.1). Phleboliths are thought to form due to intermittent episodes of thrombosis in the irregular flow channels in a low flow lesion. Ultrasound

DOI: 10.1201/9781003316626-22

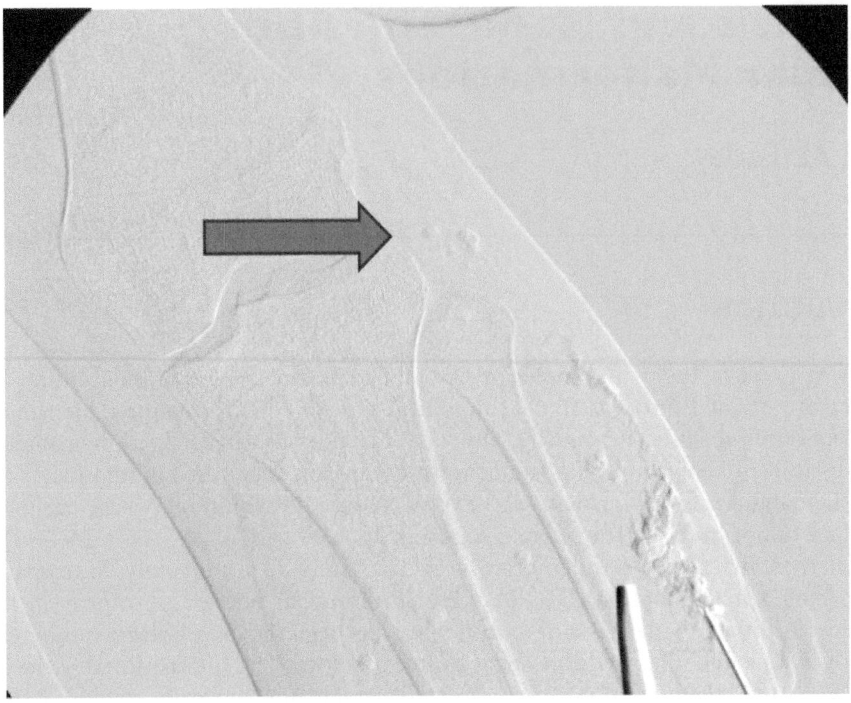

Figure 19.1 Phleboliths in a low flow vascular malformation. Fluoroscopy of the right leg, arrow points to phleboliths.

duplex can identify low flow lesions. On B-mode, compressible vascular channels and lakes can be seen. On color mode and Doppler, chaotic and multidirectional low velocity flow is seen within the vascular channels. Phleboliths can demonstrate post-acoustic shadowing and post-phlebitic vessel wall thickening is often present. Computed tomography (CT) imaging is not generally helpful except to exclude a high flow lesion. Magnetic resonance imaging (MRI) is the primary modality to fully characterize a low flow lesion. MRI provides excellent soft tissue resolution with the ability to differentiate bone, muscle, tendon, fat, skin and malformation. Contrast-assisted, dynamic MRA can also help determine if a vascular malformation is a high flow lesion through evaluation of the arterial system.

Treatment

Conservative management with elevation, compression garments and non-steroidal anti-inflammatories remain the first-line therapy. Low flow lesions do not grow, and symptoms are often mild to moderate. Phlebitis can develop intermittently and present with periods of more intense pain, but these symptoms will alleviate in a few weeks.

Patients with daily pain, difficulty sleeping or working will often request treatment. Malformations are often insinuated into the deeper structures such as muscle, tendon, nerves and near bone. Surgical excision is often not curative, and symptoms recur. The morbidity of surgery often does not justify the treatment; therefore, embolization is the generally preferred invasive treatment option.

Choice of liquid embolic agents varies among providers. Embolic agents can be categorized by the efficacy compared to the side effect profile. Absolute alcohol is considered the most powerful agent with a mechanism of direct denaturation of proteins. The potency of alcohol is balanced by its higher side effect profile characterized by damage to nearby structures such as nerves, tendons and skin. If injected superficially, alcohol can blister and ulcerate the skin. A further concern regarding alcohol use relates to total dose or volume. Higher doses can result in alcohol intoxication and sudden pulmonary venous hypertension.

Detergents are another class of liquid embolic agents. These chemicals, such as sodium tetradecyl sulfate and polidocanol, are commonly used for the treatment of varicose veins. Detergent agents come in varying concentrations with higher concentrations more associated with complications such as skin damage or deep vein thrombosis. Detergent agents can be delivered as liquid or can be foamed to expand the volume and displace the blood, allowing for more endothelial contact with the detergent. Hand foam is generated using air by the Tessari method.[3] A low nitrogen formulation of polidocanol is available commercially but not FDA approved for treatment of vascular malformations.[4] Detergent agents are most commonly delivered by direct needle puncture of the malformation as seen in Figure 19.2.

Digital subtraction angiogram of a low flow vascular malformation, Blue arrow points to the needle used for access. Red arrow points to the low flow vascular malformation. White arrow point to normal draining veins

Liquid to solid polymerizing agents can also be utilized for embolization. Cyanoacrylate is commonly used for GI bleeding and is rapidly polymerizing glue. It is generally injected transcatheter but can be used through a direct needle puncture. It rapidly solidifies and does not generally allow for repeat treatments through the same catheter. Ethylene vinyl alcohol, tradename Onyx, is another polymerizing agent approved for treatment of brain AVMs. It can also be injected by a transcatheter or direct needle injections. Advantages include a slower polymerization rate of 30 to 60 seconds. It also comes in two different densities to allow for different flow and penetration rates. Both liquid embolic agents require careful use to prevent

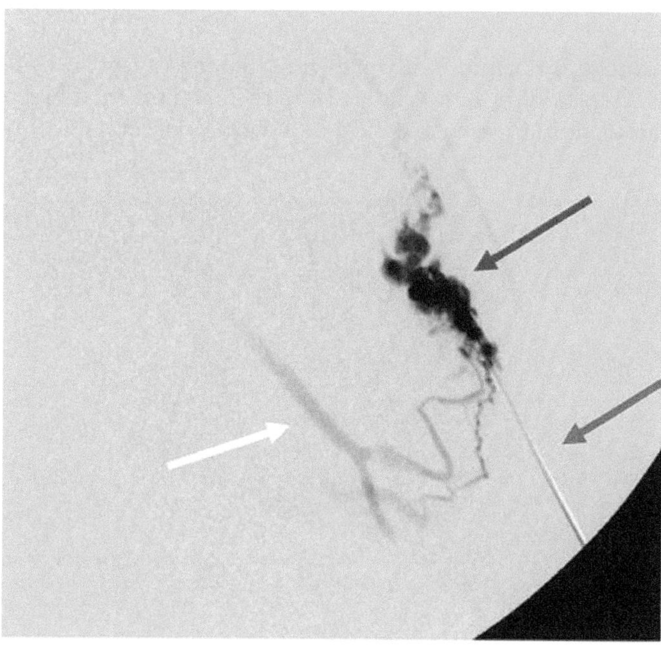

Figure 19.2 Direct needle puncture of a low flow vascular malformation.

non-target embolization and "trapping" or gluing the catheter into the patient. Onyx remains radiodense and can obscure further imaging by angiography or CT scanning. Surgical excision of Onyx with electrocautery can create sparks due to the rare earth element tantalum used in Onyx.[5] Bipolar electrocautery can reduce the fire risk during surgery. In general, the use of liquid embolic agents for venous malformations in clinical practice has been associated with only partial occlusion or recanalization of the treated areas. Also, many low malformations present in superficial locations, and some patients will complain of the firmness of the glue under the skin.

Mechanical agents can also be used for low flow embolization. Large embryonal veins and larger diameter vascular channels can be filled with a variety of coils or plugs. However, most low flow malformations are not well managed with mechanical occlusions devices.

Surgery for extensive malformations involving muscle layers or deeper are rarely curative as complete removal of the malformation is not possible. Symptom improvement can be seen with incomplete, debulking-type surgery; however, over the course of years, most patients have recurrent symptoms. Curative surgery is more likely in lesions confined to the skin and subcutaneous layers.

HIGH FLOW MALFORMATIONS

Presentation

High flow lesions can be symptomatic or asymptomatic. Anatomically, these lesions can present anywhere on the body with the highest rates in the brain. These lesions are more likely to grow, to be destructive of local anatomy and to present with bleeding (at times life threatening) and tissue loss (Figure 19.3) than their low flow counterparts.

IMAGING

Plain radiographs rarely are helpful with high flow lesions except to evaluate long bone length or bone loss. Duplex ultrasound can assist in the diagnosis of a high flow lesion. On B-mode, duplex can identify a vascular lesion and map blood vessels. On color flow and

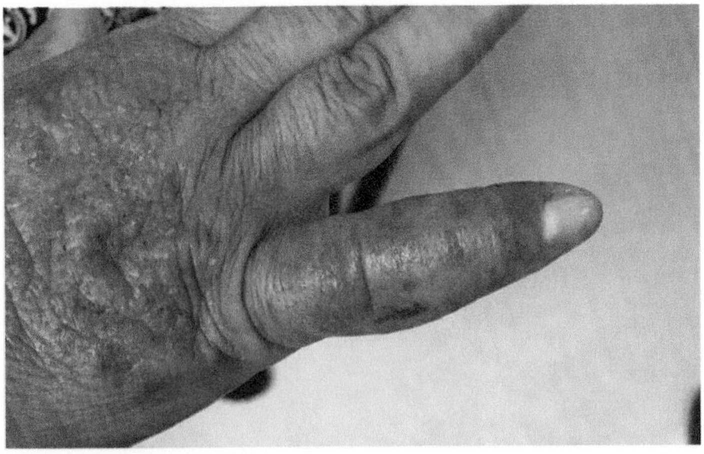

Figure 19.3 High flow malformation on physical exam. Localized swelling of the fifth digit, skin changes with early ulceration.

Doppler, high flow lesions will demonstrate mosaicism and high flow, low resistance arterial flow. Unlike low flow lesions, CT imaging can be helpful with high flow lesions. Arterial ectasia and early contrast filling of the venous system is often seen with high flow lesions. Similar to CT, MRI and contrast-enhanced, dynamic MRI will demonstrate arterial ectasia, the nidus filling and early venous drainage of contrast (Figure 19.4). Digital subtraction trans arterial angiography is diagnostic, demonstrating arterial feeding vessels, nidus filling and early venous filling as seen in Figure 19.5.

Digital subtraction angiogram of the right foot. Ectatic tibial arteries feed the AVM nidus centrally.

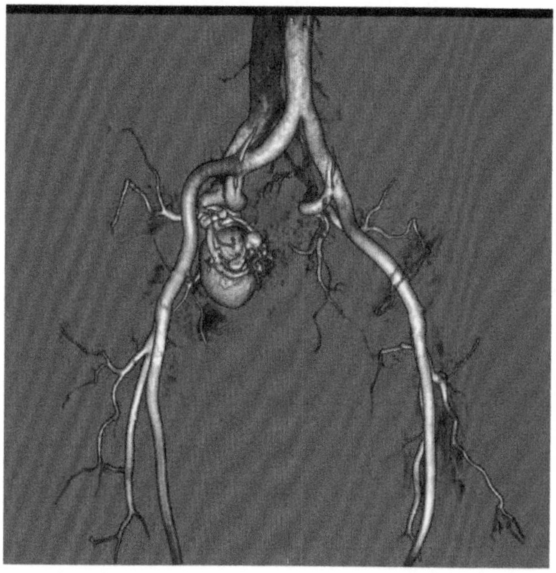

Figure 19.4 Magnetic resonance angiography reconstruction of a high flow pelvic AVM.

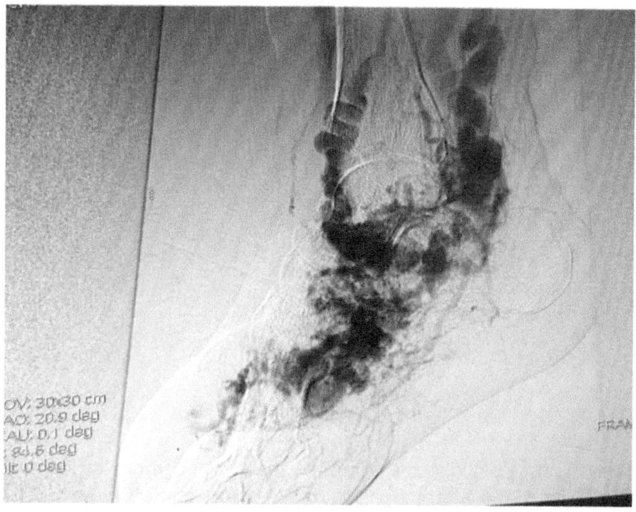

Figure 19.5 Angiogram of a high flow vascular malformation.

MANAGEMENT

Conservative management of a high flow malformation is not generally recommended. High flow lesions will grow with time and can cause thrombocytopenia, pulmonary hypertension and high output cardiac failure.[6] Watching a high flow malformation maybe reserved for high-risk patients or lesions in high-risk anatomic locations in which the risk of a complication outweighs the risk of watching the lesion. The most common group of patients who do not undergo treatment are patients with minimal to no symptoms who elect no treatment.

The primary treatment of high flow vascular malformations is embolization. Surgical excision, similar to low flow lesions, is technically difficult, unlikely to be curative and has the additional risk of significant bleeding. More superficial and smaller lesions can more reliably undergo surgical excisions. Reports of combined preoperative embolization followed by surgical excision have been documented in the literature.

Embolization of high flow lesions targets the nidus of the malformation with the goal of disconnecting the arterial system from the venous system. In other words, the goal is to stop the flow of blood through the low resistance circuit provided by the nidus. On imaging, most high flow malformations demonstrate ectatic feeding arterial vessels, which provide access to the nidus. Visualization of the nidus can be challenging due to the irregular, non-anatomic, three-dimensional nature of the nidus. Moreover, the flow rate of blood or contrast through

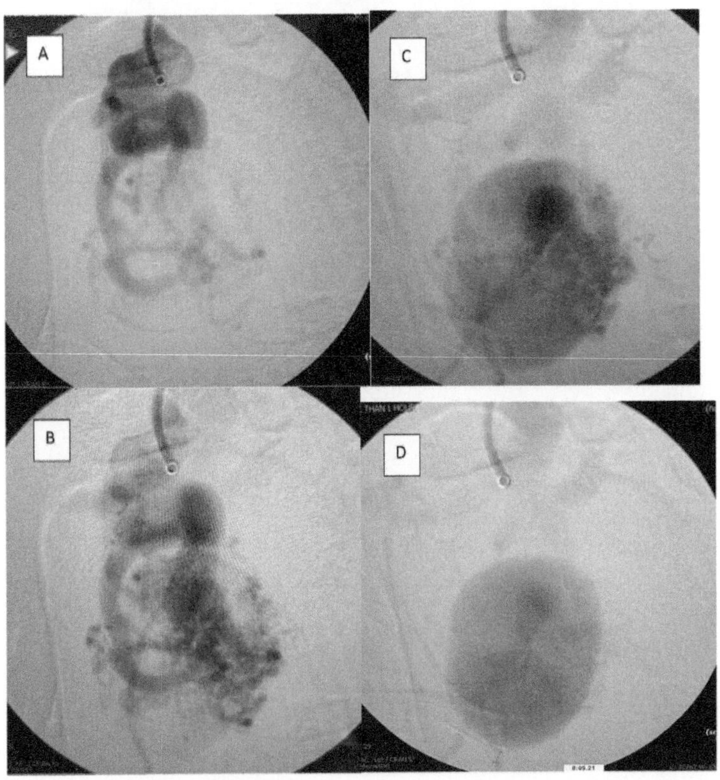

Figure 19.6 (A) Early arterial phase of a digital subtraction angiogram demonstrating feeding arteries; (B) nidus identification; (C) venous phase of the subtraction angiogram demonstrating nidus and filling of a venous aneurysm; (D) delayed imaging demonstrated pooling of contrast in a large pelvic venous aneurysm.

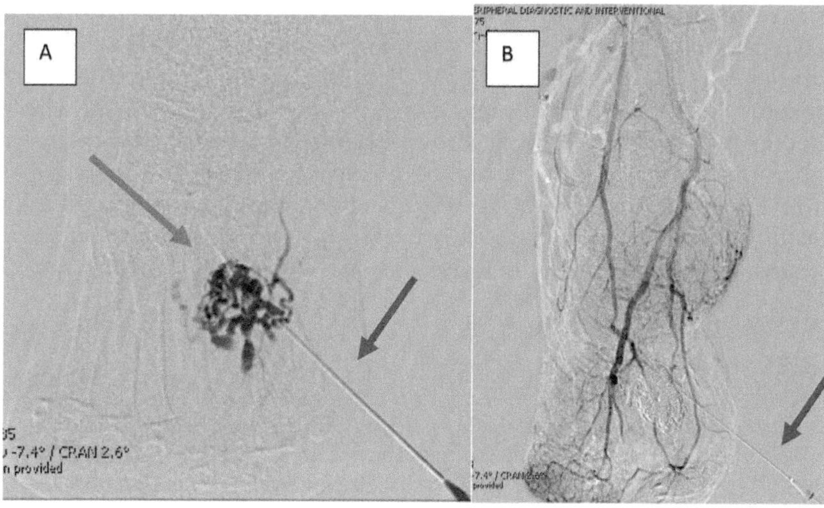

Figure 19.7 Combined direct puncture and transcatheter angiography of a high flow AVM of the foot. (A) Direct needle puncture angiography of a right foot AVM, red arrow points to needle, blue arrow to AVM. (B) Transcatheter angiogram of the same AVM after embolization, red arrow points to needle.

the nidus is high so that visualization is momentary. With large high flow AVM, the venous drainage is often dilated and can also distract from the actual nidus location. The draining veins fill after the nidus during an angiogram (Figure 19.6).

With the goal of treating the nidus, accessing it can be considered through a variety of routes. Traditionally, nidus access is done by a trans arterial, transcatheter route. For many malformations, this requires super selective catheterization of numerous feeding vessels. Some lesions do not allow for easy trans arterial access, and direct needle puncture is an option. Advantages of direct needle access are the ease of access, little to no risk of catheter entrapment with liquid embolic agents and bypassing small or tortuous feeding vessels for direct nidus access. A major drawback is the inability to image the malformation in its entirety with direct needle access. This can be managed with a hybrid approach of trans arterial angiography for imaging and direct needle access for treatment as shown in Figure 19.7. At times, a high flow connection lacks an accessible nidus and can look more like an arteriovenous fistula. Retrograde treatment via a transvenous route is another viable option.

Choices of embolic agents depends on the size and access of the nidus. A large volume nidus can be treated with mechanical agents such as plugs or coils. Also, a shorter length or a direct arterial-venous connection can be well managed with plugs as commonly seen with a renal AVM. Generally, most AVM have numerous feeding vessels, which can be catheterized for the delivery of liquid polymerizing agents. As previously described, cyanoacrylate and Onyx are common choices for treatment.

CONCLUSIONS

Vascular malformations are best described as embryologic errors in angiogenesis. They are not tumors like hemangiomas, a benign vascular tumor. Clinical management of vascular malformations is best informed by identifying a lesion as low or high flow. Low flow lesions are often symptomatic with localized swelling, heaviness, throbbing and intermittent phlebitis.

Conservative treatment with elevation, compression and an anti-inflammatory is generally safe and recommended. The treatment goal is to improve the quality of life as low flow lesions rarely bleed, grow or result in wounds. Complications of ulceration, nerve injuries or bleeding should be low for these lesions. High flow lesions are more likely to present with bleeding, ulceration and more severe pain. Treatment to reduce flow is recommended to prevent future growth, high output cardiac failure, thrombocytopenia and bleeding. Cure can be difficult with numerous arterial feeding vessels and recruitment of new vessels to the nidus. Both high flow and low flow lesions are most commonly treated with embolization techniques as surgical excision often cannot offer a cure but risks bleeding and surgical morbidity.

REFERENCES

1. Sharma CS, Bhandari SN, Rai M. Successful management of a rare manifestation of intramuscular venous malformation in a young adult: A case report. Cureus. 2023;15:e37812.
2. Andrews L, Shope C, Lee LW, Hochman M. Vascular anomalies: Nomenclature and Diagnosis. Dermatol Clin. 2022;40:339–343.
3. Shi X, Liu Y, Li D, Tursun M, Azmoun S, Liu S. The stability of physician-compounded foam is influenced by the angle of the connector. Ann Vasc Surg. In Press.
4. Redondo P, Cabrera J. Microfoam sclerotherapy. Semin Cutan Med Surg. 2005;24:175–183.
5. Schirmer CM, Zerris V, Malek AM. Electrocautery-induced ignition of spark showers and self sustained combustion of onyx ethylene-vinyl alcohol copolymer. Neurosurgery. 2006;59:413–418.
6. Chakkarapani AA, Gupta S, Jamil A, Yadav SK, Subhedar N, Hummler HD. Effects of inhaled nitric oxide in pulmonary hypertension secondary to arteriovenous malformations: A retrospective cohort study from the European iNO registry. Eur J Pediatr. 2022;181:3915–3922.

Chapter 20

Contemporary and Evidence-Based Medical Therapy for VTE

Oscar Y. Moreno-Rocha, Andrea T. Obi, and Thomas W. Wakefield

Venous thrombosis is a unique vascular pathology affecting the venous circulation and can cause local and systemic consequences of primary thrombus and subsequent emboli.[1] It is predisposed by stasis, venous wall injury, and hypercoagulability. Furthermore, the composition of venous thrombi can differ according to the timing, etiology, and shear stress, which, to a lesser extent, is responsible for increasing platelet recruitment.[2, 3] The sum of all these processes converges in thrombosis characterized by endothelial injury and activation, platelet-endothelial cell interaction, leukocyte-leukocyte interactions, leukocyte-endothelial and leukocyte-platelet interactions, and the release of tissue factor (TF).

EPIDEMIOLOGY

Venous thromboembolism (VTE) can affect more than 900,000 patients per year, including deep venous thrombosis (DVT) 378,623 (42%) and pulmonary embolism (PE) 531,370 (58%), resulting in up to 300,000 deaths per year, primary related to PE 294,112 (99%) and a lesser extent DVT 2,258 (1%).[4] A European ancestry database reported an annual VTE rate of 104 to 183 per 100,000 person-years.[5] The incidence of PE diagnosis in the United States has increased from 62 per 100,000 in 1998 to 112 per 100,000 in 2006 and 120 per 100,000 in 2016. The increase in incidence may be due to the rise in the diagnosis of smaller PEs.[6–9] VTE incidence increases with age but can vary regarding the population assessed, being higher in Black populations and lower in Asian and Native American populations. The most common location for acute DVT is the calf (posterior tibial [PT] and peroneal are more common than anterior tibial [AT], which are rare), followed by the femoral, popliteal, and iliac veins. Also, an increasing prevalence of obesity, cancer, and surgery accounts in part for the persistent VTE incidence. It's related annual incident cost to the US healthcare system is from $7 to $10 billion each year. Acute VTE treatment is associated with an incremental direct medical cost of $12,000 to $15,000 (2014 US dollars) with subsequent cumulative costs up to $18,000 to $23,000 per incident case from complications including recurrent VTE, chronic venous disease (CVD), post-thrombotic syndrome (PTS), venous ulcers (VU), and venous varicosities (VV).[10] These complications can increase the incident cost by an average of 75%,[5, 11] and it is established that DVT and PE are amongst the most common preventable causes of hospital death.[12]

RISK FACTORS

VTE risk factors are classified as acquired and genetic. Acquired factors are aging, gender (female), active malignancy (higher in patients with active chemotherapy), surgery, immobilization, trauma, oral contraceptives use and estrogen hormone replacement therapy

DOI: 10.1201/9781003316626-23

(independent of its duration), pregnancy due to the compression of the iliac veins and the puerperium, neurologic disease, cardiovascular disease, obesity, sepsis, pneumonia, calf muscle pump dysfunction, and inflammatory bowel disease.[10, 13] Genetic factors include antithrombin deficiency, protein C deficiency and protein S deficiency, factor V Leiden, prothrombin 20210A, blood group non-O, abnormalities in fibrinogen and plasminogen, elevated levels of clotting factors (e.g., factors XI, IX, VII, VIII, X, and II), and elevation in plasminogen activator inhibitor 1 (PAI-1).[10, 14] Up to 25% of patients presenting with acute DVT can have a history of a previous DVT.[15] Following an episode of DVT, 20 to 50% of patients experience permanent damage to the venous valves or vein walls, leading to incompetent valves, persistent obstruction, and increased venous pressure, called post-thrombotic syndrome (PTS).[16] COVID-19 infection has also been associated with the development of VTE due to the multiorgan endothelial dysfunction related to an exacerbated coagulopathy overlapping inflammatory pathways that lead to a hypercoagulable state, micro thrombosis, large vessel thrombosis, and death. VTE in COVID-19 ICU critically ill patients has a reported rate between 25% and 30%.[17–19]

Family history of chronic venous insufficiency (CVI) in both parents, osteoarticular disease of the lower limbs, truncal varicose veins, involvement of the great saphenous vein, lymphedema, and thrombophlebitis have been associated with the development and severity of CVI.[20] In cases of unprovoked VTE, family history of thrombosis, recurrent thrombosis, or thrombosis in unusual locations, a hypercoagulability workup may be indicated, although routine testing for hypercoagulable pathologies does not alter the medical management in the acute setting. Other diseases associated with VTE include hematologic (heparin-induced thrombocytopenia, thrombotic microangiopathy, antiphospholipid syndrome, hemolytic uremic syndrome [HUS], atypical HUS [aHUS], thrombotic thrombocytopenic purpura [TTP]), disseminated intravascular coagulation, myeloproliferative disorders, and COVID-19 associated coagulopathy.[21] The Caprini risk score is the most common risk prediction score for VTE in surgical patients, and prophylaxis is based on the risk of thrombosis defined by the score. Recommendations include early ambulation (scores 1–2), intermittent compression (scores 3–4), and pharmacological prophylaxis + intermittent compression (scores 5 or greater), but the score also can identify very high-risk patients above 8 points for whom continuation of VTE prophylaxis post discharge for at least 30 days is recommended.[22, 23]

Roger's score assesses the risk of postoperative VTE among non-cardiac surgery patients with a low risk from 1 to 6, a moderate risk from 7–10, and a high risk > 10.[24] In hospitalized patients, the IMPROVE risk score predicts the 3-month risk of VTE from 0 to 10 (a score of 10 is a 7.2% 3-month VTE risk).[25, 26] The Padua prediction score determines the anticoagulation needed in hospitalized patients by risk of VTE. With a Padua Score ≥4 points, pharmacologic prophylaxis is indicated. If there is a high risk of bleeding, mechanical prophylaxis is recommended. With a Padua Score <4 points, pharmacologic prophylaxis is not indicated, but mechanical prophylaxis should be used.[27, 28] In cancer patients, the Khorana score, endorsed by the American Society of Clinical Oncology and the National Comprehensive Cancer Network, is used to select ambulatory cancer patients for thromboprophylaxis. In outpatients, the 2.5-month rate of VTE risk remains relatively low even in the highest score groups (Low 0: 0.3–0.8%, Intermediate 1–2: 1.8–2.0%, High ≥3: 6.7–7.1%).[29, 30]

PATHOGENESIS

In addition to Virchow's 19th-century triad of stasis, vein wall injury, and hypercoagulability, our current understanding of the vein wall and thrombus interactions supports the significance of the inflammatory response and its resolution to the subsequent changes in the vein wall and valves, leading to pain and swelling in the limb (PTS). These hallmarks of thrombosis also offer new insights for novel therapeutic targets in the future. Perhaps by decreasing vascular inflammation and leukocyte-endothelium interactions, both thrombogenesis and its adverse sequelae on the vein wall can be diminished or even practically eliminated.[31]

DIAGNOSIS

Lower extremity DVT presents with unilateral calf pain and swelling symptoms and can be ruled out with the negative Wells score and a negative D-dimer.[10] The Wells score estimates the likelihood of DVT emphasizing physical presentation (where edema is the most common physical finding), the presence of active cancer, paralysis or paresis, recent plaster/cast immobilization of the lower extremity, being recently bedridden for three days or more, localized tenderness along the distribution of the deep venous system, swelling of the entire leg, calf swelling that is at least 3 cm larger on the involved side than on the non-involved side, pitting edema in the symptomatic leg, collateral superficial veins (nonvaricose), and a history of previous DVT.[10] Extensive proximal iliofemoral DVT may present with significant swelling, cyanosis, and dilated superficial collateral veins.[10] The negative predictive value of a low- or intermediate-risk Wells score with a negative D-dimer is nearly 100%, and DVT can be practically ruled out with an incidence of DVT over the next 3 months of 0% to 0.6%.

Duplex ultrasound imaging is the gold standard for ruling in the diagnosis of DVT because it is non-invasive, painless, widely available, requires no contrast, can be repeated, and is safe during pregnancy. It has sensitivity and specificity rates greater than 95% with a 1B level of evidence, depending on the pretest probability for DVT. Duplex ultrasound can also detect other potential causes of a patient's symptoms, which can help to rule out other possible diagnoses. It can also be used in symptomatic patients at the calf level. If the results of duplex ultrasound are inconclusive or if the patient has certain risk factors that make it difficult to interpret the ultrasound results (DVT in unusual locations such as the central pelvic veins or inferior vena cava [IVC]), an MRI or CTV should be obtained.

A negative duplex scan of the lower extremities is accurate enough to not require anticoagulation therapy, with minimal risk of long-term adverse thromboembolic complications. All leg veins must be examined using a duplex scan to make this decision. If the scan is inconclusive due to technical problems or swelling, treatment may be based on other factors, such as biomarkers, and the scan may be repeated in 24 to 72 hours. Using a combination of clinical characteristics and a high-sensitivity D-dimer test can reduce the number of duplex scans needed in patients who are at low risk. Although clinical features and D-dimer levels help rule out thrombosis, the converse is not true. No combination of biomarkers and clinical presentation can rule in the diagnosis yet. Still, novel translational research is focused on developing new biomarkers based on the body's inflammatory response to DVT. Our data suggest that a combination of the protein-soluble P-selectin and the Wells score can help confirm the diagnosis of DVT.[32] A D-dimer test and the Wells score should be repeated if duplex imaging is unavailable.

The differential diagnosis for DVT includes lymphedema, muscle strain, muscle contusion, and underlying systemic problems such as cardiac, renal, or hepatic abnormalities. These systemic issues often cause bilateral edema.[33] In rare cases, severe iliofemoral DVT can cause phlegmasia alba dolens (swollen white leg) or phlegmasia cerulea dolens (swollen blue leg).[34] If phlegmasia is not treated promptly, it can lead to venous gangrene when the arterial inflow is blocked by venous hypertension. This condition is often associated with underlying malignancy and always develops after phlegmasia cerulea dolens. Venous gangrene is associated with significant amputation rates, PE, and mortality.

Pulmonary Embolism

The diagnosis of PE has traditionally involved ventilation-perfusion scanning and pulmonary angiography. However, the most up-to-date techniques include spiral CT scanning, MRI, and assessments of pretest probability and high-sensitivity D-dimer levels. Furthermore, age-adjusted D-dimer measurements may improve the diagnostic value of these measurements. CT scanning has high specificity and sensitivity and can detect emboli as small as the subsegmental level. Its sensitivity can be improved by clinical analysis and lower extremity imaging. However, using higher-resolution multidetector-row CT imaging has called into question the need for lower extremity imaging in combination with CT. Alternative techniques for cases with contraindications to CT include MRI and ventilation-perfusion imaging. In low risk individuals, a score of 0 on the PE Rule-out Criteria indicates that further testing (D-dimer and CT) is unnecessary. The PE Rule-out Criteria include pulse oximetry of 94% or less, heart rate of 100 beats/min or higher, age of 50 years or older, unilateral leg swelling, hemoptysis, recent trauma or surgery, previous PE or DVT, and exogenous estrogen use.(10)

VTE Treatment

Anticoagulation is recommended for all patients who are candidates for anticoagulation with symptomatic proximal DVT, PE, and some cases of distal DVT. The need for anticoagulation is particularly strong for patients with proximal DVT, which affects veins in the thigh or pelvis, because these patients are at higher risk of complications such as PE and death, as more than 90% of cases of acute PE are caused by proximal DVT.(35, 36) When considering anticoagulants to treat DVT, the potential benefits of preventing further clotting must be balanced against the risk of bleeding. Therefore, the main goal of anticoagulation is to prevent additional thrombosis or thrombus extension and prevent PE and death. Late complications of VTE may include recurrent thrombosis, PTS from DVT, and chronic thromboembolic pulmonary hypertension from PE. It is crucial to start treatment with anticoagulants as soon as possible, as the risk of recurrent thrombosis is highest during the first month, followed by 3 months after the VTE event.(37–47) In the case of DVT, tests are often performed before starting treatment, and for PE, it is typical to start the medication and then test. However, even with proper treatment, up to one-third of patients may experience a recurrence of DVT over an 8-year period.(48)

The first line of treatment for venous thromboembolism (VTE) is anticoagulation, traditionally with heparin or low-molecular-weight heparin (LMWH) followed by oral anticoagulation with a vitamin K antagonist (warfarin). LMWH is the standard for initial treatment when an anticoagulant bridge is needed. It is administered subcutaneously, requires no monitoring (except with renal insufficiency or morbid obesity), and is associated with a lower risk of bleeding. Heparin or LMWH is stopped as soon as anticoagulation is therapeutic. When using warfarin, the international normalized ratio is recommended to be therapeutic for two consecutive days before stopping heparin or LMWH. Today, direct oral anticoagulants (DOACs) are now preferred to warfarin (Table 20.1). There are currently four DOACs that are approved by the US Food and Drug Administration (FDA) for the treatment of DVT and one for the prophylaxis of VTE. These include rivaroxaban (Xarelto) and apixaban (Eliquis), both requiring a loading dose period followed by a lower dose; dabigatran (Pradaxa) and edoxaban (Savaysa), both requiring a heparin or LMWH bridge; and betrixaban (Bevyxxa) for prophylaxis.(10) Dabigatran targets activated factor II (factor IIa), while rivaroxaban, apixaban, edoxaban, and betrixaban target activated factor X (factor Xa). The DOACs are preferred over warfarin for the treatment of acute DVT and PE, except with concomitant severe renal insufficiency, hemodynamically unstable PE, massive iliofemoral DVT (phlegmasia cerulea dolens), pregnancy, or antiphospholipid syndrome (APLS) (Figure 20.1).

Table 20.1 Initial Doses in Patients with Normal Renal Function

Anticoagulant	*Dose*
Rivaroxaban	15 mg by mouth twice daily for 21 days, followed by 20 mg once daily.
Apixaban	10 mg twice daily for seven days, followed by 5 mg twice daily (2.5 mg twice daily for extended treatment beyond 6 months).
Edoxaban	60 mg once daily.
Dabigatran	150 mg twice daily.

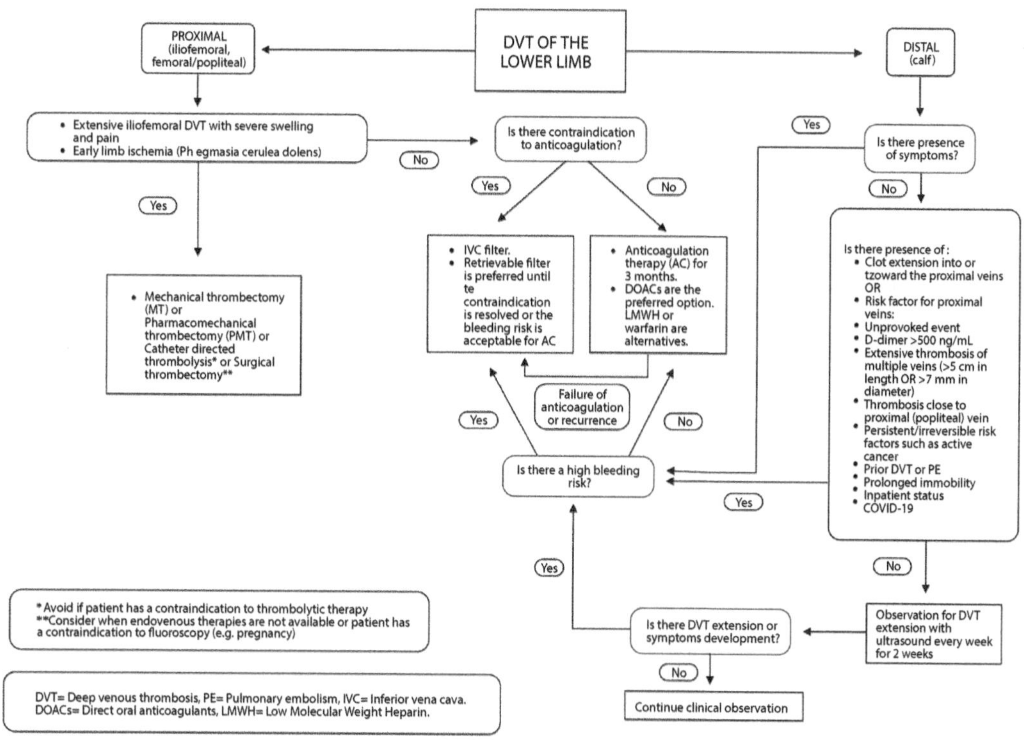

Figure 20.1 Algorithm for the treatment of deep venous thrombosis of the lower extremity.

For those rare patients with phlegmasia alba dolens or phlegmasia cerulea dolens, aggressive thrombolysis/thrombectomy is definitely indicated for limb salvage. In patients with significant symptomatic iliofemoral DVT, aggressive pharmacomechanical thrombolysis (PMT) or mechanical thrombectomy (MT) may be indicated to lessen long-term PTS. In patients with PE and systolic blood pressure of 90 mmHg or higher, first-line therapy consists of DOACs, such as apixaban, edoxaban, rivaroxaban, or dabigatran, that are as effective as heparin combined with a vitamin K antagonist followed by warfarin alone and have a 0.6% lower rate of bleeding.[6] In patients with PE and systolic blood pressure lower than 90 mmHg, systemic thrombolysis, PMT, or MT is recommended and is associated with a 1.6% absolute reduction in mortality (from 3.9% to 2.3%). However, it is controversial whether thrombolysis should be used when there is no hemodynamic compromise, but there is evidence of right heart dysfunction or positive biomarkers. Anticoagulation with heparin, including UFH and LMWH, is contraindicated with VTE and a diagnosis of heparin-induced thrombocytopenia (HIT), where a non-heparin anticoagulant should be administered. Finally, it is recommended that patients with antiphospholipid syndrome receive extended anticoagulation treatment with warfarin rather than DOACs.

Fondaparinux (Arixtra) is also approved for the treatment of VTE. It is a synthetic pentasaccharide that targets factor Xa. It has been approved for thrombosis prophylaxis in patients undergoing total hip replacement, total knee replacement, hip fracture surgery, as well as extended prophylaxis in patients with hip fractures and those undergoing abdominal surgery. It is administered subcutaneously and has a 17-hour half-life. Dosage is based on body weight and has a more predictable pharmacokinetic profile than LMWH since it does not bind to endothelial cells or protein, nor does it cause thrombocytopenia. However, there is currently no antidote for fondaparinux. Regarding effectiveness for treating VTE, fondaparinux is as effective as LMWH for DVT, and for PE, it is equivalent to standard heparin. Although LMWH has been the standard treatment for cancer-associated VTE, direct oral anticoagulants such as edoxaban and rivaroxaban are effective but with a higher risk of bleeding. A recent study found that apixaban at therapeutic doses was non-inferior to LMWH dalteparin (Fragmin) with no increased risk of major bleeding for the treatment of cancer-associated VTE.(10)

Regarding COVID-19-associated thrombosis, the ISTH has published guidelines recommending the use of therapeutic-dose heparin (with LMWH preferred) for patients with a high D-dimer level, low flow oxygen requirements, and no increased risk of bleeding.(49) Prophylactic-dose heparin is recommended for patients receiving intensive care. There are ongoing studies evaluating the use of anticoagulants in COVID-19 patients to treat both macro- and micro thrombosis with previously used and novel anticoagulants like the RECOVERY, ACTIV-4a, REMAP-CAP, CRITICAL, and GARDEN trials.(50) Some guidelines also suggest post-discharge anticoagulation for COVID-19 patients. These recommendations may change as more data becomes available.(10, 51, 52)

Surveillance without anticoagulation is recommended for patients with isolated distal DVT who are at high risk of bleeding or have a strong preference against taking anticoagulants. This approach is supported by several studies that have found that limited thrombosis confined to the calf veins has a low risk of extension without treatment compared to extensive thrombosis of multiple calf veins (about 3% versus 15%). In addition, natural history studies suggest that if the thrombosis does not extend within 2 weeks of diagnosis, it is unlikely to do so. Ultrasound is used to check for thrombus extension or resolution once a week for 2 weeks or earlier if the patient develops new or worsening symptoms. For surveillance, it is preferred to use proximal ultrasound because it is sufficient for detecting proximal DVT, for which the need for anticoagulation is strong.(53–64) Anticoagulation is preferred for patients with risk factors (Table 20.2), with proximal DVT extension, extensive thrombosis of multiple veins (>5 cm in length OR >7 mm in diameter), or thrombosis close to proximal (popliteal) vein (1 to 2 cm).(48) New studies have also shown that smaller PEs that are not life-threatening could be left untreated without adverse outcomes.(6, 65)

Nonpharmacologic treatments for DVT include using compression stockings to control symptoms of pain, swelling, and leg fatigue. Walking with optimal compression does not increase the risk of PE. Although compression therapy is essential in managing the pain and swelling of DVT, there is controversy whether it can decrease the development of PTS.(66–68) The ACCP guidelines suggest that compression stockings may not prevent the development of PTS after a first proximal DVT based on the SOX trial.(69) However, the immediate application of compression therapy has been found to lessen surrogate PTS markers reducing residual vein obstruction.(70) Thus, the main issue for preventing PTS may be the immediate application of compression.

Table 20.2 Factors Favoring Anticoagulation or Surveillance in Calf DVT

Factors Favoring Anticoagulation	*Factors Favoring Surveillance*
• Symptoms (other than minor ones) • Thrombus extension into or close to (1–2 cm) the proximal popliteal vein • Extensive thrombosis involving multiple veins (>5 cm in length, >7 mm in diameter) • D-dimer ≥500 ng/mL • Unprovoked DVT • Persistent/irreversible risk factors, such as active cancer or prolonged immobility • Previous DVT or PE • Inpatient status • COVID-19	• No symptoms (or minor symptoms) • High-risk features of proximal extension are absent (refer to the "Factors Favoring Anticoagulation" column) • Minor thrombosis in the muscular veins • A negative D-dimer level (i.e., <500 ng/mL) • Nondiagnostic ultrasonography results • High risk of, or contraindications due to bleeding

Duration of Treatment

Anticoagulation therapy duration should be individualized according to the presence of provoking events, risk factors, and risk for recurrence and bleeding. After the first episode of provoked VTE, anticoagulation is recommended for 3 months for both proximal and distal thrombi (if symptomatic). If the course of treatment is shortened to 4 or 6 weeks, it is associated with an increased risk of recurrent thrombosis.[25, 29, 30] If a patient has a second episode of VTE, it is usually recommended that they take oral anticoagulants indefinitely unless they are at high risk for bleeding as calculated by VTE-BLEED score or if they are very young at the time of their presentation.[71, 72] If a patient has a homozygous factor V Leiden or prothrombin 20210A mutation, protein C or protein S deficiency, antithrombin deficiency, antiphospholipid antibodies, or cancer, their risk of VTE recurrence is increased. As a result, long-term oral anticoagulation is usually recommended in these situations. However, if a patient has a heterozygous factor V Leiden or prothrombin 20210A mutation, their risk is not as high, the length of oral anticoagulation treatment can be shortened, and lifetime anticoagulation is not needed (unless these heterozygous states are combined in the same individual).[10]

In patients with unprovoked DVT and a low or moderate risk of bleeding, extended therapy (treatment lasting more than 3 months) is recommended. Patients at high risk of bleeding should be treated for 3 months and reevaluated. Tools such as thrombosis risk factors, residual thrombus burden, and coagulation system activation can help determine whether to continue or discontinue anticoagulation. The VIENNA[73, 74] and the DASH[75, 76] scores are prediction models to identify individuals at low risk for VTE recurrence after an unprovoked VTE in whom anticoagulation therapy could be discontinued after 3 months. These scores take into account the patient's sex, age, DVT location, D-dimer level, and the use of hormones in women at the time of the DVT onset to calculate the recurrence predicted probability within 12 to 60 months.[75, 76] The HERDOO2 score has been suggested to identify women at low risk of recurrent VTE who can stop taking anticoagulants.[77]

For the general patient population, extended therapy with low-dose DOACs is recommended when the risk-benefit relationship favors continued treatment. Studies have shown that an extended low dose of rivaroxaban can significantly decrease the rate of recurrent VTE without increasing the risk of major bleeding compared to aspirin. Additionally, extended treatment with low-dose apixaban has been found to provide long-term protection against recurrent VTE. In patients who cannot continue taking DOACs after initial treatment for VTE and do not have contraindications, aspirin should be given to prevent recurrent thrombosis.[78]

The use of bridging (temporary interruption and restarting of anticoagulation) during surgical procedures has been controversial. Bridging has been found to be associated with no decrease in thrombotic events but with a higher risk of bleeding and should only be used in high-risk patients. Currently, bridging therapy is only recommended for patients with atrial fibrillation and a recent stroke, atrial fibrillation and a high CHADS2 score,[5, 6] a recent VTE within the past 3 months, or mechanical cardiac valves, especially mitral valves.[79] The availability of DOACs with short half-lives has decreased the need for heparin or LMWH-based bridging. In most cases, DOACs only need to be stopped for 1 day for minor procedures and 2 days for major procedures and can be restarted as soon as it is safe from a surgical or procedural perspective. All patients taking anticoagulant medications should be monitored for therapeutic efficacy (recurrence prevention), bleeding, the development of conditions that can affect the half-life of the medications (renal failure, pregnancy, weight gain/loss), as well as for adverse effects of the medications (such as skin necrosis, thrombocytopenia, or osteoporosis).

In patients with active cancer, using LMWH is superior to LMWH converted to warfarin in patients with a renal clearance of ≥30 mL/min, and anticoagulation should be given for a minimum of 6 months or until the cancer is no longer active. Edoxaban, rivaroxaban, or apixaban are recommended in cancer patients with creatinine clearance is ≥30 mL/min in the absence of strong pharmacological interactions or gastrointestinal absorption impairment. Edoxaban and rivaroxaban should be used with caution in patients with a GI malignancy due to an increased risk of GI bleeding.[80]

Complications

Bleeding is the most common complication of anticoagulation. Tools available, such as the HAS-BLED score, can help estimate a patient's risk of bleeding while taking anticoagulant medications.[81–83] Risk factors for bleeding while on anticoagulation include age >65 (1 point), age >75 (2 points), previous bleeding, cancer and metastatic cancer, renal or liver failure, thrombocytopenia, prior stroke, diabetes, anemia, concurrent antiplatelet therapy, poor anticoagulant control, reduced functional capacity, recent surgery (within 3 months from index event), frequent falls (two or more in the last year), alcohol abuse, and non-steroidal anti-inflammatory drug use (NSAIDs).[10, 84] The presence of zero risk factors for major bleeding confers an absolute risk of 0.8% per year. Patients with one risk factor have a risk of 1.6% per year, and those with two or more have a 6.5% risk or higher per year. Standard heparin is associated with a bleeding rate of 10% over the first 5 days of treatment. Warfarin has a major bleeding rate of 1–2% per year. DOACs may have a total bleeding rate of 5–10%, although the risk of intracerebral bleeding appears to be lower than warfarin. However, the DOACs have their own challenges, including difficulty reversing their anticoagulant effects and difficulties with laboratory monitoring.

Heparin-induced thrombocytopenia (HIT) can occur in 0.6 to 30% of patients taking heparin or LMWH, which is associated with high morbidity and mortality rates. Still, early diagnosis and appropriate treatment can decrease these rates. HIT usually develops 3–14 days after starting unfractionated heparin, although it can occur earlier in patients who have previously been exposed to heparin. Even small exposures to heparin, such as heparin coating on indwelling catheters, can cause HIT. This exposure leads to the formation of antibodies that bind to platelets and activate them, releasing procoagulant microparticles and leading to increased thrombocytopenia and thrombosis. LMWHs have high cross-reactivity with standard heparin antibodies. Both UFH and LMWH have been associated with HIT, although the incidence and severity of thrombosis are lower with LMWH. The HIT diagnosis might be suspected with a 50% or greater drop in platelet count below 100,000/uL or when thrombosis occurs during heparin or LMWH therapy. There are two laboratory tests for HIT. The enzyme-linked immunosorbent assay (ELISA) can detect the anti-heparin antibody in the plasma, but this test is highly sensitive but not very specific. The serotonin release assay can be used as a confirmatory test and is more specific but less sensitive than the enzyme-linked immunosorbent assay. Heparin must be discontinued, and oral anticoagulation should not be started until an alternative anticoagulant has been established and the platelet count has normalized. Argatroban is FDA-approved for prophylaxis and treatment of thrombosis in patients with HIT and HITTS (heparin-induced thrombocytopenia and thrombosis syndrome).[85, 86] Non-FDA-approved alternatives include fondaparinux (Arixtra).[10]

New Novel Therapies for VTE

The goals of treating DVT are to prevent the extension or recurrence of DVT, prevent PE, and minimize the long-term effects of thrombosis, such as CVI. Standard anticoagulants can achieve the first two goals but not the third. PTS can occur in up to 30–50% of patients with DVT and even more frequently in patients with iliofemoral DVT. Reopening the vein is thought to alleviate venous hypertension and prevent PTS, a concept known as the "open vein hypothesis". [87] There is evidence to support more aggressive treatments for extensive thrombosis, including the fact that prolonged contact of the thrombus with the vein wall can increase damage and that the thrombus can initiate an inflammatory response in the vein wall that can lead to vein wall fibrosis and valvular dysfunction. The longer a thrombus is in contact with a vein valve, the less likely it is to function correctly.[10]

With the previous comments in mind, alternative forms of therapy with improved efficacy and decreased bleeding are needed to address these limitations. Factor XII and XI have been identified as potential targets for such agents.[88] Selectins, a family of glycoproteins that facilitate and augment thrombosis, have also been studied as potential biomarkers for thrombosis and as targets for agents to limit thrombosis and subsequent vein wall fibrosis that leads to PTS. Inhibition of P-selectin and E-selectin has been shown to decrease thrombosis and vein wall fibrosis without increasing bleeding in multiple different animal models (and E-selectin inhibition in two patients with calf vein thrombosis).[86] Selectin inhibition is a promising area of future study for treating VTE, either as a standalone therapy or as an adjunct to standard anticoagulation. Additionally, novel therapies to enhance fibrinolysis and decrease inflammation in PE and DVT patients are under development. These novel VTE therapies offer opportunities for improving treatment outcomes.[89–99] Finally, another new development (specifically in the treatment of PE) is the use of PE response teams (PERTs), which have become common. They allow for a coordinated and rapid treatment of PE by a multidisciplinary group of providers, such as non-invasive clinicians, emergency physicians, clinical pharmacists, endovascular proceduralists, and cardiac, thoracic, and vascular surgeons. The effectiveness of the PERT team for the treatment of PE is an area of active investigation.[10]

REFERENCES

1. Loscalzo J, Fauci AS, Kasper DL, Hauser SL, Longo DL, Jameson JL (Eds.). Harrison's Principles of Internal Medicine (21st ed., p. 1). New York: McGraw-Hill, 2022.
2. Quadros AS, Cambruzzi E, Sebben J, David RB, Abelin A, Welter D, et al. Red versus white thrombi in patients with ST-elevation myocardial infarction undergoing primary percutaneous coronary intervention: Clinical and angiographic outcomes. Am Heart J. 2012 Oct;164(4):553–60.
3. Jackson SP. Arterial thrombosis – insidious, unpredictable and deadly. Nat Med. 2011 Nov;17(11):1423–36.

4. Barnes DM, Wakefield TW, Rectenwald JE. Novel biomarkers associated with deep venous thrombosis: A comprehensive review. Biomark Insights. 2008 Jan;3.
5. Heit JA, Spencer FA, White RH. The epidemiology of venous thromboembolism. J Thromb Thrombolysis. 2016 Jan;41(1):3–14.
6. Freund Y, Cohen-Aubart F, Bloom B. Acute pulmonary embolism: A review. JAMA. 2022 Oct 4;328(13):1336.
7. Virani SS, Alonso A, Benjamin EJ, Bittencourt MS, Callaway CW, Carson AP, et al. Heart disease and stroke statistics – 2020 update: A report from the American Heart Association. Circulation. 2020 Mar 3 [cited 2022 Dec 10];141(9). Retrieved from www.ahajournals.org/doi/10.1161/CIR.0000000000000757
8. Wiener RS, Schwartz LM, Woloshin S. When a test is too good: How CT pulmonary angiograms find pulmonary emboli that do not need to be found. BMJ. 2013 Jul 3;347(2):f3368.
9. Wiener RS, Schwartz LM, Woloshin S. Time trends in pulmonary embolism in the United States: Evidence of overdiagnosis. Arch Intern Med. 2011 May 9;171(9). Retrieved from http://archinte.jamanetwork.com/article.aspx?doi=10.1001/archinternmed.2011.178
10. Kellerman RD, Rakel D. Conn's Current Therapy 2021(pp. 161–65). Phildelphia, PA: Elsevier, 2020.
11. Heit JA, Ashrani AA, Crusan DJ, McBane RD, Petterson TM, Bailey KR. Reasons for the persistent incidence of venous thromboembolism. Thromb Haemost. 2017;117(2):390–400.
12. Jha AK, Larizgoitia I, Audera-Lopez C, Prasopa-Plaizier N, Waters H, Bates DW. The global burden of unsafe medical care: Analytic modelling of observational studies. BMJ Qual Saf. 2013 Oct;22(10):809–15.
13. Kindell DG, Marulanda K, Caruso DM, Duchesneau E, Agala C, Farber M, et al. Incidence of venous thromboembolism in patients with peripheral arterial disease after endovascular intervention. J Vasc Surg Venous Lymphat Disord. 2023 Jan;11(1):61–9.
14. Lutsey PL, Zakai NA. Epidemiology and prevention of venous thromboembolism. Nat Rev Cardiol. 2022 Oct 18 [cited 2022 Dec 16]; Retrieved from www.nature.com/articles/s41569-022-00787-6
15. Thaler J, Pabinger I, Ay C. Anticoagulant treatment of deep vein thrombosis and pulmonary embolism: The present state of the art. Front Cardiovasc Med. 2015 Jul 14 [cited 2022 Dec 10];2. Retrieved from http://journal.frontiersin.org/Article/10.3389/fcvm.2015.00030/abstract
16. Eberhardt RT, Raffetto JD. Chronic venous insufficiency. Circulation. 2014 Jul 22;130(4):333–46.
17. Llitjos J, Leclerc M, Chochois C, Monsallier J, Ramakers M, Auvray M, et al. High incidence of venous thromboembolic events in anticoagulated severe COVID-19 patients. J Thromb Haemost. 2020 Jul;18(7):1743–46.
18. Klok FA, Kruip MJHA, van der Meer NJM, Arbous MS, Gommers DAMPJ, Kant KM, et al. Incidence of thrombotic complications in critically ill ICU patients with COVID-19. Thromb Res. 2020 Jul;191:145–47.
19. Longchamp A, Longchamp J, Manzocchi-Besson S, Whiting L, Haller C, Jeanneret S, et al. Venous thromboembolism in critically Ill patients with COVID-19: Results of a screening study for deep vein thrombosis. Res Pract Thromb Haemost. 2020 Jul;4(5):842–47.
20. Mota-Capitão L, Menezes JD, Gouveia-Oliveira A. Clinical predictors of the severity of chronic venous insufficiency of the lower limbs: A multivariate analysis. Phlebology: The Journal of Venous Disease. 1995 Dec;10(4):155–59.
21. Merrill JT, Erkan D, Winakur J, James JA. Emerging evidence of a COVID-19 thrombotic syndrome has treatment implications. Nat Rev Rheumatol. 2020 Oct;16(10):581–89.
22. Caprini JA, Arcelus JI, Hasty JH, Tamhane AC, Fabrega F. Clinical assessment of venous thromboembolic risk in surgical patients. Semin Thromb Hemost. 1991;17(Suppl 3):304–12.
23. Obi AT, Pannucci CJ, Nackashi A, Abdullah N, Alvarez R, Bahl V, et al. Validation of the caprini venous thromboembolism risk assessment model in critically ill surgical patients. JAMA Surg. 2015 Oct 1;150(10):941.
24. Rogers SO, Kilaru RK, Hosokawa P, Henderson WG, Zinner MJ, Khuri SF. Multivariable predictors of postoperative venous thromboembolic events after general and vascular surgery: Results from the patient safety in surgery study. J Am Coll Surg. 2007 Jun;204(6):1211–21.

25. Spyropoulos AC, Anderson FA, Fitzgerald G, Decousus H, Pini M, Chong BH, et al. Predictive and associative models to identify hospitalized medical patients at risk for VTE. Chest. 2011 Sep;140(3):706–14.
26. Rosenberg D, Eichorn A, Alarcon M, McCullagh L, McGinn T, Spyropoulos AC. External validation of the risk assessment model of the international medical prevention registry on venous thromboembolism (IMPROVE) for medical patients in a tertiary health system. JAHA. 2014 Dec 17;3(6):e001152.
27. Barbar S, Noventa F, Rossetto V, Ferrari A, Brandolin B, Perlati M, et al. A risk assessment model for the identification of hospitalized medical patients at risk for venous thromboembolism: The padua prediction score. J Thromb Haemost. 2010 Nov;8(11):2450–57.
28. Vardi M, Ghanem-Zoubi NO, Zidan R, Yurin V, Bitterman H. Venous thromboembolism and the utility of the padua prediction score in patients with sepsis admitted to internal medicine departments. J Thromb Haemost. 2013 Mar;11(3):467–73.
29. Khorana AA, Kuderer NM, Culakova E, Lyman GH, Francis CW. Development and validation of a predictive model for chemotherapy-associated thrombosis. Blood. 2008 May 15;111(10):4902–7.
30. Dutia M, White RH, Wun T. Risk assessment models for cancer-associated venous thromboembolism: VTE risk in cancer. Cancer. 2012 Jul 15;118(14):3468–76.
31. Henke P, Sharma S, Wakefield T, Myers D, Obi A. Insights from experimental post-thrombotic syndrome and potential for novel therapies. Transl Res. 2020 Nov;225:95–104.
32. Vandy FC, Stabler C, Eliassen AM, Hawley AE, Guire KE, Myers DD, et al. Soluble P-selectin for the diagnosis of lower extremity deep venous thrombosis. J Vasc Surg: Venous Lymphat Disord. 2013 Apr;1(2):117–25.
33. Mulholland MW. Greenfield's Surgery: Scientific Principles and Practice [Internet]. Wolters Kluwer Health; 2016. Retrieved from https://books.google.com/books?id=MayADQAAQBAJ
34. Wakefield TW, Caprini J, Comerota AJ. Thromboembolic diseases. Curr Probl Surg. 2008 Dec;45(12):844–99.
35. Browse NL, Thomas ML. Source of non-lethal pulmonary emboli. Lancet. 1974 Feb 16;1(7851):258–59.
36. Havig O. Deep vein thrombosis and pulmonary embolism. An autopsy study with multiple regression analysis of possible risk factors. Acta Chir Scand Suppl. 1977;478:1–120.
37. Baglin T, Bauer K, Douketis J, Buller H, Srivastava A, Johnson G. Duration of anticoagulant therapy after a first episode of an unprovoked pulmonary embolus or deep vein thrombosis: Guidance from the SSC of the ISTH: Unprovoked VTE: Duration of anticoagulation. J Thromb Haemost. 2012 Apr;10(4):698–702.
38. Hull R, Delmore T, Genton E, Hirsh J, Gent M, Sackett D, et al. Warfarin sodium versus low-dose heparin in the long-term treatment of venous thrombosis. N Engl J Med. 1979 Oct 18;301(16):855–58.
39. Hull R, Delmore T, Genton E, Hirsh J, Gent M, Sackett D, et al. Warfarin sodium versus low-dose heparin in the long-term treatment of venous thrombosis. N Engl J Med. 1979 Oct 18;301(16):855–58.
40. Research Committee of the British Thoracic Society. Optimum duration of anticoagulation for deep-vein thrombosis and pulmonary embolism. Lancet. 1992 Oct 10;340(8824):873–76.
41. Lagerstedt CI, Olsson CG, Fagher BO, Oqvist BW, Albrechtsson U. Need for long-term anticoagulant treatment in symptomatic calf-vein thrombosis. Lancet. 1985 Sep 7;2(8454):515–18.
42. Levine MN, Hirsh J, Gent M, Turpie AG, Weitz J, Ginsberg J, et al. Optimal duration of oral anticoagulant therapy: A randomized trial comparing four weeks with three months of warfarin in patients with proximal deep vein thrombosis. Thromb Haemost. 1995 Aug;74(2):606–11.
43. Schulman S, Granqvist S, Holmström M, Carlsson A, Lindmarker P, Nicol P, et al. The duration of oral anticoagulant therapy after a second episode of venous thromboembolism. The duration of anticoagulation trial study group. N Engl J Med. 1997 Feb 6;336(6):393–98.
44. Schulman S, Rhedin AS, Lindmarker P, Carlsson A, Lärfars G, Nicol P, et al. A comparison of six weeks with six months of oral anticoagulant therapy after a first episode of venous

thromboembolism. Duration of anticoagulation trial study group. N Engl J Med. 1995 Jun 22;332(25):1661–65.
45. Boutitie F, Pinede L, Schulman S, Agnelli G, Raskob G, Julian J, et al. Influence of preceding length of anticoagulant treatment and initial presentation of venous thromboembolism on risk of recurrence after stopping treatment: Analysis of individual participants' data from seven trials. BMJ. 2011 May 24;342:d3036.
46. Pinede L, Ninet J, Duhaut P, Chabaud S, Demolombe-Rague S, Durieu I, et al. Comparison of 3 and 6 months of oral anticoagulant therapy after a first episode of proximal deep vein thrombosis or pulmonary embolism and comparison of 6 and 12 weeks of therapy after isolated calf deep vein thrombosis. Circulation. 2001 May 22;103(20):2453–60.
47. Kearon C, Akl EA, Comerota AJ, Prandoni P, Bounameaux H, Goldhaber SZ, et al. Antithrombotic therapy for VTE disease: Antithrombotic therapy and prevention of thrombosis, 9th ed: American College of Chest Physicians evidence-based clinical practice guidelines. Chest. 2012 Feb;141(2 Suppl):e419S–96S.
48. Lip GY, Hull RD. Overview of the treatment of proximal and distal lower extremity deep vein thrombosis (DVT). UpToDate (p. 50), 2022. Retrieved from https://www.uptodate.com/contents/overview-of-the-treatment-of-proximal-and-distal-lower-extremity-deep-vein-thrombosis-dvt
49. Spyropoulos AC, Levy JH, Ageno W, Connors JM, Hunt BJ, Iba T, et al. Scientific and Standardization Committee communication: Clinical guidance on the diagnosis, prevention, and treatment of venous thromboembolism in hospitalized patients with COVID-19. J Thromb Haemost. 2020 Aug;18(8):1859–65.
50. Connors JM, Ridker PM. Thromboinflammation and antithrombotics in COVID-19: Accumulating evidence and current status. JAMA. 2022 Apr 5;327(13):1234.
51. The ATTACC, ACTIV-4a, and REMAP-CAP Investigators. Therapeutic anticoagulation with heparin in noncritically ill patients with covid-19. N Engl J Med. 2021 Aug 26;385(9):790–802.
52. The REMAP-CAP, ACTIV-4a, and ATTACC Investigators. Therapeutic Anticoagulation with heparin in critically ill patients with covid-19. N Engl J Med. 2021 Aug 26;385(9):777–89.
53. Stevens SM, Woller SC, Kreuziger LB, Bounameaux H, Doerschug K, Geersing GJ, et al. Antithrombotic therapy for VTE disease: Second update of the CHEST guideline and expert panel report. Chest. 2021 Dec;160(6):e545–608.
54. Kearon C, Akl EA, Comerota AJ, Prandoni P, Bounameaux H, Goldhaber SZ, et al. Antithrombotic therapy for VTE disease: Antithrombotic therapy and prevention of thrombosis, 9th ed: American College of Chest Physicians evidence-based clinical practice guidelines. Chest. 2012 Feb;141(2 Suppl):e419S–e496S.
55. Kearon C. Natural history of venous thromboembolism. Circulation. 2003 Jun 17;107(23 Suppl 1):I22–30.
56. Masuda EM, Kistner RL. The case for managing calf vein thrombi with duplex surveillance and selective anticoagulation. Dis Mon. 2010 Oct;56(10):601–13.
57. Righini M, Paris S, Le Gal G, Laroche JP, Perrier A, Bounameaux H. Clinical relevance of distal deep vein thrombosis. Review of literature data. Thromb Haemost. 2006 Jan;95(1):56–64.
58. Schwarz T, Schmidt B, Beyer J, Schellong SM. Therapy of isolated calf muscle vein thrombosis with low-molecular-weight heparin. Blood Coagul Fibrinolysis. 2001 Oct;12(7):597–99.
59. Macdonald PS, Kahn SR, Miller N, Obrand D. Short-term natural history of isolated gastrocnemius and soleal vein thrombosis. J Vasc Surg. 2003 Mar;37(3):523–27.
60. Gillet JL, Perrin MR, Allaert FA. Short-term and mid-term outcome of isolated symptomatic muscular calf vein thrombosis. J Vasc Surg. 2007 Sep;46(3):513–19; discussion 519.
61. Lautz TB, Abbas F, Walsh SJN, Chow C, Amaranto DJ, Wang E, et al. Isolated gastrocnemius and soleal vein thrombosis: Should these patients receive therapeutic anticoagulation? Ann Surg. 2010 Apr;251(4):735–42.
62. Schwarz T, Buschmann L, Beyer J, Halbritter K, Rastan A, Schellong S. Therapy of isolated calf muscle vein thrombosis: A randomized, controlled study. J Vasc Surg. 2010 Nov;52(5):1246–50.
63. Sales CM, Haq F, Bustami R, Sun F. Management of isolated soleal and gastrocnemius vein thrombosis. J Vasc Surg. 2010 Nov;52(5):1251–54.

64. Palareti G, Cosmi B, Lessiani G, Rodorigo G, Guazzaloca G, Brusi C, et al. Evolution of untreated calf deep-vein thrombosis in high risk symptomatic outpatients: The blind, prospective CALTHRO study. Thromb Haemost. 2010 Nov;104(5):1063–70.
65. Dobler CC. Overdiagnosis of pulmonary embolism: Definition, causes and implications. Breathe (Sheff). 2019 Mar;15(1):46–53.
66. Kahn SR. How I treat postthrombotic syndrome. Blood. 2009 Nov 19;114(21):4624–31.
67. Cohen JM, Akl EA, Kahn SR. Pharmacologic and compression therapies for postthrombotic syndrome: A systematic review of randomized controlled trials. Chest. 2012 Feb;141(2): 308–20.
68. Lattimer CR, Azzam M, Kalodiki E, Makris GC, Geroulakos G. Compression stockings significantly improve hemodynamic performance in post-thrombotic syndrome irrespective of class or length. J Vasc Surg. 2013 Jul;58(1):158–65.
69. Kahn SR, Shapiro S, Wells PS, Rodger MA, Kovacs MJ, Anderson DR, et al. Compression stockings to prevent post-thrombotic syndrome: A randomised placebo-controlled trial. Lancet. 2014 Mar;383(9920):880–88.
70. Amin EE, Bistervels IM, Meijer K, Tick LW, Middeldorp S, Mostard G, et al. Reduced incidence of vein occlusion and postthrombotic syndrome after immediate compression for deep vein thrombosis. Blood. 2018 Nov 22;132(21):2298–304.
71. Klok FA, Hösel V, Clemens A, Yollo WD, Tilke C, Schulman S, et al. Prediction of bleeding events in patients with venous thromboembolism on stable anticoagulation treatment. Eur Respir J. 2016 Nov;48(5):1369–76.
72. Klok FA, Barco S, Turpie AGG, Haas S, Kreutz R, Mantovani LG, et al. Predictive value of venous thromboembolism (VTE)-BLEED to predict major bleeding and other adverse events in a practice-based cohort of patients with VTE: Results of the XALIA study. Br J Haematol. 2018 Nov;183(3):457–65.
73. Eichinger S, Heinze G, Jandeck LM, Kyrle PA. Risk assessment of recurrence in patients with unprovoked deep vein thrombosis or pulmonary embolism: The Vienna prediction model. Circulation. 2010 Apr 13;121(14):1630–36.
74. Tritschler T, Méan M, Limacher A, Rodondi N, Aujesky D. Predicting recurrence after unprovoked venous thromboembolism: Prospective validation of the updated Vienna prediction model. Blood. 2015 Oct 15;126(16):1949–51.
75. Tosetto A, Iorio A, Marcucci M, Baglin T, Cushman M, Eichinger S, et al. Predicting disease recurrence in patients with previous unprovoked venous thromboembolism: A proposed prediction score (DASH). J Thromb Haemost. 2012 Jun;10(6):1019–25.
76. Tosetto A, Testa S, Martinelli I, Poli D, Cosmi B, Lodigiani C, et al. External validation of the DASH prediction rule: A retrospective cohort study. J Thromb Haemost. 2017 Oct;15(10):1963–70.
77. Rodger MA, Le Gal G, Anderson DR, Schmidt J, Pernod G, Kahn SR, et al. Validating the HERDOO2 rule to guide treatment duration for women with unprovoked venous thrombosis: Multinational prospective cohort management study. BMJ. 2017 Mar 17;356:j1065.
78. Vasanthamohan L, Boonyawat K, Chai-Adisaksopha C, Crowther M. Reduced-dose direct oral anticoagulants in the extended treatment of venous thromboembolism: A systematic review and meta-analysis. J Thromb Haemost. 2018 Jul;16(7):1288–95.
79. Douketis JD, Spyropoulos AC, Kaatz S, Becker RC, Caprini JA, Dunn AS, et al. Perioperative bridging anticoagulation in patients with atrial fibrillation. N Engl J Med. 2015 Aug 27;373(9):823–33.
80. Farge D, Frere C, Connors JM, Khorana AA, Kakkar A, Ay C, et al. 2022 International clinical practice guidelines for the treatment and prophylaxis of venous thromboembolism in patients with cancer, including patients with COVID-19. Lancet Oncol. 2022 Jul;23(7):e334–47.
81. Brown JD, Goodin AJ, Lip GYH, Adams VR. Risk stratification for bleeding complications in patients with venous thromboembolism: Application of the HAS-BLED bleeding score during the first 6 months of anticoagulant treatment. J Am Heart Assoc. 2018 Mar 7;7(6):e007901.
82. Rief P, Raggam RB, Hafner F, Avian A, Hackl G, Cvirn G, et al. Calculation of HAS-BLED score is useful for early identification of venous thromboembolism patients at high risk for

major bleeding events: A prospective outpatients cohort study. Semin Thromb Hemost. 2018 Jun;44(4):348–52.

83. Kooiman J, van Hagen N, Iglesias Del Sol A, Planken EV, Lip GYH, van der Meer FJM, et al. The HAS-BLED score identifies patients with acute venous thromboembolism at high risk of major bleeding complications during the first six months of anticoagulant treatment. PLoS One. 2015;10(4):e0122520.
84. Palareti G, Antonucci E, Mastroiacovo D, Ageno W, Pengo V, Poli D, et al. The American College of Chest Physician score to assess the risk of bleeding during anticoagulation in patients with venous thromboembolism. J Thromb Haemost. 2018 Oct;16(10):1994–2002.
85. Jeske W, Walenga JM, Lewis BE, Fareed J. Pharmacology of argatroban. Expert Opin Investig Drugs. 1999 May;8(5):625–54.
86. Hassan Y, Awaisu A, Al-Meman AA, Aziz NA. The pharmacotherapy of heparin-induced thrombocytopenia (HIT): A review of contemporary therapeutic challenges in clinical practice. Malays J Med Sci. 2008 Apr;15(2):3–13.
87. Aday AW, Beckman JA. The open vein hypothesis and postthrombotic syndrome: Not dead yet. Circulation. 2021 Mar 23;143(12):1239–41.
88. Weitz JI, Fredenburgh JC. Factors XI and XII as targets for new anticoagulants. Front Med [Internet]. 2017 Feb 24 [cited 2023 Jan 23];4. Retrieved from: http://journal.frontiersin.org/article/10.3389/fmed.2017.00019/full
89. Purdy M, Obi A, Myers D, Wakefield T. P- and E-selectin in venous thrombosis and non-venous pathologies. J Thromb Haemost. 2022 May;20(5):1056–66.
90. Devata S, Angelini DE, Blackburn S, Hawley A, Myers DD, Schaefer JK, et al. Use of GMI-1271, an E-selectin antagonist, in healthy subjects and in 2 patients with calf vein thrombosis. Res Pract Thromb Haemost. 2020 Feb;4(2):193–204.
91. Weitz JI, Chan NC. Novel antithrombotic strategies for treatment of venous thromboembolism. Blood. 2020 Jan;135(5):351–59.
92. Gorog DA, Storey RF, Gurbel PA, Tantry US, Berger JS, Chan MY, et al. Current and novel biomarkers of thrombotic risk in COVID-19: A consensus statement from the international COVID-19 thrombosis biomarkers colloquium. Nat Rev Cardiol. 2022 Jul;19(7):475–95.
93. Myers DD, Henke PK, Diaz JA, Wrobleski SK, Hawley AE, Slack D, et al. Pan-selectin antagonist, GMI-1070 decreases venous thrombosis in a mouse model. Blood. 2011 Nov;118(21):3273–73.
94. Culmer DL, Dunbar ML, Hawley AE, Sood S, Sigler RE, Henke PK, et al. E-selectin inhibition with GMI-1271 decreases venous thrombosis without profoundly affecting tail vein bleeding in a mouse model. Thromb Haemost. 2017 Jan;117(6):1171–781.
95. Peterson J, Baek MG, Locatelli-Hoops S, Lee JW, Deng L, Stewart DA, et al. A novel and potent inhibitor of e-selectin, GMI-1687, attenuates thrombus formation and augments chemotherapeutic intervention of AML in preclinical models following subcutaneous administration. Blood. 2018 Nov;132(Suppl 1):4678–78.
96. Peterson J, Vohra Y, Myers DD, Locatelli-Hoops S, Lee JW, Deng L, et al. A Novel glycomimetic compound (GMI-1757) with dual functional antagonism to e-selectin and galectin-3 demonstrates inhibition of thrombus formation in an inferior vena cava model. Blood. 2018 Nov;132(Suppl 1):2211–11.
97. Myers D, Lester P, Adili R, Hawley A, Durham L, Dunivant V, et al. A new way to treat proximal deep venous thrombosis using E-selectin inhibition. J Vasc Surg: Venous Lymphat Disord. 2020 Mar;8(2):268–78.
98. Myers DD, Ning J, Lester P, Adili R, Hawley A, Durham L, et al. E-selectin inhibitor is superior to low-molecular-weight heparin for the treatment of experimental venous thrombosis. J Vasc Surg: Venous Lymphat Disord. 2022 Jan;10(1):211–20.
99. Smith BAH, Bertozzi CR. The clinical impact of glycobiology: Targeting selectins, siglecs and mammalian glycans. Nat Rev Drug Discov. 2021 Mar;20(3):217–43.

Chapter 21

Endovascular Management of Deep Venous Thrombosis

Tyler Callese, Savannah Fletcher, Aniket Joglekar, Lucas Cusumano, John Moriarty, and Justin McWilliams

INTRODUCTION

Endovascular treatment of deep venous thrombosis (DVT) is largely based on the "open vein hypothesis," which suggests that the proactive removal of thrombus improves flow within the deep venous system, prevents chronic venous hypertension, venous reflux and decreases the risk of post-thrombotic syndrome (PTS).[1] While conservative management, including anticoagulation and compression stockings, is effective at preventing thrombus propagation and decreasing risk of pulmonary embolism, in almost half of all patients it does not restore baseline quality of life or prevent PTS.[2]

Catheter-directed therapies are effective at rapidly removing thrombus and restoring in-line flow with randomized trials supporting the implementation of these techniques in certain populations. Patient selection and procedure technique depend on the location, extent, etiology, and clinical presentation of DVT. This chapter reviews methods of endovascular thrombus removal and management recommendations based on clinical presentation.

ENDOVASCULAR TECHNIQUES AND DEVICES

Catheter-Directed Thrombolysis

Catheter-directed thrombolysis (CDT) most commonly involves straight, multiple side-hole infusion catheters (Table 21.1), which are placed across the thrombosed segment for direct administration of fibrinolytic agents into the thrombus.[3] Fibrinolytic agents include urokinase, streptokinase, reteplase, tenecteplase, and tissue plasminogen activator (tPA).[2, 4] CDT requires lower doses of lytic agents compared to systemic thrombolysis, minimizing the risk of systemic bleeding.[4] Contraindications to thrombolytic agents include recent or active hemorrhagic event (cerebral, gastrointestinal, trauma, etc.) or major surgery.[5]

In the first stage of CDT, infusion catheters are placed across the thrombus and lytic agents are administered for 12 to 36 hours.[5] tPA is commonly used and generally administered at 0.01 mg/kg/hr mg/hr up to a max dose of 20 mg/24 hours or fixed dose of 0.25–1 mg/hr.[12] Systemic anticoagulation is held during thrombolysis, but subtherapeutic (300–500 Units/hour) unfractionated heparin is typically administered through the sheath side-arm(s) to prevent additional thrombus formation.[13] Patients are monitored closely in the intensive care unit or specialty surgical ward for evidence of complications associated with bleeding.[5]

In the second stage, venography is performed to evaluate for thrombus resolution and any underlying anatomy and pathology that may indicate adjunctive procedures, such as venoplasty and stenting.[14] There is no consensus regarding the necessity of, or a standardized protocol for, fibrinogen monitoring during thrombolysis and significant practice variability exists.[15]

DOI: 10.1201/9781003316626-24

Table 21.1 Endovascular Devices for Deep Venous Thrombosis Interventions

Manufacturer	*Device Name*	*Size (Fr)*	*Device Components*	*Mechanism of Action*	*Relevant Clinical Trials*
Angiodynamics	AlphaVac System	25	22 Fr funnel-tip catheter (20- or 180-degree tip) Aspiration handle 250 cc waste canister	Mechanical Aspiration Thrombectomy	
Argon Medical Devices, Inc.	Cleaner 15	7	Handheld battery-driven motor with atraumatic sinusoidal wire tip	Mechanical Thrombectomy	
	Cleaner XT	6			
Boston Scientific Corporation	AngioJet ZelanteDVT	8	AngioJet Ultra Console (monitors and energizes pump) Optional Clothunter device compatible with ZelanteDVT device facilitates wall-to-wall contact	Rheolytic Thrombectomy	ATTRACT (6) PEARL I Registry (7) PEARL II Registry (8)
	AngioJet Solent Omni	6			
	AngioJet Solent Proxi	6			
	Ekos+ Endovascular System	8	Ekos Control Unit CU 4.0 (current generation) able to control two Ekos+ catheters Single-use 7.8 Fr catheter with ultrasonic core and varying infusion lengths (8–20 cm)	Ultrasound-Assisted Thrombolysis	CAVA (9) ACCESS PTS (10)
Inari Medical	FlowTriever System	16,20,24	Triever Aspiration catheter Optional Intri24 introducer sheath Optional Protrieve introducer sheath Optional FlowTriever nitinol disk for clot disruption FlowSaver blood salvage system	Mechanical Aspiration Thrombectomy	PEERLESS (NCT05111613)
	ClotTriever System	13, 16	ClotTriever catheter Optional ClotTriever sheath Optional Protrieve sheath	Mechanical Thrombectomy	CLOUT (11) DEFIANCE (NCT05701917)
Medtronic	Cragg-McNamara Valved Infusion Catheter	4, 5	Single-use single lumen catheter with variable infusion lengths (5–50 cm) Standard intravenous hospital infusion pump.	Catheter-Directed Thrombolysis	
Penumbra, Inc	Indigo System	3,5,6,7,8,12,16	Penumbra Engine aspiration source Engine aspiration canister Intelligent Aspiration Tubing Aspiration catheter Optional Separator wire	Mechanical Aspiration Thrombectomy	BOLT (NCT05003843)

Ultrasound-Assisted Thrombolysis

Ultrasound-assisted thrombolysis (USAT) combines CDT with intravascular ultrasound energy to simultaneously fragment and dissolve thrombus.[16, 17] The EkoSonic endovascular system (Ekos) utilizes an infusion catheter containing a core wire that emits pulsed high frequency, low intensity ultrasound waves to theoretically increase thrombus permeability to the thrombolytic agent, reduce infusion times, and decrease thrombolytic dose.[18] While USAT is associated with high rates of substantial lysis (>50%), it does not demonstrate improvements in clinical outcomes and is associated with much higher costs than conventional CDT.[19, 20]

Mechanical Thrombectomy

Mechanical thrombectomy (MT) involves physical fragmentation of thrombus (Table 21.1) and may be performed concomitantly with thrombolysis administration.[21] The Cleaner device (Argon Medical) is low profile (6–7 F) and handheld with a rotating atraumatic sinusoidal vortex wire that macerates the thrombus.[22] There are currently several devices on the market with a similar mechanism.

The ClotTriever (Inari Medical) is a novel large-bore mechanical thrombectomy device (11 F device requiring a 13–16 F sheath) and contains a nitinol coring element and braided collection bag designed to core and extract thrombus (Table 21.1).

Mechanical Aspiration Thrombectomy

Mechanical aspiration thrombectomy (MAT) involves aspiration of thrombus with or without fragmentation (Table 21.1).

The AlphaVac (Angiodynamics) is a large-bore aspiration thrombectomy device with an angled cannula tip and negative pressure generated by a handle-actuated syringe (Table 21.1).[22] This device is targeted for larger thrombus including iliocaval thrombus and right atrial thrombus.[23]

The Triever device (Inari Medical) is a large-bore aspiration catheter available in multiple sizes (Table 21.1).[22] Negative pressure is created by an attached syringe. Adjunctive MT can be performed through this device with the FlowTriever nitinol disk catheter, which engages and fragments thrombus facilitating retrieval through the Triever catheter.

The Indigo system (Penumbra) is a family of mechanical aspiration catheters that use computer-aided aspiration for thrombectomy (Table 21.1).[22] Catheters are available in a wide array of sizes and lengths allowing use throughout the vascular system. Negative pressure is supplied via the Penumbra ENGINE, which senses when the aspiration catheter is in freely flowing blood or thrombus. Intermittent aspiration is initiated when thrombus is detected (Figure 21.1). Aspirated material is collected in a canister attached to the ENGINE. Thrombus can be manipulated by advancing the separator wire (Penumbra) through the aspiration catheter helping to clear the catheter tip.

Large-bore aspiration catheters are efficient at removing thrombus within larger vessels (e.g., iliofemoral and caval thrombus); however, their use requires the consideration of sheath size and operative blood loss.[2] Common femoral vein or internal jugular vein access is often required, although many physicians are increasing their comfort with large-bore popliteal vein access. With sheath sizes greater than 12 Fr, a venous access site closure technique, such as a preclose technique or retention suture, should be considered.[24]

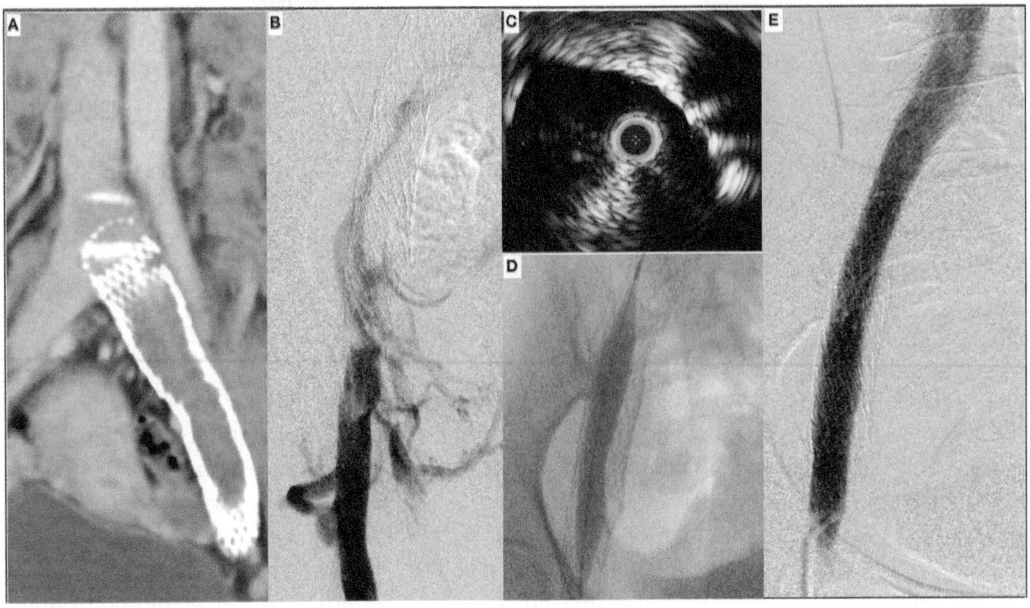

Figure 21.1 A 36-year-old female with past medical history of left iliofemoral DVT status post prior endovascular interventions including stent placement at an outside hospital presented with acute left lower extremity swelling and pain with ambulation for 1 day. She had been compliant on warfarin with no missed doses. CT venogram demonstrated left common and external iliac vein in-stent thrombosis (A). Initial venogram confirmed in-stent stenosis of the left common and external iliac stent (B). Systemic therapeutic heparin was administered and mechanical thrombectomy was performed using the Penumbra Lightning Flash device with removal of large volume acute and chronic thrombus. Follow-up intravascular ultrasound demonstrated persistent greater than 70% stenosis at the superior aspect of the stent complex, representing a residual May-Thurner compression lesion (C). Balloon venoplasty was then performed with overlapping stations to 14 mm (D). Finally, 16 mm stents were placed, relining the existing external iliac vein stents with final venography demonstrating brisk in-line flow (E).

Pharmacomechanical Thrombectomy

Pharmacomechanical catheter-directed thrombectomy (PCDT) accelerates thrombus removal by combining low-dose thrombolytics and MT and/or MAT techniques.[25]

Rheolytic thrombectomy is a distinct type of PCDT that involves thrombus fragmentation and aspiration by injecting high-pressure saline through the catheter tip.[21, 26] The AngioJet device (Boston Scientific) device (Table 21.1) includes a power pulse spray mode and can be used with heparin, saline, or tPA.[8, 27] A black box warning exists for its use in the pulmonary vasculature as the release of adenosine from disrupted platelets can cause bradycardia, pulmonary vasospasm, and hypoxia.[28]

ENDOVASCULAR MANAGEMENT

Inferior Vena Cava DVT

Isolated inferior vena cava (IVC) deep venous thrombosis (DVT) is a rare entity with a reported incidence of less than 1.7 per 100,000.[29, 30] IVC DVT is more commonly diagnosed with concomitant lower extremity DVT. Due to various reasons including non-specific presenting symptoms and lack of diagnostic and management guidelines, IVC DVT is likely underdiagnosed.[31] Acute IVC DVT can be associated with significant morbidity often related to venous hypertension, pain, swelling, pulmonary embolism, and PTS. Chronic IVC DVT can manifest as a heterogeneous spectrum from hard, organized thrombus to an obliterated, atretic vein. Primary causes include anatomic variants and inherited thrombophilias. Secondary causes include the presence of foreign bodies (e.g., IVC filters), extrinsic compression (e.g., malignancy), or outflow obstructions (Budd-Chiari Syndrome).

Management options for symptomatic patients include conservative management, with anticoagulation and compression stockings, and interventional management with catheter-directed or open surgical techniques. Anticoagulation should be initiated promptly due to risk of thrombus propagation and pulmonary embolism.[2] Management goals include symptomatic relief and resolution of underlying stenosis or occlusion. Commonly reported endovascular techniques for the removal of caval thrombus primarily involve mechanical thrombectomy with adjunctive catheter-directed thrombolysis.[29] Given the large thrombus burden typically encountered in caval thrombus, prolonged thrombolytic infusion periods of up to 36–48 hours may be required. Establishing in-line flow may require multiple vascular accesses, multiple devices, advanced filter retrieval techniques, and/or blunt or sharp recanalization and stenting, which is beyond the scope of this chapter.[29] The introduction of large-bore aspiration and mechanical thrombectomy devices has limited the number of devices needed during these procedures.

Iliofemoral DVT

Iliofemoral DVT requires careful diagnosis and management due to a heterogeneous patient population, evolving techniques and devices, and potential for severe long-term sequelae.[32–34] Acute (less than 2 weeks) iliofemoral DVT is associated with a 28% incidence of moderate-to-severe PTS in untreated patients, increased risk of recurrent DVT, and an increased risk of PTS.[6, 35, 36]

Management goals include symptomatic relief and mitigating risk of PTS. There are a variety of acceptable interventional technique options, and patient selection for intervention is crucial. Numerous retrospective and single-arm studies and few randomized trials and reports are available; however, no concrete consensus has been reached regarding optimal management strategies.[37] Several societal guidelines are available and provide management recommendations.[12, 33, 38–41]

Patient Selection

Patients with iliofemoral DVT who are likely to benefit from intervention are younger patients with good functional status, moderate-to-severe or severe symptoms and non-threatened limbs; patients with acute/subacute DVT with moderate-to-severe symptoms and decreased DVT-related functional status; and patients who have failed an initial trial of anticoagulation or who have progressive thrombosis while on anticoagulation[33, 37] (Figure 21.2). A short trial of anticoagulation alone can be considered while deciding whether to intervene.[40] Additional predictors of clinical success following endovascular intervention include increased DVT clinical severity (Villalta) at presentation and personal history of DVT.[42]

Special patient populations include pregnant women and children/adolescents. Pregnant women are at higher risk of exposure to radiation, iodinated contrast, and thrombolytics.[43–45] Thrombolysis is associated with maternal death (2.8%), loss of pregnancy (8.5%), and preterm delivery (9.9%).[46] Intervention is currently only recommended in situations involving life-limiting DVT or limb threat,[33] although advanced techniques using IVUS to

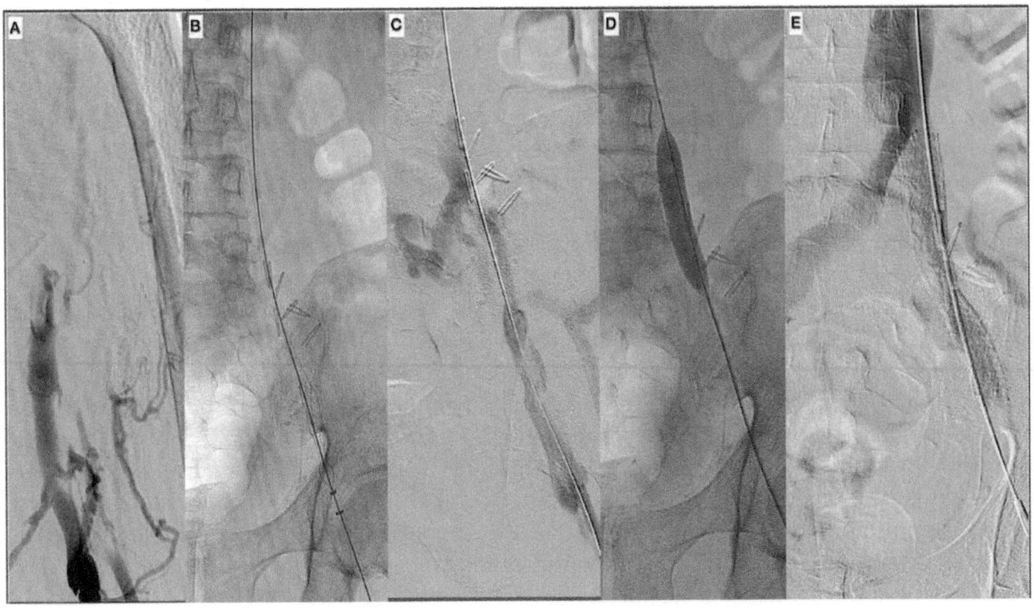

Figure 21.2 A 51-year-old man with a history of prior gunshot wound to the right lower extremity requiring arterial repair and right lower extremity DVT on enoxaparin presenting with acute on chronic right lower extremity swelling and pain. CT angiogram demonstrated narrowing of the right common femoral and external iliac veins with partial to occlusive thrombosis of the iliofemoral veins. Initial venogram via right popliteal vein access demonstrated occlusion of the right iliofemoral venous system (A). After gentle venoplasty to create a channel for passage of the ClotTriever device, mechanical thrombectomy was performed throughout the iliofemoral vein with a moderate amount of acute and chronic clot removed (B). Multistation venoplasty was performed, with persistent stenosis at the level of the sutures (C). Additional venoplasty was performed up to 12 mm (D), with persistent stenosis. A 14 mm Zilver Vena stent was placed in the common and external iliac veins and venoplasty to 12 mm. Final venogram demonstrates brisk in-line flow with re-expansion of the previous stenosis (E).

limit radiation exposure and aspiration or mechanical thrombectomy to avoid thrombolysis can be employed.

Children and adolescents are a challenging population because of the severe impact of PTS on quality of life and their expected long lifespans.[47–49] There is no high-level evidence for an optimal method of thrombus removal and considerations include high rates of early re-thrombosis, long-term effects of potential endothelial damage, stent placement in patients expected to grow, and physiologic differences in hemostasis and thrombolysis in children compared to adults.[47, 48, 50, 51]

Clinical Management

The first step is managing iliofemoral DVT is evaluation of bleeding risk and initiation of therapeutic anticoagulation in the absence of any major contraindication.[33] The goal of anticoagulation is to prevent thrombus progression and pulmonary embolism.[2] Anticoagulant choice is beyond the scope of this article, but in general low-molecular-weight heparin is favored due to its rapid onset of therapeutic anticoagulation compared to unfractionated heparin and unknown risks associated with direct-acting oral anticoagulants in the setting of concomitant thrombolytics.[33]

Phlegmasia cerula dolens is a limb-threatening emergency with high-risk of limb compromise, amputation, and mortality.[33] In these cases, CDT or PCDT are recommended.[32, 33, 39] MT alone is limited in this setting because it may remove large thrombus within the large deep veins but will not restore in-line flow from the occluded peripheral and small (perforator) veins.[33]

Beyond these two generally agreed upon management points, patient presentation, severity of symptoms, and operator experience play a large role in the decision to intervene. There are numerous interventional platforms currently available for thrombus removal (Table 21.1).

Currently, the highest-level evidence available is with CDT and PCDT.[6, 9, 12] The CAVENT trial included 209 patients with acute iliofemoral or femoral-popliteal DVT randomized 1:1 to CDT with tPA or anticoagulation alone.[12] The results of this trial demonstrated reduced rates of PTS at 2 and 5 years in patients treated with CDT.[12]

The ATTRACT trial included 692 patients with acute iliofemoral or femoral-popliteal DVT randomized to intervention or anticoagulation alone.[6] Interventions included PCDT and CDT. In the iliofemoral subgroup of the ATTRACT trial, PCDT improved early leg pain and swelling within 30 days, reduced the occurrence of moderate-to-severe PTS at 2 years, reduced the severity of PTS, and improved quality of life score. It is worth noting that the ATTRACT trial included follow-up at several time points between 6 and 24 months, therefore, participants could reach the primary endpoint at any follow-up visit regardless of progression at future visits.

The CAVA trial included 184 patients with iliofemoral DVT randomized to USAT or anticoagulation alone.[49] The results of this trial did not demonstrate a significant difference in PTS occurrence or quality of life at 1 year. In general, USAT is not recommended due lack of evidence of superiority to traditional CDT and increased costs.[9, 52]

Recurrent DVT rates were not improved in any of these trials regardless of CDT or PCDT. The iliofemoral subgroup analysis of the ATTRACT trial demonstrated increased PTS severity in patients with increased residual thrombus volume and non-compressibility of the common femoral vein on follow-up ultrasound imaging.[53] For this reason, maximizing thrombus removal is paramount to improving clinical outcomes.

MT (without thrombolytics) was investigated in a single-center randomized trial.[54] This trial included 42 patients with acute iliofemoral DVT randomized to MAT or anticoagulation alone.[54] Results at 1-year demonstrated higher venous patency and decreased clinical symptoms with MAT.

The remaining evidence for MT lies in observational studies, which are inherently limited due to study design and frequency of additional interventions (i.e., use of adjunctive PCDT or CDT).[55, 56] Another challenge pertains to the rapid development of large-bore thrombectomy technology (Table 21.1). These devices are associated with observational studies that demonstrate symptom improvement and thrombus removal; however, generalizability remains limited.[55, 56]

Additional Considerations

Intravascular ultrasound facilitates visualization of thrombus, extrinsic compression, and flow dynamics and allows for more accurate vessel sizing.[33] No high-level evidence exists demonstrating clinical benefit or cost-effectiveness; however, a growing number of operators find it to be a highly valuable adjunct.

Another important adjunct to thrombus removal and restoration of in-line flow is treatment of underlying flow-limiting lesions.[33, 37] There is a higher rate of recurrent DVT and thrombosis in patients with a residual flow-limiting lesion.[57] Stent placement can be considered in these patients. Importantly, little is known regarding which patients, lesions, and flow dynamics will be most responsive to stenting. Further, no data exists regarding the risks of long-term stent implantation, an important consideration for younger patients. Finally, the optimal stent design for use in the venous system has yet to be developed and repeat interventions for secondary patency are common.[58]

Femoral-Popliteal DVT

Infrainguinal lower extremity DVT limited to superficial femoral and popliteal segments requires a different management algorithm compared to iliofemoral DVT. The ATTRACT trial included a 300 patient femoral-popliteal DVT subgroup analysis, which found no difference in PTS, quality of life, or rates of recurrent DVT in patients who underwent intervention versus conservative management.[6, 59] PCDT was associated with higher risk of bleeding complications.[6, 59] The results from this study do not support endovascular intervention for femoral-popliteal DVT, except in patients with severe clinical symptoms or who prefer rapid restoration of flow and thrombus removal.[14]

Distal Lower Extremity DVT

Isolated distal lower extremity DVT, otherwise known as "calf" or "infrapopliteal" DVT, involves the posterior tibial, peroneal, anterior tibial, or muscular calf veins (soleus or gastrocnemius veins) and constitutes approximately 30–70% of all lower extremity DVT diagnosed with US.[60, 61] Symptoms are similar to those of more proximal DVT with pain being the predominant symptom.[61] Wells score and D-dimer may be lower than those seen in patients with proximal DVT, and D-dimer may even be within normal limits.[61] Diagnosis is typically made on venous duplex and compression ultrasound, although the accuracy for detecting distal DVT is lower than for detecting proximal DVT.[62] The utility of detecting and managing distal DVT is uncertain and debated, with institutional protocols varying widely.[60–65]

The CACTUS trial evaluated outcomes in low risk outpatients with isolated distal lower extremity DVT treated with compression stockings and placebo or anticoagulation (nadroparin) for 6 weeks.[65] The study found no significant difference in the risk of DVT extension or symptomatic PE between the two groups at 6 weeks.[65] The study did find increased risk of clinically relevant non-major bleeding events with anticoagulation.[65]

The results of this study as well as recommendations from the American College of Chest Physicians suggest that symptomatic isolated calf DVT in patients without severe symptoms or risk factors, such as active malignancy or prior DVT, may be safely managed with serial ultrasound over 2 weeks, repeat ultrasound if worsening symptoms, and no anticoagulation unless proximal extension is observed.[41, 65] In cases of severe symptoms or the presence of risk factors for thrombus extension, anticoagulation is recommended.[41] Endovascular intervention is not indicated in cases of isolated distal DVT.[66]

Axillosubclavian Vein

Upper extremity DVT (UEDVT) comprises approximately 1–5% of all DVT.[67–69] Primary upper extremity DVT includes idiopathic etiologies, venous thoracic outlet syndrome (VTOS), and Paget-Schroetter syndrome (PSS) or "effort thrombosis".[68, 69] VTOS, often referred to synonymously with PSS, is related to compression and thrombosis of the Axillosubclavian vein at the level of the first rib, clavicle, and subclavius muscle/costo-clavicular ligament.[70] Limb abduction and external rotation, muscle hypertrophy, or anatomic abnormalities may exacerbate PSS, and as such this syndrome is often seen in young, healthy males in their 30s.[71, 72] Secondary upper extremity DVT is more common and is related to the presence of central venous catheters, pacemakers, or malignancy.[68, 69] The average age of patients with secondary UEDVT is approximately 60 years.[69]

Prompt initiation of anticoagulation after diagnosis is recommended in cases of either primary or secondary UEDVT.[71, 72] Management of secondary UEDVT with anticoagulation alone is typically sufficient.[2] However, in PSS or VTOS, anticoagulation alone results in high rates of residual disability and complications such as venous gangrene and pulmonary embolism.[71, 72, 74] Further, the frequency of post-thrombotic syndrome (PTS) in the upper extremity is estimated to be between 7–46%.[68] Upper extremity PTS in the dominant arm may be particularly debilitating.[68] More aggressive interventions are recommended and result in improved patient-reported outcomes.[71, 72] Catheter-directed venography and thrombolysis should be initiated ideally within 2 weeks of symptom onset if no contraindications to thrombolysis exist.[71, 72] Duration of lysis is typically 24–48 hours.[72] A retrospective analysis of CDT in 30 patients with UEDVT demonstrated >90% lysis in 97% of patients.[75] Median symptom onset was 8 days prior to CDT initiation.[75] Major bleeding was seen in 9% of patients with no intracerebral hemorrhage, clinical pulmonary embolism, or death.[75] No severe PTS was seen at the time of follow-up (median 21 months).[75] The addition of PCDT using the AngioJet rheolytic thrombectomy catheter to CDT has been associated with shorter treatment duration and lower thrombolytic dose requirements.[76]

MT in the setting of UEDVT has not been widely studied by any large trials.[77] Few small studies evaluating the Penumbra Indigo CAT 8 and CAT D systems have shown these devices can be safely used in the setting of UEDVT with promising efficacy in thrombus burden reduction.[78, 79] A retrospective analysis of 22 patients with symptomatic UEDVT evaluated results for 10 patients treated with MAT using the Penumbra Indigo CAT8 System compared to 12 patients treated with CDT or Rheolytic PCDT.[78] Resolution of greater than 70% of thrombus burden was achieved by single-session therapy in 50% of patients who underwent MT compared to only 8.3% of patients in the CDT/PCDT group.[78] 30% of patients in the MT group did not require thrombolytics.[78] Primary and secondary patency was similar for both groups.[78] MT for UEDVT may be useful for minimizing cost, number of interventions, length of hospital stays, and bleeding risk.[78]

Delayed interventions are associated with lower rates of patient-reported symptom improvement.[72] After 2 weeks, thrombus is considered chronic and is more difficult to treat.[71] After restoration of venous patency using endovascular techniques, surgical decompression should be performed to prevent recurrent thrombosis.[72]

Superior Vena Cava

Obstruction of the superior vena cava (SVC), known as superior vena cava syndrome (SVCS), occurs in 0.005% of Americans every year and is most commonly related to malignancy and central venous catheters or other intravascular devices.[80, 81] Other causes such as fibrosing mediastinitis are rarer.[80, 81] Presenting symptoms may include cough, dyspnea, and swelling of the face, neck, and upper extremities.[2, 80] Treatment options depend on the underlying cause as well as chronicity.[2] Pre-procedure imaging with either CT venography or catheter-based venography should be obtained for adequate planning, particularly if stenting is anticipated.[80] Particular care is required for interventions in the SVC due to risk of pericardial tamponade.[80] Materials and expertise for pericardial drain placement should be readily available.[80]

Malignant obstructions may indicate stenting with most commonly self-expanding or balloon-expandable uncovered stents for palliative symptom relief.[80] Stenting in the setting of benign etiologies has been reported but should be reserved for settings in which angioplasty has already failed.[80] Complete obstructions may require various recanalization techniques, which are beyond the scope of this chapter.[80]

Acute thrombotic occlusions are managed initially with systemic anticoagulation.[80] CDT should be initiated within 2–5 days of symptom onset and becomes relatively ineffective after 10 days.[80] CDT may be particularly beneficial in cases of central venous catheter associated SVCS.[80, 82, 83] In cases where stenting is planned, reduction of thrombus burden with CDT may reduce the number of stents required, permit greater final stent expansion, and minimize the volume of potential embolic material.[80, 84]

CONCLUSIONS

Management of DVT is complex due to a heterogeneous patient population with several distinct clinical presentation subgroups carrying different management recommendations. Endovascular intervention for DVT is a rapidly evolving field with new devices and techniques entering the market. Early, proactive thrombus removal restores in-line flow within the deep venous system and can improve acute DVT-related symptoms. Long-term effects on PTS and venous-related quality of life are still not proven. Recent trials have helped to identify which patients may benefit from intervention, but more work is needed to produce more generalizable results, refine patient selection, and identify risk factors for PTS. Endovascular interventions for DVT are dependent on the location, extent, etiology, and clinical presentation of DVT and should be utilized on an individualized patient basis.

REFERENCES

1. Nathan AS, Giri J. Reexamining the open-vein hypothesis for acute deep venous thrombosis. Circulation. 2019 Feb 26;139(9):1174–76.
2. Thukral S, Vedantham S. Catheter-based therapies and other management strategies for deep vein thrombosis and post-thrombotic syndrome. Journal of Clinical Medicine. 2020 May 12;9(5):1439.
3. Tichelaar VYIG, Brodin EE, Vik A, Isaksen T, Skjeldestad FE, Kumar S, et al. A retrospective comparison of ultrasound-assisted catheter-directed thrombolysis and catheter-directed thrombolysis alone for treatment of proximal deep vein thrombosis. CardioVascular and Interventional Radiology. 2016;39:1115–21.
4. Fleck D, Albadawi H, Shamoun F, Knuttinen G, Naidu S, Oklu R. Catheter-directed thrombolysis of deep vein thrombosis: Literature review and practice considerations. Cardiovascular Diagnosis and Therapy. 2017 Dec;7(Suppl 3):S228–37.
5. Watson L, Broderick C, Armon MP. Thrombolysis for acute deep vein thrombosis. Cochrane Database of Systematic Reviews. 2016 Nov 10;2016(11):CD002783.
6. Vedantham S, Goldhaber SZ, Julian JA, Kahn SR, Jaff MR, Cohen DJ, et al. Pharmacomechanical catheter-directed thrombolysis for deep-vein thrombosis. New England Journal of Medicine. 2017 Dec 7;377(23):2240–52.
7. Leung DA, Blitz LR, Nelson T, Amin A, Soukas PA, Nanjundappa A, et al. Rheolytic pharmacomechanical thrombectomy for the management of acute limb ischemia: Results from the pearl registry. Journal of Endovascular Therapy. 2015 Aug;22(4):546–57.
8. Garcia MJ, Lookstein R, Malhotra R, Amin A, Blitz LR, Leung DA, et al. Endovascular management of deep vein thrombosis with rheolytic thrombectomy: Final report of the prospective multicenter PEARL (peripheral use of angiojet rheolytic thrombectomy with a variety of catheter lengths) registry. Journal of Vascular and Interventional Radiology. 2015 Jun;26(6):777–85; quiz 786.

9. Notten P, ten Cate-Hoek AJ, Arnoldussen CWKP, Strijkers RHW, de Smet AAEA, Tick LW, et al. Ultrasound-accelerated catheter-directed thrombolysis versus anticoagulation for the prevention of post-thrombotic syndrome (CAVA): A single-blind, multicentre, randomised trial. Lancet Haematology. 2020 Jan;7(1):e40–49.
10. Garcia MJ, Sterling KM, Kahn SR, Comerota AJ, Jaff MR, Ouriel K, et al. Ultrasound-accelerated thrombolysis and venoplasty for the treatment of the postthrombotic syndrome: Results of the ACCESS PTS Study. JAHA. 2020 Feb 4;9(3):e013398.
11. Dexter DJ, Kado H, Schor J, Annambhotla S, Olivieri B, Mojibian H, et al. Interim outcomes of mechanical thrombectomy for deep vein thrombosis from the all-comer clout registry. Journal of Vascular Surgery: Venous and Lymphatic Disorders. 2022 Jul;10(4):832–40.e2.
12. Enden T, Haig Y, Kløw NE, Slagsvold CE, Sandvik L, Ghanima W, et al. Long-term outcome after additional catheter-directed thrombolysis versus standard treatment for acute iliofemoral deep vein thrombosis (the CaVenT study): A randomised controlled trial. Lancet. 2012 Jan;379(9810):31–38.
13. Joffe HV, Goldhaber SZ. Upper-extremity deep vein thrombosis. Circulation. 2002 Oct;106(14):1874–80.
14. Huang MH, Benishay ET, Desai KR. Endovascular management of acute iliofemoral deep vein thrombosis. Seminars in Interventional Radiology. 2022 Oct;39(5):459–63.
15. Kaufman C, Kinney T, Quencer K. Practice trends of fibrinogen monitoring in thrombolysis. Journal of Clinical Medicine. 2018 May 10;7(5):111.
16. Soltani A, Volz KR, Hansmann DR. Effect of modulated ultrasound parameters on ultrasound-induced thrombolysis. Physics in Medicine and Biology. 2008 Dec 7;53(23):6837–47.
17. Francis CW, Blinc A, Lee S, Cox C. Ultrasound accelerates transport of recombinant tissue plasminogen activator into clots. Ultrasound in Medicine & Biology. 1995;21(3):419–24.
18. Shi Y, Shi W, Chen L, Gu J. A systematic review of ultrasound-accelerated catheter-directed thrombolysis in the treatment of deep vein thrombosis. Journal of Thrombosis and Thrombolysis. 2018 Apr;45(3):440–51.
19. Engelberger RP, Stuck A, Spirk D, Willenberg T, Haine A, Périard D, et al. Ultrasound-assisted versus conventional catheter-directed thrombolysis for acute iliofemoral deep vein thrombosis: 1-year follow-up data of a randomized-controlled trial. Journal of Thrombosis and Haemostasis. 2017 Jul 1;15(7):1351–60.
20. Engelberger RP, Spirk D, Willenberg T, Alatri A, Do DD, Baumgartner I, et al. Ultrasound-assisted versus conventional catheter-directed thrombolysis for acute iliofemoral deep vein thrombosis. Circulation: Cardiovascular Interventions. 2015 Jan;8(1):e002027.
21. Shamaki GR, Soji-Ayoade D, Adedokun SD, Kesiena O, Favour M, Bolaji O, et al. Endovascular venous interventions- A state-of-the-art review. Current Problems in Cardiology. 2022 Dec;101534.
22. Endovascular Today United States Device Guide [Internet]. Endovascular Today; 2023 [cited 2023 Apr 12]. Retrieved from https://evtoday.com/device-guide/us
23. Ranade M, Moriarty JM. Use of the AlphaVac system for the removal of right atrial thrombus. Endovascular Today. 2022 May;21(5):3.
24. Mohammed M, Nona P, Abou Asala E, Chiang M, Lemor A, O'Neill B, et al. Preclosure of large bore venous access sites in patients undergoing transcatheter mitral replacement and repair. Catheterization and Cardiovascular Interventions. 2022;100(1):163–68.
25. Sudheendra D, Vedantham S. Catheter-directed therapy options for iliofemoral venous thrombosis. Surgical Clinics of North America. 2018 Apr;98(2):255–65.
26. Hubbard J, Saad WEA, Sabri SS, Turba UC, Angle JF, Park AW, et al. Rheolytic thrombectomy with or without adjunctive indwelling pharmacolysis in patients presenting with acute pulmonary embolism presenting with right heart strain and/or pulseless electrical activity. Thrombosis. 2011 Dec 28;2011:e246410.
27. Cynamon J, Stein EG, Dym RJ, Jagust MB, Binkert CA, Baum RA. A new method for aggressive management of deep vein thrombosis: Retrospective study of the power pulse technique. Journal of Vascular and Interventional Radiology. 2006 Jun;17(6):1043–49.

28. Kuo WT, Hofmann LV. Letter to the Editor. Journal of Vascular and Interventional Radiology. 2010 Nov;21(11):1776–77.
29. Harrison B, Hao F, Koney N, McWilliams J, Moriarty JM. Caval thrombus management: The data, where we are, and how it's done. Techniques in Vascular and Interventional Radiology. 2018 Jun;31;21(20).
30. Stein PD, Matta F, Yaekoub AY. Incidence of vena cava thrombosis in the United States. The American Journal of Cardiology. 2008 Oct;102(7):927–29.
31. Alkhouli M, Morad M, Narins CR, Raza F, Bashir R. Inferior vena cava thrombosis. JACC: Cardiovascular Interventions. 2016 Apr 11;9(7):629–43.
32. Liu D, Peterson E, Dooner J, Baerlocher M, Zypchen L, Gagnon J, et al. Diagnosis and management of iliofemoral deep vein thrombosis: Clinical practice guideline. Canadian Medical Association Journal. 2015 Nov 17;187(17):1288–96.
33. Vedantham S, Desai KR, Weinberg I, Marston W, Winokur R, Patel S, et al. Society of interventional radiology position statement on the endovascular management of acute iliofemoral deep vein thrombosis. Journal of Vascular and Interventional Radiology. 2023 Feb;34(2):284–99.e7.
34. Mastoris I, Kokkinidis DG, Bikakis I, Archontakis-Barakakis P, Papanastasiou CA, Jonnalagadda AK, et al. Catheter-directed thrombolysis vs. anticoagulation for the prevention and treatment of post-thrombotic syndrome in deep vein thrombosis: An updated systematic review and meta-analysis of randomized trials. Phlebology. 2019 Dec 1;34(10):675–82.
35. Douketis JD, Crowther MA, Foster GA, Ginsberg JS. Does the location of thrombosis determine the risk of disease recurrence in patients with proximal deep vein thrombosis? American Journal of Medicine. 2001 May;110(7):515–19.
36. Kahn SR, Shbaklo H, Lamping DL, Holcroft CA, Shrier I, Miron MJ, et al. Determinants of health-related quality of life during the 2 years following deep vein thrombosis. Journal of Thrombosis and Haemostasis. 2008 Jul;6(7):1105–12.
37. Desai KR. Endovascular management of acute iliofemoral deep vein thrombosis: Who benefits? Journal of Vascular and Interventional Radiology. 2022 Oct;33(10):1171–72.
38. National Institute for Health and Care Excellence. Venous thromboembolic diseases: Diagnosis, management and thrombophilia testing. NICE Guidelines [Internet]. 2020 Mar 26 [cited 2023 Feb 23]; Retrieved from www.nice.org.uk/guidance/ng158
39. Kakkos SK, Gohel M, Baekgaard N, et al. Editor's Choice – European Society for Vascular Surgery (ESVS) 2021: Clinical practice guidelines on the management of deep venous thrombosis. European Journal of Vascular and Endovascular Surgery. 2021;61:9–82.
40. Ortel TL, Neumann I, Ageno W, Beyth R, Clark NP, Cuker A, et al. American Society of Hematology 2020 guidelines for management of venous thromboembolism: Treatment of deep vein thrombosis and pulmonary embolism. Blood Advances. 2020 Oct 13;4(19):4693–738.
41. Stevens SM, Woller SC, Baumann Kreuziger L, Bounameaux H, Doerschug K, Geersing GJ, et al. Executive summary. Chest. 2021 Dec;160(6):2247–59.
42. Thukral S, Salter A, Lancia S, Kahn SR, Vedantham S. Predictors of clinical outcomes of pharmacomechanical catheter-directed thrombolysis for acute iliofemoral deep vein thrombosis: Analysis of a multicenter randomized trial. Journal of Vascular and Interventional Radiology. 2022 Oct;33(10):1161–70.e11.
43. Herrera S, Comerota AJ, Thakur S, Sunderji S, DiSalle R, Kazanjian SN, et al. Managing iliofemoral deep venous thrombosis of pregnancy with a strategy of thrombus removal is safe and avoids post-thrombotic morbidity. Journal of Vascular Surgery. 2014 Feb;59(2):456–64.
44. Bloom AI, Farkas A, Kalish Y, Elchalal U, Spectre G. Pharmacomechanical catheter-directed thrombolysis for pregnancy-related iliofemoral deep vein thrombosis. Journal of Vascular and Interventional Radiology. 2015 Jul;26(7):992–1000.
45. Huegel U, Surbek D, Mosimann B, Kucher N. Radiation- and contrast medium-free catheter-directed thrombolysis for early pregnancy-related massive iliocaval deep venous thrombosis. Journal of Vascular Surgery: Venous and Lymphatic Disorders. 2019 Jan;7(1):122–25.
46. Sousa Gomes M, Guimarães M, Montenegro N. Thrombolysis in pregnancy: A literature review. Journal of Maternal-Fetal & Neonatal Medicine. 2019 Jul 18;32(14):2418–28.

47. Goldenberg NA, Branchford B, Wang M, Ray C, Durham JD, Manco-Johnson MJ. Percutaneous mechanical and pharmacomechanical thrombolysis for occlusive deep vein thrombosis of the proximal limb in adolescent subjects: Findings from an institution-based prospective inception cohort study of pediatric venous thromboembolism. Journal of Vascular and Interventional Radiology. 2011 Feb;22(2):121–32.
48. Goldenberg NA, Durham JD, Knapp-Clevenger R, Manco-Johnson MJ. A thrombolytic regimen for high-risk deep venous thrombosis may substantially reduce the risk of postthrombotic syndrome in children. Blood. 2007 Jul 1;110(1):45–53.
49. Avila L, Cullinan N, White M, Gaballah M, Cahill AM, Warad D, et al. Pediatric May-Thurner Syndrome – systematic review and individual patient data meta-analysis. Journal of Thrombosis and Haemostasis. 2021 May;19(5):1283–93.
50. Andrew M, Vegh P, Johnston M, Bowker J, Ofosu F, Mitchell L. Maturation of the hemostatic system during childhood. Blood. 1992 Oct 15;80(8):1998–2005.
51. Gupta AA, Leaker M, Andrew M, Massicotte P, Liu L, Benson LN, et al. Safety and outcomes of thrombolysis with tissue plasminogen activator for treatment of intravascular thrombosis in children. Journal of Pediatrics. 2001 Nov 1;139(5):682–88.
52. Callese TE, Moriarty JM, Maehara C, Cusumano L, Mathevosian S, Enzmann D, et al. Cost drivers in endovascular pulmonary embolism interventions. Clinical Radiology. 2023 Feb;78(2):e143–49.
53. Weinberg I, Vedantham S, Salter A, Hadley G, Al-Hammadi N, Kearon C, et al. Relationships between the use of pharmacomechanical catheter-directed thrombolysis, sonographic findings, and clinical outcomes in patients with acute proximal DVT: Results from the ATTRACT Multicenter Randomized Trial. Vascular Medicine. 2019 Oct;24(5):442–51.
54. Cakir V, Gulcu A, Akay E, Capar AE, Gencpinar T, Kucuk B, et al. Use of percutaneous aspiration thrombectomy vs. anticoagulation therapy to treat acute iliofemoral venous thrombosis: 1-year follow-up results of a randomised, clinical trial. CardioVascular and Interventional Radiology. 2014 Aug;37(4):969–76.
55. Quinn E, Arndt M, Capanegro J, Sherard D. Successful removal of an acute deep vein thrombosis by the INARI clottriever system. Radiology Case Reports. 2021 Apr 10;16(6):1433–37.
56. Shah NG, Wible BC, Paulisin JA, Zaki M, Lamparello P, Sista A, et al. Management of inferior vena cava thrombosis with the Flowtriever and Clottriever systems. Journal of Vascular Surgery Venous and Lymphatic Disorders. 2021 May;9(3):615–20.
57. Joh M, Desai KR. Treatment of nonthrombotic iliac vein lesions. Seminars in Interventional Radiology. 2021 Jun;38(2):155–59.
58. Li N, Mendoza F, Rugonyi S, Farsad K, Kaufman JA, Jahangiri Y, et al. Venous biomechanics of angioplasty and stent placement: Implications of the Poisson effect. Journal of Vascular and Interventional Radiology. 2020 Aug;31(8):1348–56.
59. Kearon C, Gu CS, Julian J, Goldhaber S, Comerota A, Gornik H, et al. Pharmacomechanical catheter-directed thrombolysis in acute femoral – popliteal deep vein thrombosis: Analysis from a stratified randomized trial. Thrombosis and Haemostasis. 2019 Apr;119(4):633–44.
60. Robert-Ebadi H, Righini M. Management of distal deep vein thrombosis. Thrombosis Research. 2017 Jan 1;149:48–55.
61. Heller T, Becher M, Kröger JC, Beller E, Heller S, Höft R, et al. Isolated calf deep venous thrombosis: Frequency on venous ultrasound and clinical characteristics. BMC Emergency Medicine. 2021 Oct 30;21:126.
62. Kearon CA, Julian J, Math ME, Newman TS, Ginsberg J. Noninvasive diagnosis of deep venous thrombosis. Annals of Internal Medicine. 2000 Aug 15 [cited 2023 Jan 20]. Retrieved from www.acpjournals.org/doi/10.7326/0003-4819-128-8-199804150-00011
63. Righini M. Is it worth diagnosing and treating distal deep vein thrombosis? No. Journal of Thrombosis and Haemostasis. 2007 Jul;5:55–59.
64. Robert-Ebadi H, Righini M. Should we diagnose and treat distal deep vein thrombosis? Hematology. 2017 Dec 8;2017(1):231–36.

65. Righini M, Galanaud JP, Guenneguez H, Brisot D, Diard A, Faisse P, et al. Anticoagulant therapy for symptomatic calf deep vein thrombosis (CACTUS): A randomised, double-blind, placebo-controlled trial. Lancet Haematology. 2016 Dec 1;3(12):e556–62.
66. Kim KA, Choi SY, Kim R. Endovascular treatment for lower extremity deep vein thrombosis: An overview. Korean Journal of Radiology. 2021 Jun;22(6):931–43.
67. Ageno W, Haas S, Weitz JI, Goldhaber SZ, Turpie AGG, Goto S, et al. Characteristics and management of patients with venous thromboembolism: The Garfield-VTE registry. Thrombosis and Haemostasis. 2019 Feb;119(2):319–27.
68. Elman EE, Kahn SR. The post-thrombotic syndrome after upper extremity deep venous thrombosis in adults: A systematic review. Thrombosis Research. 2006;117(6):609–14.
69. Bosch FTM, Nisio MD, Büller HR, van Es N. Diagnostic and therapeutic management of upper extremity deep vein thrombosis. Journal of Clinical Medicine. 2020 Jul;9(7):2069.
70. Moore R, Lum YW. Venous thoracic outlet syndrome. Vascular Medicine. 2015 Apr 1;20(2):182–89.
71. Hangge P, Rotellini-Coltvet L, Deipolyi AR, Albadawi H, Oklu R. Paget-Schroetter syndrome: Treatment of venous thrombosis and outcomes. Cardiovascular Diagnosis and Therapy. 2017 Dec;7(Suppl 3):S285–90.
72. Taylor JM, Telford RJ, Kinsella DC, Watkinson AF, Thompson JF. Long-term clinical and functional outcome following treatment for Paget – Schroetter syndrome. British Journal of Surgery. 2013 Oct 1;100(11):1459–64.
73. Kearon C, Akl EA, Ornelas J, Blaivas A, Jimenez D, Bounameaux H, et al. Antithrombotic therapy for VTE disease. Chest. 2016 Feb;149(2):315–52.
74. AbuRahma AF, Sadler D, Stuart P, Khan MZ, Boland JP. Conventional versus thrombolytic therapy in spontaneous (effort) axillary-subclavian vein thrombosis. The American Journal of Surgery. 1991 Apr 1;161(4):459–65.
75. Vik A, Holme PA, Singh K, Dorenberg E, Nordhus KC, Kumar S, et al. Catheter-directed thrombolysis for treatment of deep venous thrombosis in the upper extremities. CardioVascular and Interventional Radiology. 2009 Sep 1;32(5):980–87.
76. Kim HS, Patra A, Paxton BE, Khan J, Streiff MB. Catheter-directed thrombolysis with percutaneous rheolytic thrombectomy versus thrombolysis alone in upper and lower extremity deep vein thrombosis. CardioVascular and Interventional Radiology. 2006;29(6):1003–7.
77. Koury JP, Burke CT. Endovascular management of acute upper extremity deep venous thrombosis and the use of superior vena cava filters. Seminars in Interventional Radiology. 2011 Mar;28(1):3–9.
78. Fuller T, Neville E, Shapiro J, Muck AE, Broering M, Kulwicki A, et al. Comparison of aspiration thrombectomy to other endovascular therapies for proximal upper extremity deep venous thrombosis. Journal of Vascular Surgery: Venous and Lymphatic Disorders. 2022 Mar 1;10(2):300–5.
79. Teter K, Arko F, Muck P, Lamparello PJ, Khaja MS, Huasen B, et al. Aspiration thrombectomy for the management of acute deep venous thrombosis in the setting of venous thoracic outlet syndrome. Vascular. 2020 Apr;28(2):183–88.
80. Rachapalli V, Boucher LM. Superior Vena Cava Syndrome: Role of the Interventionalist. Canadian Association of Radiologists Journal. 2014 May 1;65(2):168–76.
81. Sfyroeras GS, Antonopoulos CN, Mantas G, Moulakakis KG, Kakisis JD, Brountzos E, et al. A review of open and endovascular treatment of superior vena cava syndrome of benign aetiology. European Journal of Vascular and Endovascular Surgery. 2017 Feb;53(2):238–54.
82. Cui J, Kawai T, Irani Z. Catheter-directed thrombolysis in acute superior vena cava syndrome caused by central venous catheters. Seminars in Dialysis. 2015;28(5):548–51.
83. Ghanavati R, Amiri A, Ansarinejad N, Hajsadeghi S, Riahi Beni H, Sezavar SH. Successful treatment of a catheter-induced superior vena cava syndrome through catheter-directed thrombolysis: A case report. Journal of Tehran University Heart Center. 2017 Oct;12(4):188–91.
84. Kee ST, Kinoshita L, Razavi MK, Nyman UR, Semba CP, Dake MD. Superior vena cava syndrome: Treatment with catheter-directed thrombolysis and endovascular stent placement. Radiology [Internet]. 1998 Jan 1 [cited 2023 Feb 26]; Retrieved from https://pubs.rsna.org/doi/10.1148/radiology.206.1.9423671

Section 4

Special Topics

Chapter 22

Indications, Techniques, and Retrieval of Inferior Vena Cava Filters

Charles A. Banks and Marc A. Passman

INTRODUCTION

In the United States, the annual incidence of deep venous thrombosis (DVT) with pulmonary thromboembolism (PTE) is approximately 900,000 cases according to the Center for Disease Control and Prevention (CDC). Mortality ranges from 6–10% in patients presenting with DVT/PTE with an estimated 25% of patients with PTE experiencing sudden death as initial symptom.[1] Due to the relatively high morbidity and mortality associated with PTE, prompt initiation of therapeutic anticoagulation has remained the standard of treatment in patients presenting with DVT. Additionally, chemoprophylaxis with prophylactic-dose anticoagulation has been used in patients at high-risk for developing DVT such as polytrauma patients, orthopedic patients requiring prolonged immobility, and major surgical patients.

A minority of patients with contraindications to therapeutic or prophylactic anticoagulation require alternative means of therapy. Inferior vena cava filters (IVCF) were initially introduced in 1969 as a mechanical modality for prevention of PTE.[2] After initial market approval, annual utilization of IVCFs increased rapidly with peak in the early 2000s and gradual downtrend after 2010.[3,4] In recent years, an estimated 65,000–94,000 IVCFs are deployed annually as a therapeutic or prophylactic measure in patients unable to be therapeutically anticoagulated.[3,5] Utilizing the available data in the literature, multiple academic societies have established evidence-based guidelines for IVCF utilization. In this chapter, we provide an overview of current indications, deployment, and retrieval of IVCFs.

CLINICAL INDICATIONS

Practice patterns regarding IVCF utilization have varied widely based upon institutional utilization, geographical location, and patient population.[6–8] Multiple sub-specialty academic societies have developed guidelines concerning appropriate use of IVCFs.[2,9] The primary consensus among these specialties is to reserve IVCF placement for thromboembolic protection in patients presenting with DVT or PTE who have absolute contraindications to therapeutic anticoagulation or have experienced a complication or recurrent DVT/PTE despite therapeutic anticoagulation.[2,10] Therapeutic anticoagulation is absolutely contraindicated in patients with severe coagulopathy or thrombocytopenia, active hemorrhage, recent hemorrhagic stroke, high risk intracranial lesions, or poorly controlled hypertension (SBP > 230).[2,10,11] Therapeutic anticoagulation may also be contraindicated in patients with significant hepatic or renal dysfunction due to inability to adequately metabolize anticoagulants. Lastly, patients with severely compromised pulmonary capacity secondary to PTE are considered primary candidates for IVCF placement due to increased mortality with potential recurrent PTE.[2,10]

DOI: 10.1201/9781003316626-26

There are few prospective randomized controlled trials (RCTs) validating the efficacy of IVCF deployment. Guidelines and practice paradigms are largely derived from reported clinical experience and retrospective cohort studies evaluating the efficacy of IVCF placement in different patient populations.[10] The initial development of IVCF guidelines were primarily based upon the early RCT known as the PREPIC trial (Prevention du Risqué d'Embolie par Interruption Cave).[12,13] This trial randomized patients experiencing acute DVT to anticoagulation alone and anticoagulation combined with IVCF. This trial successfully demonstrated the efficacy of IVCF placement in preventing PTE with 4.8% of no-IVCF patients compared to 1.1% of IVCF patients experiencing PTE at 12 days and 20.8% compared to 11.6% experienced recurrent DVT at 2 years, respectively.[12] This pattern was demonstrated in a subsequent study evaluating the same patient cohort at 8-years follow-up revealing long-term PTE protection. However, the study demonstrated an increased risk of DVT and no survival benefit in the IVCF group.[13] To date, the PREPIC trials remain the largest RCT conducted regarding IVCF utilization. However, it is difficult to generalize the findings from the PREPIC trial because the clinical decision regarding IVCF utilization is primarily in patients without the ability to be anticoagulated.

Multiple, small RCTs have corroborated the original findings of the PREPIC trial.[11,14–17] These studies primarily focused on specific patient groups such as cancer patients, trauma patients, and patients with prior PTE. A meta-analysis of these RCTs including 1,274 patients revealed an overall decrease in the incidence of PTE in patients receiving IVCF placement without a significant increase in recurrent DVTs (11.9% vs 9.1%; $p = 0.58$). Conglomerate results from the RCTs failed to demonstrate a statistically significant overall mortality difference between the IVCF group and anticoagulation alone group at 3 months (9.22% vs 6.73%, respectively; $p = 0.13$). Overall, no current study has demonstrated a survival benefit related to IVCF placement when therapeutic anticoagulation alone is feasible.[11,18]

As endovascular techniques evolved and IVCF technology expanded to retrievable IVCFs (rIVCF), practice paradigms incorporated extended or relative indications for IVCF placement including prophylactic deployment. The development of rIVCFs in the early 2000s resulted in an exponential increase (3-fold) in rIVCF deployment as prophylactic thromboembolic protection specifically in polytrauma patients.[4,19,20] However, an associated increase in adverse events and relatively low attempted removal rate (<50%) prompted an issuance from the FDA in 2010 that intensified scrutiny and reduced excessive utilization of rIVCF over subsequent years.[19] An additional FDA warning was issued in 2014 regarding the need for improved post-market approval surveillance and filter retrieval.[21]

Although results have been mixed, studies focusing on prophylactic IVCF placement have demonstrated some efficacy of IVCF placement in certain selective scenarios.[17,18,22] In a large propensity-matched study investigating effects of prophylactic IVCF placement in patients with high bleeding risk, Muriel and colleagues demonstrated a trend toward lower overall mortality in the IVCF group (6.6% vs 10.2%; $p = 0.12$) as well as a significantly lower PTE-related mortality in the IVCF group compared to no-IVCF (1.7% vs 4.9%; $p = 0.03$).[22] As a patient population at relatively high risk for DVT and subsequent PTE, prophylactic IVCF placement has been well studied in trauma patients.[23] In the multicenter RCT conducted by Ho and colleagues, prophylactic IVCF placement failed to provide significant benefit in terms of PTE prevention or death when compared to pharmaco-prophylaxis alone.[17] However, in a subset of patients primarily with head or spinal cord injuries precluding prophylactic anticoagulation, prophylactic IVCF placement was associated with 0% incidence of PTEs compared to 14.7% in the no-IVCF group. A meta-analysis of multiple observational studies conducted in 2011 revealed significant reduction in PTE events in trauma patients undergoing prophylactic IVCF placement compared to prophylactic anticoagulation alone.[23] This meta-analysis was unable to provide conclusive evidence regarding the survival benefit provided by IVCF placement.[23]

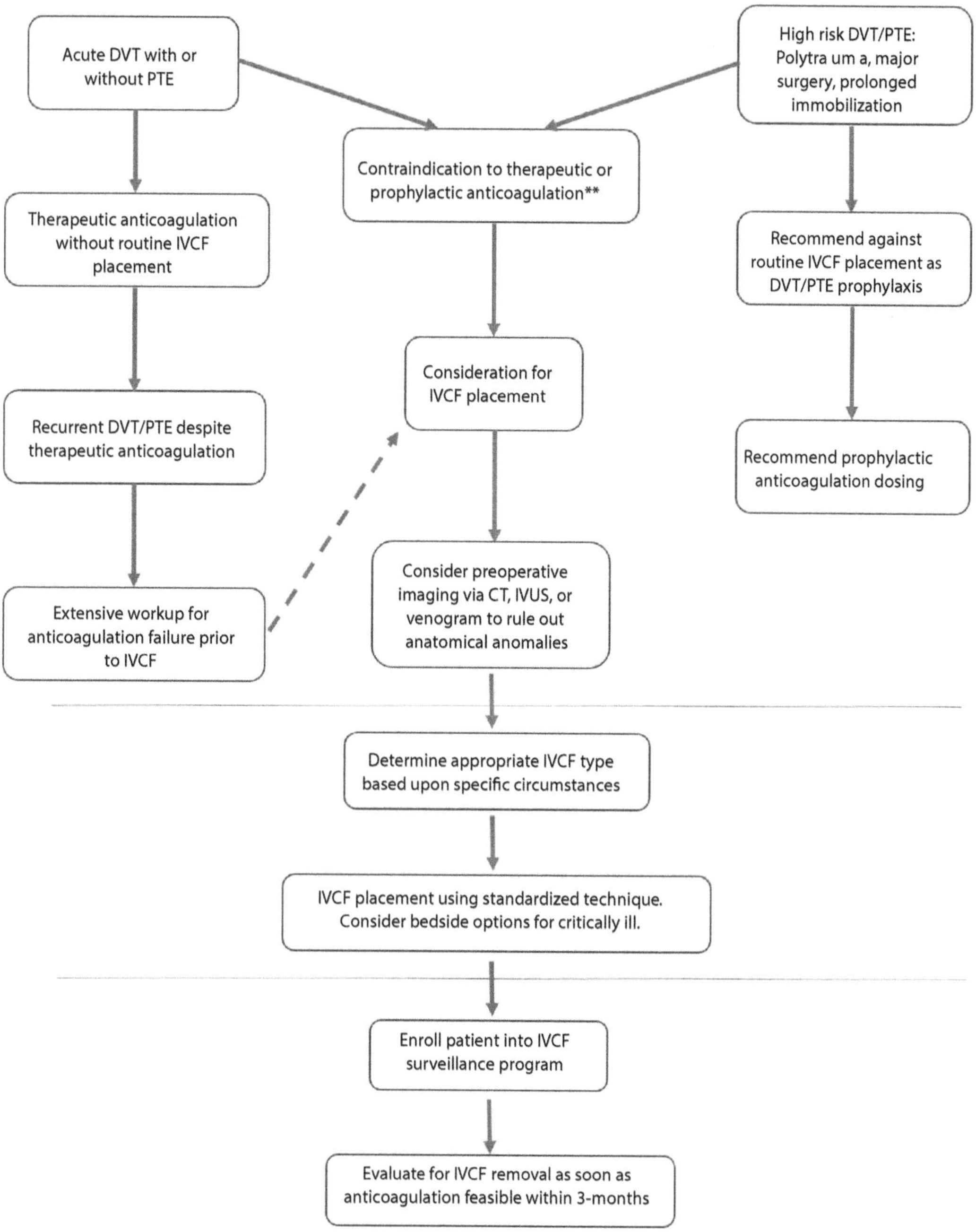

Figure 22.1 Algorithm based on evidence-based recommendations regarding the use of inferior vena cava (IVC) filters in the treatment of patients with or at substantial risk of venous thromboembolic disease. * IVCF = Inferior vena cava filter; DVT = Deep venous thrombosis; PTE = Pulmonary thromboembolism; IVUS = intravascular ultrasound. ** Therapeutic anticoagulation is absolutely contraindicated in patients with severe coagulopathy or thrombocytopenia, active hemorrhage, recent hemorrhagic stroke, high risk of intracranial lesions, or poorly controlled hypertension [SBP > 230]. Therapeutic anticoagulation may also be contraindicated in patients with significant hepatic or renal dysfunction due to inability to adequately metabolize anticoagulants.

Recently, the PRESERVE trial (Predicting the Safety and Effectiveness of Inferior Vena Cava Filters) was completed.[24] This study was a large, nonrandomized trial consisting of 1429 patients with contraindications to anticoagulation undergoing IVCF placement (71.7% with current DVT/PTE and 8.9% prophylactic). Despite the lack of randomization in this study, the authors demonstrated the efficacy and safety of IVCF utilization with a 2.2% significant adverse event rate and 98.3% freedom from clinically significant PTE. In patients with prophylactic indication for IVCF placement, no patients experienced PTE, 3.9% experienced DVTs, and 0.7% experienced caval thrombosis. Of the cohort, 44.5% underwent IVCF retrieval with median time from implantation to retrieval of 86 days. Adverse events related to IVCF retrieval procedures occurred in 1.95% of patients.[24]

The quality of evidence from all studies have been evaluated and combined to generate evidence-based guidelines for the utilization of IVCFs.[2] The current guidelines established by the Society of Interventional Radiology in collaboration with multiple other academic societies including the Society for Vascular Surgery are represented as an algorithm in Figure 22.1.

IVC FILTER DEVICES

The most critical design feature of an IVCF is to minimize embolic events while maximizing IVC patency and prevent IVC occlusion. Many different IVCF designs are available and are utilized in a variety of patient scenarios. Different materials have been employed in manufacturing of IVCFs including nitinol, stainless steel, titanium, and cobalt. Although makeup and size differ between filter types, most IVCFs preserve the traditional conical shape as utilized in the initial Greenfield IVCF.[25] The conical design preserves IVC patency while providing excellent thromboembolic protection.[25] The conical filter can maintain nearly 50% of IVC luminal patency despite being filled to 70% capacity. The excellent success of the early Greenfield IVCF models provided a framework for the evolution of IVCF technology and deployment strategies.

Overall, IVCFs are divided into two primary categories, permanent and retrievable. Permanent IVCFs (pIVCFs) are intended as lifelong mechanical thromboembolic protection modality in at risk patients and are designed without a percutaneous retrieval method. Retrievable or optional IVCFs (rIVCFs) are designed with features allowing for endovascular removal should the need for mechanical thromboembolic protection resolve. The utilization of rIVCFs allows for temporary thromboembolic prophylaxis and provides a delay in determining permanent requirement for thromboembolic protection. All rIVCFs are also FDA approved for permanent deployment providing enhanced flexibility compared to permanent filters.[19] Currently available FDA approved IVCFs are listed and imaged in Table 22.1.

Few studies have been conducted comparing the outcomes of pIVCFs and rIVCFs. A retrospective study consisting of 702 patients receiving IVCF (60.8% rIVCF and 39.2% pIVCF) demonstrated similar rates of DVT and symptomatic IVC thrombosis at 1 year. Currently, no randomized controlled trial has been performed appraising the outcomes of pIVCFs and rIVCFs. However, in a large evaluation of the MAUDE (Manufacturer and User Facility Device Experience) registry, Andreoli and colleagues revealed significantly higher frequency of all adverse events in patients receiving rIVCF.[27] These adverse events included device fracture, migration, IVC thrombus, and limb embolization. Studies have indicated that risk of adverse events related to rIVCFs are directly related to dwell time.[19,25–28] Additionally, prolonged dwell time of greater than 7-months is associated with a high failure rate of conventional retrieval techniques at 40.9%.[28] Other studies focusing on specific rIVCF designs have

Table 22.1 Currently Available Inferior Vena Cava Filters and Device Information

Device		Manufacturer	Material	Design	Approach	Delivery Sheath (Fr)	Maximum Caval Diameter	Maximum Deployed Length	FDA-Approved Use
Greenfield Filter	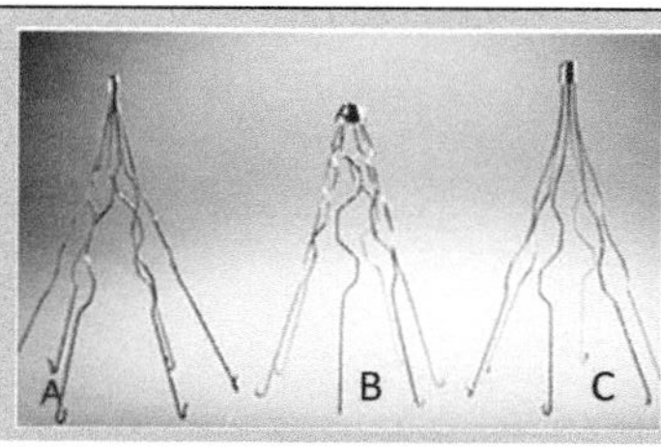	Boston Scientific Natick, MA	**A.** Stainless steel **B.** Titanium **C.** Low profile Stainless steel	Conical; Single Trapping	Femoral or Jugular	12	28	49	Permanent
Bird's Nest Filter	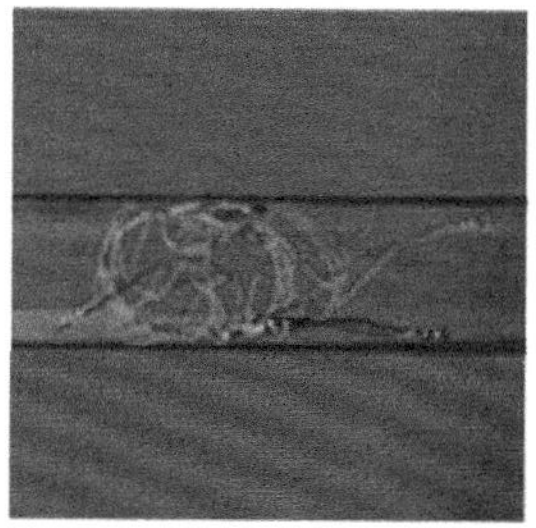	Cook Inc. Bloomington, IN	Stainless Steel	Variable	Femoral or Jugular	12	40	80	Permanent
Simon Nitinol Filter	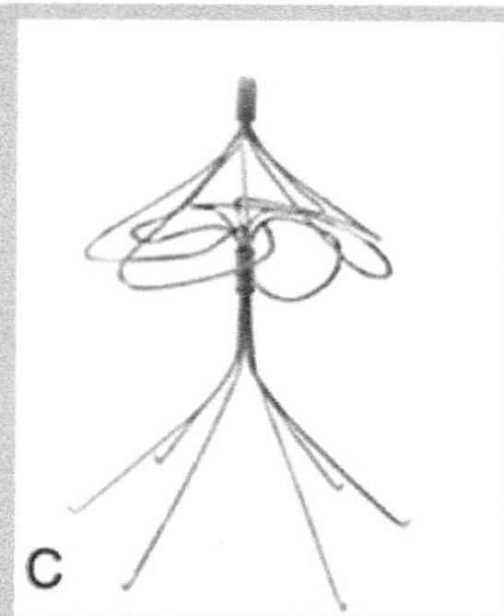	Bard Peripheral Vascular Tempe, AZ	Nitinol	Conical Bilevel	Femoral or Jugular	7	28	38	Permanent

(Continued)

Table 22.1 Currently Available Inferior Vena Cava Filters and Device Information *(Continued)*

Device		Manufacturer	Material	Design	Approach	Delivery sheath (Fr)	Maximum Caval Diameter	Maximum Deployed Length	FDA-Approved Use
Denali	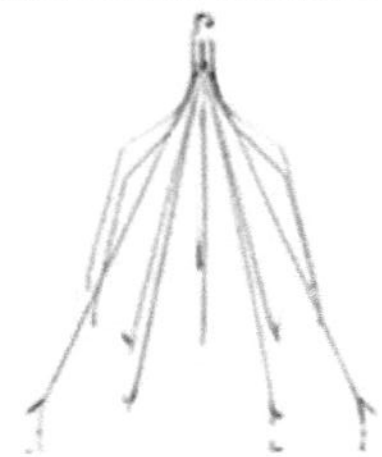	Bard Peripheral Vascular Tempe, AZ	Nitinol	Conical Bilevel	Femoral or Jugular	8.4	28	43	Permanent
VenaTech LP Filter	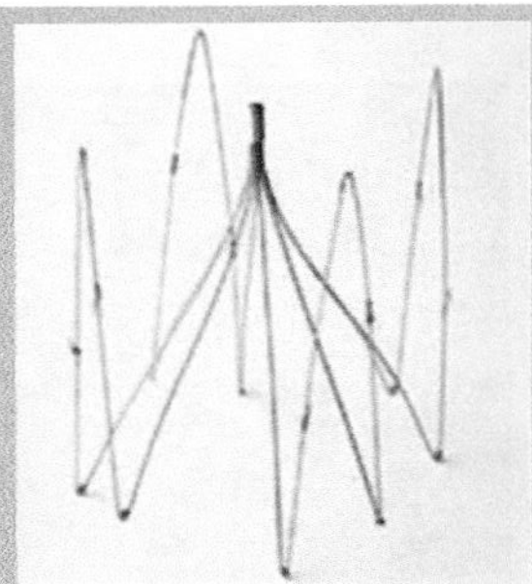	Braun/Vena Tech, Bethlehem, PA	Cobalt Chromium	Conical Single Trapping	Femoral or Jugular	7	28	43	Permanent
VenaTech Convertible	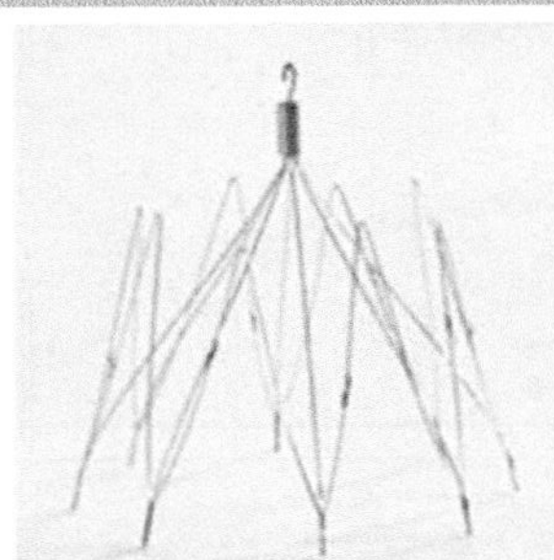	Braun/Vena Tech, Bethlehem, PA	Cobalt Chromium	Conical Single Trapping	Femoral or Jugular	12.9	28	--	Convertible

Option Elite Filter	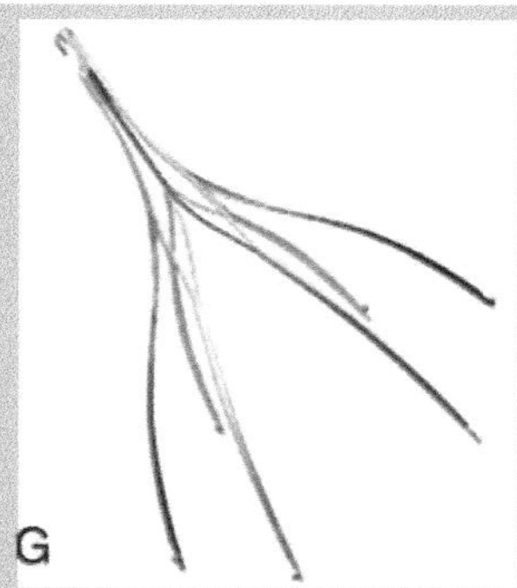 G	Argon Medical Devices Inc., Plano, TX	Nitinol	Conical	Femoral, Jugular, or Brachial	6.5	30	56.5	Optional
Gunther Tulip Filter	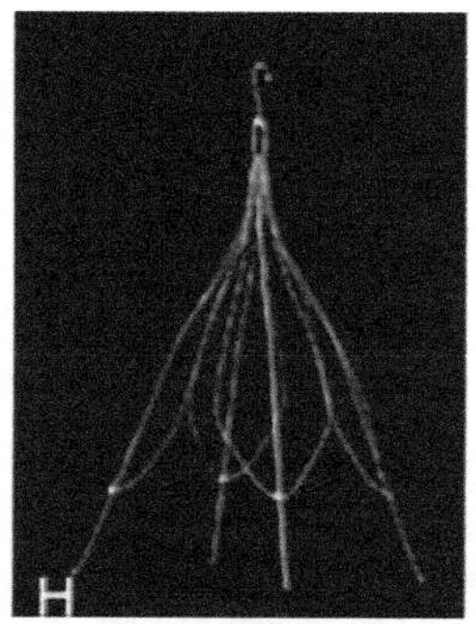 H	Cook Inc., Bloomington, IN	Conichrome	Conical, Single trapping	Femoral or Jugular	Femoral 8.5 Jugular 7	30	50	Optional
Celect Platinum	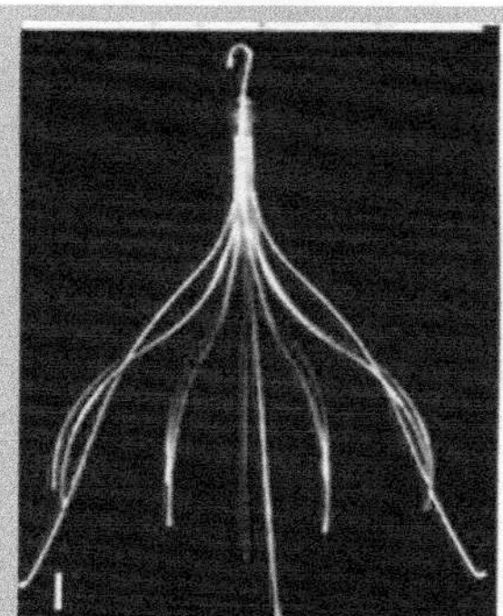 I	Cook Inc., Bloomington, IN	Conichrome	Conical, Single trapping	Femoral or Jugular	7	30	51	Optional

(Continued)

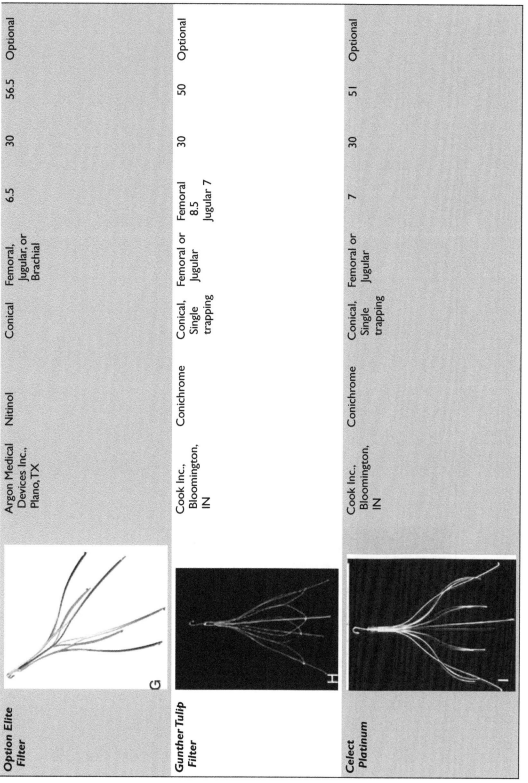

Table 22.1 Currently Available Inferior Vena Cava Filters and Device Information *(Continued)*

Device		*Manufacturer*	*Material*	*Design*	*Approach*	*Delivery sheath (Fr)*	*Maximum Caval Diameter*	*Maximum Deployed Length*	*FDA-Approved Use*
OptEase Filter	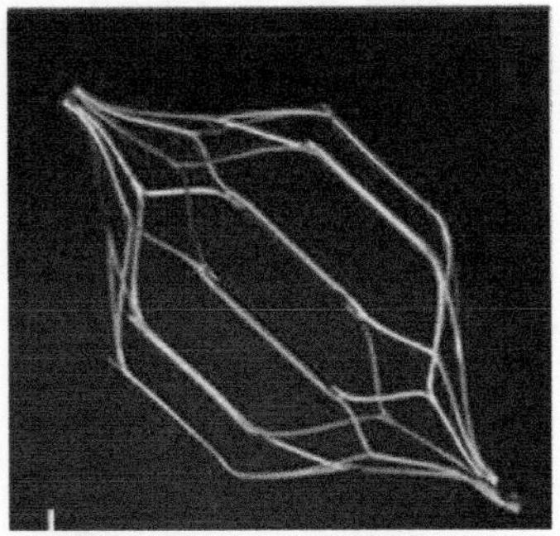	Cordis Endovascular, Miami, FL	Nitinol	Double basket	Femoral, Jugular, or antecubital	6	30	44	Optional
ALN Optional Filter	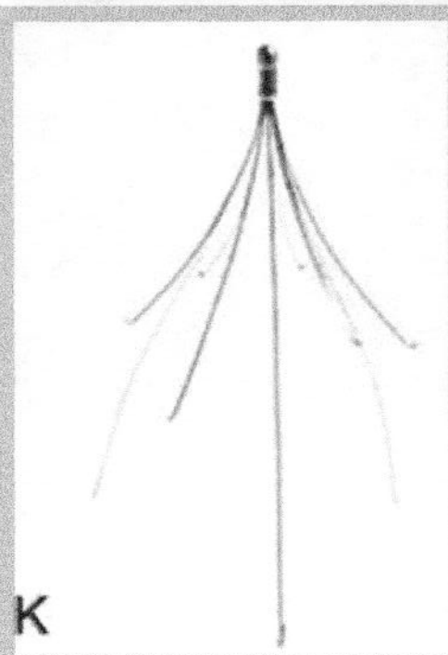 K	ALN, Bormes Les Mimosas, France	Stainless Steel	Conical	Femoral, Jugular, or brachial	7	28	55	Optional

Sentry	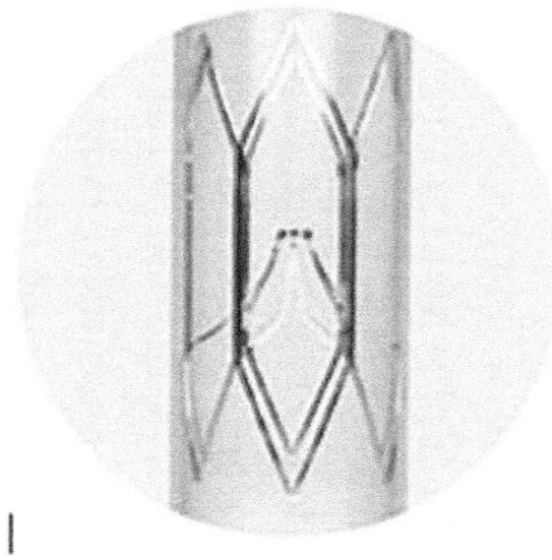	Boston Scientific Natick, MA	Nitinol frame, Bioabsorbable filament	Conical	Femoral or Jugular	7	16–28	57.7	Convertible
Angel Catheter	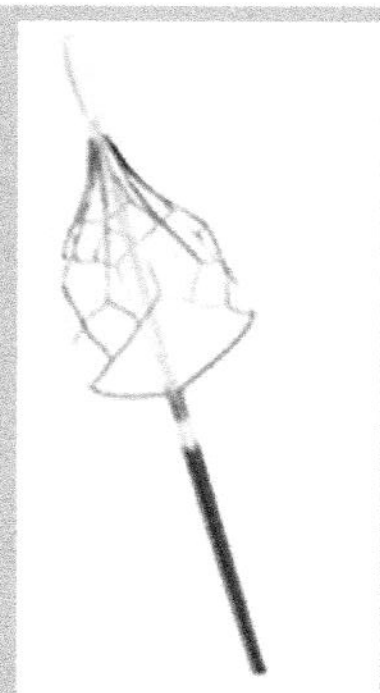	Mermaid Medical	Nitinol	Conical	Femoral	8	15–30	50	Temporary

Source: Adapted from: Passman M. Vena Cava Interruption. In: Perler SSaB, editor. Rutherford's Vascular Surgery and Endovascular Therapy. Philidelphia, PA: Elsevier; 2020. pp. 2013–30.[26]

corroborated this finding.[28–30] However, these studies demonstrated a much earlier association of failed standard retrieval techniques and rIVCF dwell time of greater than 90 days.[29,30] Based on currently available evidence, rIVCFs should be promptly removed once the indication for deployment has resolved.

Convertible IVCFs are a newer subtype of IVCFs that are designed with a mechanism to convert from a thromboembolic filtration system to non-filtration state while remaining implanted. These convertible IVCFs are primarily intended for short-term thromboembolic prophylaxis without requiring retrieval. There are currently three FDA approved convertible IVCF designs. The VenaTech convertible IVCF (B. Braun Interventional Systems, Bethlehem, PA) has a conical design with a removable central component that leaves behind a functional IVC stent once removed.[11] Results from this filter at 6 months have been excellent in patients with converted filters with low adverse event rates.[31] The VenaTech system, however, requires an additional endovascular procedure for removal of the filtration component. Other convertible IVCFs such as the Sentry (BTG Vascular, Bothell, Washington) are designed with a bioconvertible central filament that hydrolyzes after 60 days leaving behind only nitinol scaffolding. The Sentry IVCF has demonstrated high rates of successful bioconversion and low adverse event rates.[32] The Angel IVCF (Bio2 Medical, San Antonio, Texas) consists of a multi-lumen central venous catheter that remains attached to the IVCF. This provides for removal at the bedside in critically ill patients without an additional endovascular procedure.[33]

IVC ANATOMICAL CONSIDERATIONS

In the vast majority of patients (97%), the IVC is a retroperitoneal venous structure that is positioned to the right of the vertebral column. The confluence of the iliac veins forms the inferior aspect of the IVC with direct drainage into the right atrium superiorly.[2,34,35] The IVC consists of four primary segments: infrarenal, renal, suprarenal, and hepatic. Although rare, there are several anatomic variants to be aware of prior to attempting deployment of an IVCF. Retroaortic or circumaortic left renal vein is the most common anomaly with a prevalence of approximately 3.0–7.0%.[2,35] In these patients, the confluence of the left renal vein and IVC may occur more caudally, which may affect IVCF deployment site. Duplicated IVC is present in 0.2–3.0% of patients and exists with multiple anatomical subtypes primarily affecting renal vein drainage.[34] The most generally accepted IVCF deployment strategy in these patients is bilateral infrarenal IVCF deployment.[35] This anatomical variant predisposes patients to increased risk of PTE despite IVCF deployment.[35] Left-sided IVC is a rare anatomical anomaly (0.5% of patients) that creates difficult determination of anatomical landmarks during IVCF deployment.[33,35] Typically, the IVC will cross midline via the left renal vein or hemiazygos venous system. This creates difficulty in recognizing anatomical landmarks for deployment and may prohibit a transjugular approach.[36] An interrupted IVC or IVC agenesis occurs in 0.6% of patients and is highly associated with concomitant cardiovascular anomalies.[34,36] In these patients, the infrahepatic IVC is interrupted with primary IVC drainage occurring through the hemiazygos and azygos systems.[36] Although these anomalies are uncommon, detailed imaging should be strongly considered prior to attempting IVCF deployment.

IVC FILTER PLACEMENT TECHNIQUES

There are multiple techniques designed for IVCF deployment that accommodate different clinical scenarios. These range from IVCF placement in an interventional imaging suite, at the bedside of critically ill patients under transabdominal duplex ultrasound-guidance, utilization of intravascular ultrasound (IVUS), and deployment using a fixed or mobile C-arm in the operating room or hybrid suite. Percutaneous venous access is obtained through either femoral vein, jugular vein (right preferred over left), or brachial vein (for lower profile devices).[25] IVCF deployment using conventional venography is the mainstay of current deployment options. Venography allows for optimal IVCF sizing, precise measurements of anatomical landmarks, and identification of aberrant anatomy to avoid inadvertent IVCF deployment into venous tributaries in the infrarenal IVC. Some studies indicate that pre-deployment selective venography identified unsuspected anatomical variants that altered deployment anatomical location or technique in 18–26% of cases.[37,38] Venography also allows for direct visualization of the IVCF post-deployment to confirm optimal placement and ensure IVCF tilt along the IVC axis is <15°. The optimal positioning of IVCFs in the general population is just inferior to the lowest renal vein and superior to the iliac veins.

Deployment approaches specific to different filter devices are generally similar but may vary with specific filter designs. For femoral access, the patient is supine, and both groins are prepped. For jugular access, positioning the patient supine with head rotation to the contralateral side. Ultrasound-guided access with a micropuncture 5-French sheath is performed followed by an 0.035 wire advanced into the IVC. A pigtail catheter is advanced over the 0.035 wire and an ascending digital subtraction venography of the IVC is obtained (Figure 22.2A). Diameter of the IVC is confirmed and anatomical landmarks such as the iliac vein confluence and renal veins are identified (Figure 22.2A). After sequential venous dilations, the 5-French sheath is exchanged for a 10-French delivery sheath. Once optimal location is established, the IVCF is deployed, and location is confirmed by digital subtraction venography (Figure 22.2B and C). After sheath removal, manual pressure is held to achieve hemostasis.

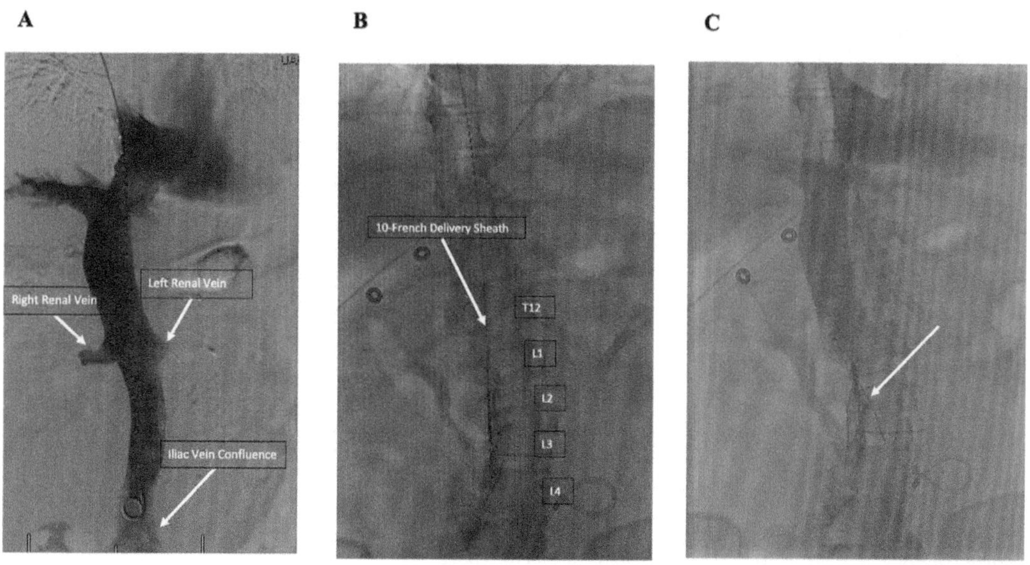

Figure 22.2 Inferior vena cava filter deployment by venography. (A) Pre-deployment digital subtraction angiogram. (B) Positioning of IVC deployment sheath with bony anatomic landmarks indicated. (C) IVCF deployed.

Other deployment techniques include transabdominal ultrasound guidance and IVUS. These modalities are typically employed during bedside deployment in critically ill patients or in patients with contraindications to intravenous contrast or fluoroscopy such as renal insufficiency and pregnancy. In duplex ultrasound-guided placement, pre-deployment ultrasound is utilized to map and measure the IVC and the lowest renal vein junction. The deployment process involving serial dilations to upsize to a larger sheath are similar to that described previously. At time of deployment, a transverse image of the renal vein-IVC junction is generated, and the IVC deployment catheter is visualized. The catheter is retracted inferiorly until the echogenic catheter tip is no longer visualized indicating appropriate deployment position. The catheter is then visualized in the longitudinal view and deployed under direct observation.[39] Technical success rate using transabdominal ultrasonography is 97%.[40]

The deployment of IVCF using IVUS alone or as an adjunct to venography has been performed with success. Utilizing IVUS alone for IVCF placement can be performed by dual or single venous access.[39] Dual venous access can be obtained contralaterally or ipsilaterally and allows for IVUS to be utilized until the moment of deployment. In the single venous access technique, IVUS is used to obtain precise measurements of the IVC and location of the renal veins. These measurements are then applied to the deployment sheath, and the IVCF

Table 22.2 Comparison of Vena Cava Filter Types for the Prevention of Pulmonary Embolism and Complications Rates Based on Systematic Reviews

Filter Device	*PTE Overall (%)*	*PTE Fatal (%)*	*Insertion Site Thrombosis*	*Vena Cava Thrombosis*	*Filter Migration*	*Tilt >15*	*Filter Leg Penetration (%)*
STAINLESS STEEL GREENFIELD	3.5	1.3	8.6	3.5	2.0	*	2–15
TITANIUM GREENFIELD	3.4	1.8	13.1	4.4	7.5–15	*	13–50
PERCUTANEOUS STAINLESS STEEL GREENFIELD	2.7	0.3	4.3	3	2.6	*	1.0
SIMON NITINOL	3.3	1.8	11.5	5.2	0–5	*	25–95
BIRD'S NEST	3.4	1.5	7.4	2.8	1.1	*	85
VENA TECH LP OR LGM	3.6	0.9	15.3	9.5	6–18.4	*	*
TRAPEASE	0.9	*	0.4	2	0.9	*	*
OPTEASE	1.6	*	0.8	3.7	0.3	5.6	1.9
G2	3.4	*	--	3.7	4.5	*	44
RECOVERY G2	1.0	*	10.4	1.0	0.8	15.5	15.1
GUNTHER TULIP	0.9	0.4	*	2.3	0.7	5.9	22–78
CELECT	1.1	*	1.2	0.6	0.6	12.1	22–93
ALN OPTIONAL	0.7	*	14.0	1.8	0.5	*	3.4
REX OPTION	4.0	*	18.0	1.0	2.0	*	2.9–10
DENALI	*	*	*	*	*	*	2.5

*Limited or insufficient systemically reviewed published data to report.

Abbreviation: PTE = Pulmonary thromboembolism.

Source: Adapted from table from: Passman M. Vena Cava Interruption. In: Perler SSaB, editor. Rutherford's Vascular Surgery and Endovascular Therapy. Philidelphia, PA: Elsevier; 2020. p. 2013–30.[26]

is deployed after removal of the IVUS probe. The IVUS technique has been performed with technical success of 95–96%.[40,41] A large systematic review of 21 studies containing 2166 cases revealed similar technical success rates and procedural complication rates when comparing ultrasound guidance, IVUS, and venography.[42] Some studies have suggested that IVUS alone can be more accurate than venography in determining venous anatomy and optimal deployment location.[43] Regardless of IVCF placement strategy, pre-deployment and post-deployment imaging are necessary for optimal filter placement.

Overall, the technical success rate of IVCF deployment is 98% with rare overall incidence of procedural-related complications.[25] Procedural and postoperative complications vary by IVCF design (Table 22.2). Vascular access complications are most common with a rate of 4–11%.[44] Arteriovenous fistulas have also been demonstrated at a low rate (0.02%).[44] Malpositioning at time of placement and air embolism are other uncommon procedural complications occurring in 1.3% and 0.2% of cases, respectively. Procedural mortality is rare ranging from 0.13–0.34% and is usually associated with patients succumbing to other comorbidities.[26] Filter-related complications include filter tilt >15° (5%), filter migration (<1.0%) and incomplete filter deployment (0.7–13.9%).[44]

In certain cases, such as infrarenal IVC thrombus, pregnancy, and previously malpositioned IVCF, suprarenal IVCF placement may be necessary. Currently, suprarenal deployment of IVCFs is considered off-label and has not been approved by the FDA. Due to the larger diameter of the suprarenal IVC and the more dynamic vessel wall secondary to proximity to the cardiopulmonary systems, there have been concerns for filter migration. Initial studies revealed significant IVCF migration as high as 27%.[45] More recent appraisal demonstrated that filters deployed in the suprarenal IVC can be performed with excellent technical success and complication rates similar to infrarenal IVCF.[45] In patients with a contraindication to anticoagulation in the setting of an obliterated infrarenal IVC secondary to compression by a gravid uterus or pelvic mass, thrombosed infrarenal IVC, or malpositioned infrarenal IVC, suprarenal IVC deployment and retrieval are safe and efficacious.[45,46]

IVC FILTER RETRIEVAL

Although procedural-related complications are rare, long-term outcomes after IVCF placement are of significant concern. Long-term complications following IVCF deployment are directly correlated with prolonged IVCF dwell time (>90 days) or non-retrieval.[28,47] These complications include IVC perforation with or without associated organ perforation (12.4%–20%), device fracture (21%), delayed migration (11.8%), DVT (1.9–14.5%), and PTE (0.5–12%).[44,47,48] Device fracture has almost exclusively involved rIVCFs comprising 95% of fracture events.[49] After FDA-approval, rIVCFs comprised 75% of the filters utilized in the United States.[44]

Filter thrombosis, device fracture, and IVC perforation may complicate and, in some cases, prevent successful percutaneous filter retrieval. Nationally, rIVCF retrieval remain relatively rare at an estimated 12–18% aggregate rate.[47,50] The long-term outcomes associated with prolonged IVCF dwell time and low retrieval rates highlight the importance of active clinical surveillance and prompt retrieval of IVCFs when clinically appropriate. Currently, IVCF removal is indicated in patients whose risk for PTE is mitigated, contraindications to anticoagulation have resolved, and the device is eligible for retrieval.[2]

The development of institutional databases and registries to promote active clinical surveillance models is critical to promote IVCF removal and prevent delayed complications.

Previously, institutions followed a passive surveillance paradigm in which information was provided to the referring physicians and the patients regarding the importance of eventual filter retrieval.[47] However, follow-up with the interventionalist was not structured. At our institution, 2926 rIVCFs were deployed between 2000–2018 with initial retrieval rates of 10–15% from 2007–2015.[51] After implementation of active surveillance programs, we observed a near 4-fold increase to 40.3% rIVCF retrieval rates in 2018.[51] Other institutions have implemented active surveillance protocols with similar success.[47,52,53] In Sterbis' and colleagues' study, they demonstrated superior retrieval rates in patients followed by active surveillance (58.1%) compared to passive surveillance (46.4%) after rIVCF placement ($p = 0.003$).[47] Another study utilizing an active institutional registry of patients undergoing rIVCF placement demonstrated a retrieval rate as high as 92.5% in eligible patients.[52] The Cardiovascular and Interventional Radiology Society of Europe (CIRSE) developed a societal registry (CIRSE Registry) for rIVCF placement that demonstrated a similar retrieval rate of 92%.[54] Other institutions have employed dedicated clinics for IVCF surveillance, which have also improved IVCF retrieval rates.[19]

Generally, standard retrieval techniques are technically successful in 82% of cases with 18% requiring advanced endovascular techniques.[28] Prolonged rIVCF dwell time has been significantly associated with standard retrieval technique failure.[28] When extended to 7-months of implantation time, risk of standard retrieval technique failure is over 40%.[28] The requirement of advanced retrieval techniques predisposes patients to increased rates of procedural complications.

Standard retrieval modalities vary among different IVC models and are mostly related to the shape of the device. Each manufacturer provides a retrieval kit that is specific to the previously deployed IVCF. The most common technique is an endovascular snare that allows for the collapsing of the filter into a large retrieval sheath. Our experience has primarily been with the Cook Celect IVCF Retrieval kit. Retrieval is primarily performed through internal jugular venous access over an 0.035 wire. A pigtail catheter is utilized to perform pre-retrieval venography to confirm absence of caval thrombus (Figure 22.3A). The initial 6-French micropuncture sheath is then upsized to an 11-French sheath. An endovascular snare is used under fluoroscopic guidance to capture the hook at the cranial extent of the IVCF (Figure 22.3B). Once the device is snared, it is collapsed into the retrieval sheath by gentle retraction. A completion venogram is performed post-retrieval and the filter is examined for any device fracture or missing filter components (Figure 22.3C).

ADVANCED IVC FILTER RETRIEVAL TECHNIQUES

Most IVCFs are equipped with struts and barbs that are designed to prevent filter migration or tilt. However, prolonged IVCF dwell time may lead to extensive endothelization of these components or caval wall penetration that may require advanced endovascular retrieval techniques.[52] Other indications for advanced retrieval techniques include filter fracture, thrombosis, and caval perforation. When employed, advanced endovascular techniques for IVCF retrieval are successful in 85–98% of cases.[5,28,53,56] Overall, risk factors predictive of complex filter retrieval include excessive IVCF transverse tilt, embedded tip, leg penetration (>3 mm), thrombosis (>20%), and dwell time >90 days.[5,56]

In cases of excessive IVCF tilt or embedded struts precluding routine retrieval, multiple advanced techniques have been described. The guidewire loop and snare technique involves single venous access with passage of a guidewire through the IVCF struts and with

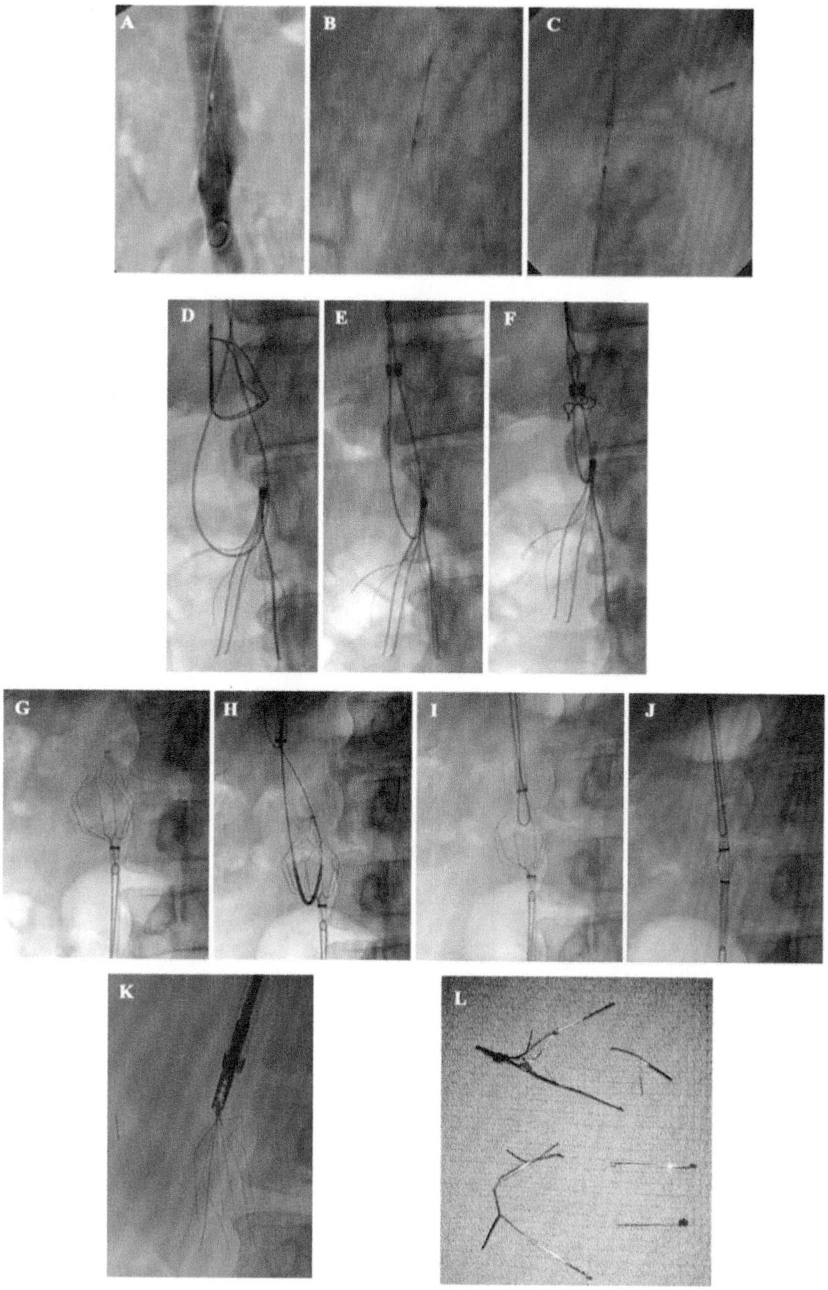

Figure 22.3 Endovascular IVCF retrieval techniques. (A) Pre-retrieval venogram to confirm absence of filter thrombus. (B) and (C) Standard snare retrieval with IVCF collapsed into the retrieval sheath. (D–F) Represents the single venous access loop and snare technique with passage of a wire through the struts and redirected superiorly for snare placement. (G–J) Demonstrates dual venous access advanced retrieval technique. The filter is snared inferiorly and superiorly and then collapsed into the sheaths. (K) Off-label utilization of endobronchial forceps for complex retrieval. (L) Fragmented IVCF after retrieval by endobronchial forceps. (Images from Kuyumcu G, Walker TG. Inferior vena cava filter retrievals, standard and novel techniques. Cardiovasc Diagn Ther. 2016;6(6):642–50.[55])

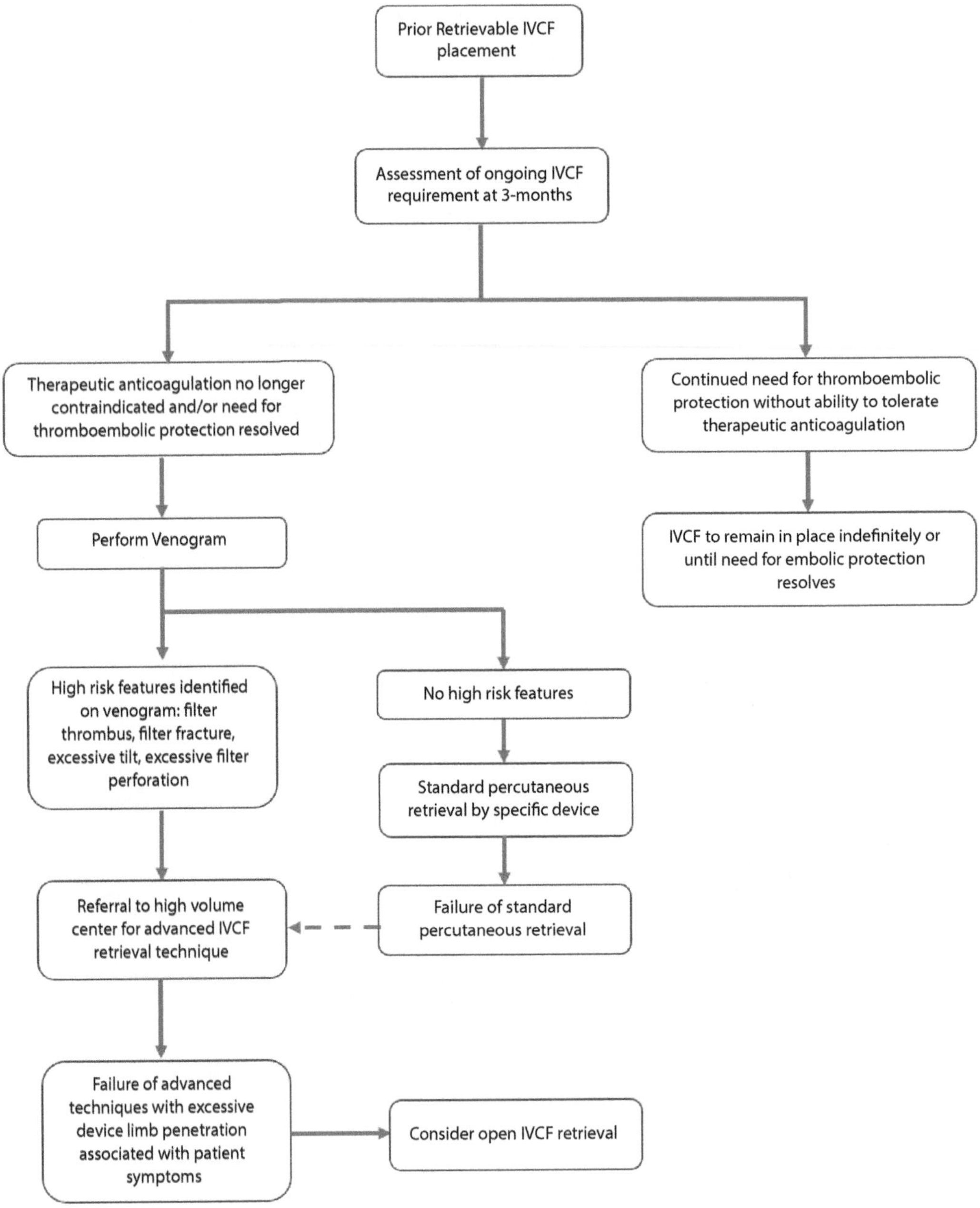

Figure 22.4 Algorithm for IVCF retrieval consideration. (Adapted from Charlton-Ouw KM, Afaq S, Leake SS, Sandhu HK, Sola CN, Saqib NU, et al. Indications and outcomes of open inferior vena cava filter removal. Ann Vasc Surg. 2018;46:205 e5–e11.[56])

redirection of the wire tip to proceed superiorly. A snare is introduced that is used to capture the wire forming a large loop around the cephalad aspect of the IVCF. This maneuver provides a traction point to free the IVCF struts from the IVCF lumen. Once freed, the IVCF can be collapsed into a retrieval sheath and removed (Figure 22.3D–F).[5,53,55] A compliant endovascular balloon can also be used as an adjunctive procedure to displace embedded IVCF struts.[55] In significantly embedded or tilted IVCFs, a dual venous access loop technique that involves internal jugular and transfemoral venous access may be required. The procedure is similar the single venous access technique. The additional guidewire in the dual venous access provides a second point of traction to assist in separating the IVCF from the vena caval wall.[53,55] This technique has been successful in retrieving permanent filters as well (Figure 22.3G–J).

Other advanced retrieval techniques include off-label use of endobronchial forceps and endovenous laser ablation. Endobronchial forceps as a method of IVCF retrieval was originally introduced by Stavropoulos et al.[57] This technique requires a larger introducer sheath ranging from 14–18 Fr.[55,58] The forceps can be used to dissect the IVCF hook or struts free from the vena caval wall. Once dissected free, the forceps can be used to grasp the IVCF hook to retract the filter into the retrieval sheath. Proceduralists should proceed with caution when utilizing the endobronchial forceps as they can result in filter fracture and embolization if excessive traction is applied.[5,55,57,58] Endovenous laser ablation was initially described by Kuo and colleagues in 2013.[59] This technique also requires a larger introducer sheath ranging from 16–18 Fr. The laser-equipped catheter is positioned near the IVCF, and photothermal energy is emitted allowing for lysis of dense fibrotic tissue adhered to the IVCF.[5,55] This technique has been associated with luminal thermal injury (7%) that can lead to IVC pseudoaneurysms and perforation.[5]

Although employed with success, utilization of advanced retrieval techniques incurs a significant increase in overall complication rates at 20%.[5] Due to low possibility of major complications during advanced retrieval techniques such as IVC rupture, rescue maneuvers including IVC occlusion balloon (i.e. CODA, Cook Medical Inc. Bloomington, IN) and endovenous stents should be readily accessible.[5] Additionally, advanced IVCF retrieval should be performed at high-volume centers that are technologically and procedurally equipped to perform these complex procedures and manage the potential complications.

Open surgical techniques for IVCF retrieval are reserved for patients in which advanced percutaneous techniques fail, presence of arterial or visceral strut perforation, or in patients with symptoms related to the filter. Depending upon surgeon preference, IVC exposure may be obtained by a transperitoneal or retroperitoneal approach. IVC exposure through the transperitoneal approach usually involves a right medial visceral rotation through mobilization of the ascending colon and duodenum to the patient's left. The IVCF is typically extracted through a longitudinal venotomy with subsequent primary vena caval repair.[56] Careful inspection of the IVCF should be performed after retrieval to ensure all components have been removed successfully. In surgically optimized patients, open IVCF retrieval can be performed with low morbidity and mortality.[56] An algorithm regarding IVCF retrieval is presented in Figure 22.4.

CONCLUSIONS

Overall, IVCF deployment and retrieval are relatively minor procedures that can be performed with low perioperative complications. However, for the most optimal benefit, IVCF placement must be reserved for appropriate patient populations and employed with discretion due to low rates of subsequent removal portending long-term complications. Patients should be closely surveilled following IVCF placement by clinical follow-up or institutional registry to ensure IVCF retrieval when clinically appropriate. The importance of close surveillance and subsequent IVCF retrieval is reflected in the long-term outcomes following prolonged IVCF dwell time and increased rate of complications in advanced retrieval techniques. As IVCFs continue to be utilized as thromboprophylaxis, mechanisms for close follow-up must be implemented.

REFERENCES

1. Centers for Disease Control and Prevention CDC 24/72023 [www.cdc.gov/ncbddd/dvt/data.html].
2. Kaufman JA, Barnes GD, Chaer RA, Cuschieri J, Eberhardt RT, Johnson MS, et al. society of interventional radiology clinical practice guideline for inferior vena cava filters in the treatment of patients with venous thromboembolic disease: Developed in collaboration with the American College of Cardiology, American College of Chest Physicians, American College of Surgeons Committee on Trauma, American Heart Association, Society for Vascular Surgery, and Society for Vascular Medicine. J Vasc Interv Radiol. 2020;31(10):1529–44.
3. Ahmed O, Patel K, Patel MV, Baadh AS, Madassery S, Turba UC, et al. Declining national annual ivc filter utilization: An analysis on the impact of societal and governmental communications. Chest. 2017;151(6):1402–4.
4. Stein PD, Kayali F, Olson RE. Twenty-one-year trends in the use of inferior vena cava filters. Arch Intern Med. 2004;164(14):1541–45.
5. Quencer KB, Smith TA, Deipolyi A, Mojibian H, Ayyagari R, Latich I, et al. Procedural complications of inferior vena cava filter retrieval, an illustrated review. CVIR Endovasc. 2020;3(1):23.
6. Meltzer AJ, Connolly PH, Kabutey NK, Jones DW, Schneider DB. Endovascular recanalization of iliocaval and inferior vena cava filter chronic total occlusions. J Vasc Surg Venous Lymphat Disord. 2015;3(1):86–89.
7. White RH, Brunson A, Romano PS, Li Z, Wun T. Outcomes after vena cava filter use in noncancer patients with acute venous thromboembolism: A population-based study. Circulation. 2016;133(21):2018–29.
8. Baadh AS, Zikria JF, Rivoli S, Graham RE, Javit D, Ansell JE. Indications for inferior vena cava filter placement: Do physicians comply with guidelines? J Vasc Interv Radiol. 2012;23(8):989–95.
9. De Gregorio MA, Guirola JA, Sierre S, Urbano J, Ciampi-Dopazo JJ, Abadal JM, et al. Ibero-American society of interventionism (sidi) and the spanish society of vascular and interventional radiology (servei) standard of practice (sop) for the management of inferior vena cava filters in the treatment of acute venous thromboembolism. J Clin Med. 2021;11(1).
10. DeYoung E, Minocha J. Inferior vena cava filters: Guidelines, best practice, and expanding indications. Semin Intervent Radiol. 2016;33(2):65–70.
11. Liu Y, Lu H, Bai H, Liu Q, Chen R. Effect of inferior vena cava filters on pulmonary embolism-related mortality and major complications: A systematic review and meta-analysis of randomized controlled trials. J Vasc Surg Venous Lymphat Disord. 2021;9(3):792–800 e2.
12. Decousus H, Leizorovicz A, Parent F, Page Y, Tardy B, Girard P, et al. A clinical trial of vena caval filters in the prevention of pulmonary embolism in patients with proximal deep-vein thrombosis. Prevention du Risque d'Embolie Pulmonaire par Interruption Cave Study Group. N Engl J Med. 1998;338(7):409–15.
13. Group PS. Eight-year follow-up of patients with permanent vena cava filters in the prevention of pulmonary embolism: The PREPIC (prevention du risque d'embolie pulmonaire par interruption cave) randomized study. Circulation. 2005;112(3):416–22.
14. Barginear MF, Gralla RJ, Bradley TP, Ali SS, Shapira I, Greben C, et al. Investigating the benefit of adding a vena cava filter to anticoagulation with fondaparinux sodium in patients with

cancer and venous thromboembolism in a prospective randomized clinical trial. Support Care Cancer. 2012;20(11):2865–72.

17. Ho KM, Rogers FB, Lipman J. A Multicenter Trial of Vena Cava Filters in Severely Injured Patients. Reply. N Engl J Med. 2019;381(15):1496–97.
18. Bikdeli B, Chatterjee S, Desai NR, Kirtane AJ, Desai MM, Bracken MB, et al. Inferior vena cava filters to prevent pulmonary embolism: Systematic review and meta-analysis. J Am Coll Cardiol. 2017;70(13):1587–97.
19. Ghatan CE, Ryu RK. Permanent versus retrievable inferior vena cava filters: Rethinking the "one-filter-for-all" approach to mechanical thromboembolic prophylaxis. Semin Intervent Radiol. 2016;33(2):75–78.
20. Morales JP, Li X, Irony TZ, Ibrahim NG, Moynahan M, Cavanaugh KJ, Jr. Decision analysis of retrievable inferior vena cava filters in patients without pulmonary embolism. J Vasc Surg Venous Lymphat Disord. 2013;1(4):376–84.
21. Removing Retrievable Inferior Vena Cava Filters: FDA Safety Communication. 2014; http://wayback.archive-it.org/7993/20170722215731/www.fda.gov/MedicalDevices/Safety/AlertsandNotices/ucm396377.htm.
22. Muriel A, Jimenez D, Aujesky D, Bertoletti L, Decousus H, Laporte S, et al. Survival effects of inferior vena cava filter in patients with acute symptomatic venous thromboembolism and a significant bleeding risk. J Am Coll Cardiol. 2014;63(16):1675–83.
23. Rajasekhar A, Lottenberg L, Lottenberg R, Feezor RJ, Armen SB, Liu H, et al. A pilot study on the randomization of inferior vena cava filter placement for venous thromboembolism prophylaxis in high-risk trauma patients. J Trauma. 2011;71(2):323–28; discussion 8–9.
24. Johnson MS, Spies JB, Scott KT, Kato BS, Mu X, Rectenwald JE, et al. Predicting the Safety and Effectiveness of Inferior Vena Cava Filters (PRESERVE): Outcomes at 12 months. J Vasc Surg Venous Lymphat Disord. 2023;11(3):573–85 e6.
25. Ha CP, Rectenwald JE. Inferior vena cava filters: Current indications, techniques, and recommendations. Surg Clin North Am. 2018;98(2):293–319.
26. Passman M. Vena Cava Interruption. In Perler SSaB (ed.), Rutherford's Vascular Surgery and Endovascular Therapy (pp. 2013–30). Philidelphia, PA: Elsevier, 2020.
27. Andreoli JM, Lewandowski RJ, Vogelzang RL, Ryu RK. Comparison of complication rates associated with permanent and retrievable inferior vena cava filters: A review of the MAUDE database. J Vasc Interv Radiol. 2014;25(8):1181–85.
28. Desai KR, Laws JL, Salem R, Mouli SK, Errea MF, Karp JK, et al. Response by desai et al to letter regarding article, "defining prolonged dwell time: When are advanced inferior vena cava filter retrieval techniques necessary? An analysis in 762 procedures". Circ Cardiovasc Interv. 2017;10(9).
29. Geisbusch P, Benenati JF, Pena CS, Couvillon J, Powell A, Gandhi R, et al. Retrievable inferior vena cava filters: Factors that affect retrieval success. Cardiovasc Intervent Radiol. 2012;35(5):1059–65.
30. Glocker RJ, Awonuga O, Novak Z, Pearce BJ, Patterson M, Matthews TC, et al. Bedside inferior vena cava filter placement by intravascular ultrasound in critically ill patients is safe and effective for an extended time. J Vasc Surg Venous Lymphat Disord. 2014;2(4):377–82.
31. Lin CY, Tung TH, Wu MY, Tseng CN, Tsai FC. Surgical outcomes of DeBakey type I and type II acute aortic dissection: A propensity score-matched analysis in 599 patients. J Cardiothorac Surg. 2021;16(1):208.
32. Dake MD, Murphy TP, Kramer AH, Darcy MD, Sewall LE, Curi MA, et al. Final two-year outcomes for the sentry bioconvertible inferior vena cava filter in patients requiring temporary protection from pulmonary embolism. J Vasc Interv Radiol. 2020;31(2):221–30.e3.
33. Tapson VF, Hazelton JP, Myers J, Robertson C, Gilani R, Dunn JA, et al. evaluation of a device combining an inferior vena cava filter and a central venous catheter for preventing pulmonary embolism among critically Ill trauma patients. J Vasc Interv Radiol. 2017;28(9):1248–54.

34. Smillie RP, Shetty M, Boyer AC, Madrazo B, Jafri SZ. Imaging evaluation of the inferior vena cava. Radiographics. 2015;35(2):578–92.
35. Doe C, Ryu RK. Anatomic and technical considerations: Inferior vena cava filter placement. Semin Intervent Radiol. 2016;33(2):88–92.
36. Petik B. Inferior vena cava anomalies and variations: Imaging and rare clinical findings. Insights Imaging. 2015;6(6):631–39.
37. Kandpal H, Sharma R, Gamangatti S, Srivastava DN, Vashisht S. Imaging the inferior vena cava: A road less traveled. Radiographics. 2008;28(3):669–89.
38. Martin KD, Kempczinski RF, Fowl RJ. Are routine inferior vena cavograms necessary before Greenfield filter placement? Surgery. 1989;106(4):647–50; discussion 50–51.
39. Hicks ME, Malden ES, Vesely TM, Picus D, Darcy MD. Prospective anatomic study of the inferior vena cava and renal veins: Comparison of selective renal venography with cavography and relevance in filter placement. J Vasc Interv Radiol. 1995;6(5):721–29.
40. Passman MA, Dattilo JB, Guzman RJ, Naslund TC. Bedside placement of inferior vena cava filters by using transabdominal duplex ultrasonography and intravascular ultrasound imaging. J Vasc Surg. 2005;42(5):1027–32.
41. MA Abusedera CK, and DM Williams. Bedside intravascular ultrasound-guided inferior vena cava filter placement in medical-surgical intensive care critically-ill patients. The Egyptian Journal of Radiology and Nuclear Medicine. 2015;46(3):659–64.
42. Sengodan P, Sankaramangalam K, Li M, Wang X, Subramaniam S, Alappan N. Comparative analysis of technical success rates and procedural complication rates of bedside inferior vena cava filter placement by intraprocedural imaging modality. J Vasc Surg Venous Lymphat Disord. 2019;7(4):601–9.
43. Ashley DW, Gamblin TC, McCampbell BL, Kitchens DM, Dalton ML, Jr., Solis MM. Bedside insertion of vena cava filters in the intensive care unit using intravascular ultrasound to locate renal veins. J Trauma. 2004;57(1):26–31.
44. Grewal S, Chamarthy MR, Kalva SP. Complications of inferior vena cava filters. Cardiovasc Diagn Ther. 2016;6(6):632–41.
45. Baheti A, Sheeran D, Patrie J, Sabri SS, Angle JF, Wilkins LR. suprarenal inferior vena cava filter placement and retrieval: Safety analysis. J Vasc Interv Radiol. 2020;31(2):231–35.
46. Harris SA, Velineni R, Davies AH. Inferior vena cava filters in pregnancy: A systematic review. J Vasc Interv Radiol. 2016;27(3):354–60.e8.
47. Sterbis E, Lindquist J, Jensen A, Hong M, Jr., Gupta S, Ryu R, et al. Inferior vena cava filter retrieval rates associated with passive and active surveillance strategies adopted by implanting physicians. JAMA Netw Open. 2023;6(3):e233211.
48. Jia Z, Wu A, Tam M, Spain J, McKinney JM, Wang W. Caval penetration by inferior vena cava filters: A systematic literature review of clinical significance and management. Circulation. 2015;132(10):944–52.
49. Ayad MT, Gillespie DL. Long-term complications of inferior vena cava filters. J Vasc Surg Venous Lymphat Disord. 2019;7(1):139–44.
50. Morris E, Duszak R, Jr., Sista AK, Hemingway J, Hughes DR, Rosenkrantz AB. National trends in inferior vena cava filter placement and retrieval procedures in the Medicare population over two decades. J Am Coll Radiol. 2018;15(8):1080–86.
51. Axley JC, May MM, Novak Z, Aucoin VJ, Spangler EL, McFarland GE, et al. Clinical practice and volume trends of inferior vena cava filter usage at a single tertiary care center during a 19-year period. J Vasc Surg Venous Lymphat Disord. 2022;10(4):887–93.
52. Sheehan M, Coppin K, O'Brien C, McGrath A, Given M, Keeling A, et al. A single center 9-year experience in IVC filter retrieval – the importance of an IVC filter registry. CVIR Endovasc. 2022;5(1):15.
53. Laws JL, Lewandowski RJ, Ryu RK, Desai KR. Retrieval of inferior vena cava filters: Technical considerations. Semin Intervent Radiol. 2016;33(2):144–8.

54. Lee MJ, Valenti D, de Gregorio MA, Minocha J, Rimon U, Pellerin O. The CIRSE retrievable IVC filter registry: Retrieval success rates in practice. Cardiovasc Intervent Radiol. 2015;38(6):1502–7.
55. Kuyumcu G, Walker TG. Inferior vena cava filter retrievals, standard and novel techniques. Cardiovasc Diagn Ther. 2016;6(6):642–50.
56. Charlton-Ouw KM, Afaq S, Leake SS, Sandhu HK, Sola CN, Saqib NU, et al. Indications and Outcomes of Open Inferior Vena Cava Filter Removal. Ann Vasc Surg. 2018;46:205 e5–e11.
57. Stavropoulos SW, Dixon RG, Burke CT, Stavas JM, Shah A, Shlansky-Goldberg RD, et al. Embedded inferior vena cava filter removal: Use of endobronchial forceps. J Vasc Interv Radiol. 2008;19(9):1297–301.
58. Stavropoulos SW, Ge BH, Mondschein JI, Shlansky-Goldberg RD, Sudheendra D, Trerotola SO. Retrieval of tip-embedded inferior vena cava filters by using the endobronchial forceps technique: Experience at a single institution. Radiology. 2015;275(3):900–7.
58. Sharifi M, Bay C, Skrocki L, Lawson D, Mazdeh S. Role of IVC filters in endovenous therapy for deep venous thrombosis: The FILTER-PEVI (filter implantation to lower thromboembolic risk in percutaneous endovenous intervention) trial. Cardiovasc Intervent Radiol. 2012;35(6):1408–13.
59. Kuo WT, Doshi AA, Ponting JM, Rosenberg JK, Liang T, Hofmann LV. Laser-assisted removal of embedded vena cava filters: A first-in-human escalation trial in 500 patients refractory to high-force retrieval. J Am Heart Assoc. 2020;9(24):e017916.
59. Mismetti P, Laporte S, Pellerin O, Ennezat PV, Couturaud F, Elias A, et al. Effect of a retrievable inferior vena cava filter plus anticoagulation vs anticoagulation alone on risk of recurrent pulmonary embolism: A randomized clinical trial. JAMA. 2015;313(16):1627–35.
60. Hann CL, Streiff MB. The role of vena caval filters in the management of venous thromboembolism. Blood Rev. 2005;19(4):179–202.
61. Deso SE, Idakoji IA, Kuo WT. Evidence-based evaluation of inferior vena cava filter complications based on filter type. Semin Intervent Radiol. 2016;33(2):93–100.

Chapter 23

Axillosubclavian Vein Thrombosis (Paget-Schroetter Syndrome)

Hugh A. Gelabert

INTRODUCTION

Acute spontaneous axillosubclavian vein thrombosis (Paget-Schroetter syndrome) is a potentially devastating condition, typically presenting with pain, discoloration and massive swelling. The condition is dramatic, alarming and disabling. Fortunately with accurate diagnosis and appropriate treatment the condition may be managed to achieve complete resolution. The objective of this chapter is to review the current management of axillosubclavian vein thrombosis in both the acute and chronic presentations.

DEFINITIONS

Paget-Schroetter Syndrome

The diagnosis of Paget-Schroetter syndrome is spontaneous thrombosis of the subclavian vein.[1] The diagnosis requires demonstration of thrombus in the subclavian vein in a patient who has had no prior interventions in the subclavian vein (no catheters, or pacemakers etc). For purposes of this chapter the terms axillosubclavian vein and subclavian vein will be used interchangeably.

Venous Thoracic Outlet Syndrome

Venous thoracic outlet syndrome refers to the subset of TOS which is characterized by extrinsic compression of the subclavian vein at the thoracic outlet.[2] In order to demonstrate extrinsic compression of the subclavian vein at the thoracic outlet, the subclavian vein must be patent and imaging should show loss of luminal dimension at the thoracic outlet. This may be accomplished with CT, MR catheter venogram or IVUS. US may be a suboptimal means of establishing this diagnosis as clear view of subclavian vein beneath the clavicle may be limited.

Paget-Schroetter Syndrome Related to Venous Thoracic Outlet Compression (PSS VTOS)

The diagnosis of PSS VTOS relies on demonstrating extrinsic compression in a vein which has thrombosed. In order to accomplish this, the vein must first be cleared of thrombus. Clearing the thrombus may be achieved by either catheter-directed therapy (CDT) or by anticoagulation and intrinsic thrombolysis. Once the thrombus is cleared the imaging may demonstrate extrinsic compression at the thoracic outlet.

DOI: 10.1201/9781003316626-27

Incidence, Etiology of Paget-Schroetter Syndrome

Paget-Schroetter syndrome is an infrequent presentation of TOS, accounting for approximately 5–10% of cases. The incidence of 1 per 100,00 population.[3] The number of new PSS cases has been estimated to be about 2000 per year.[4] Based on nationwide hospital data, the number of VTOS PSS operations done yearly is about 300 cases.[5]

The initial description indicates spontaneous thrombosis of the subclavian vein. The causes of PSS include venous thoracic outlet compression, malignancy and coagulation abnormalities.

When initially described most cases were identified in heavy laborers. Subsequently other groups were identified as developing PSS (patients with malignancy and hypercoagulable conditions conditions). Currently, PSS still affects those engaged in heavy labor however the majority of cases currently relate to exercise and athletics. These tend to be the patients with VTOS-related PSS. Body building with weightlifting is a common cause of Paget-Schroetter syndrome. Athletics also represents a significant cause of Paget-Schroetter syndrome. Overhead throwing sports such as baseball, volleyball and tennis are often counted in the ranks of Paget-Schroetter syndrome patients. Additionally, athletes who engage in upper body workouts such as crew and football are also affected. The commonality between these activities is the repetitive engagement of musculature in the upper torso with hypertrophy of the scalene and subclavius muscles in particular.

Anatomy of VTOS PSS

The pertinent anatomy of Paget-Schroetter syndrome revolves about the costo-clavicular space. This is the anterior portion of the thoracic outlet bound by the bony elements (first rib, the clavicle) and the muscular elements (anterior scalene muscle and the subclavius muscle) (Figure 23.1).

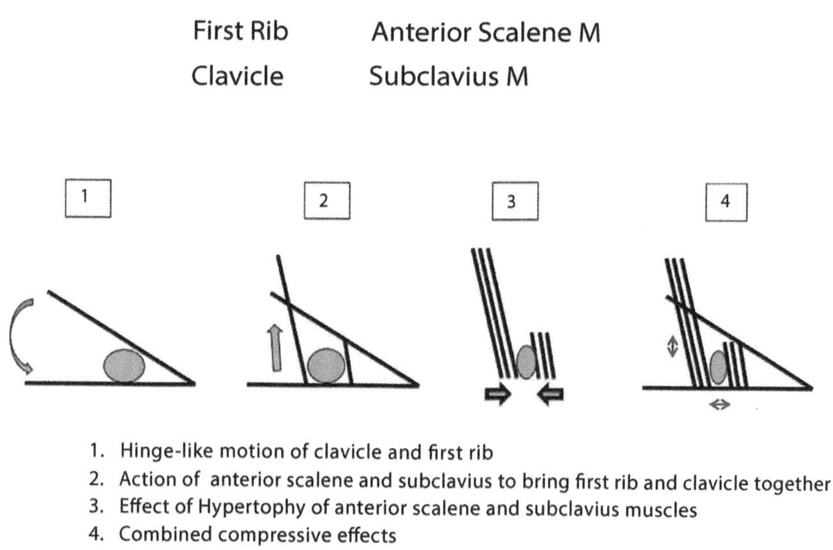
First Rib
Anterior Scalene M
Clavicle
Subclavius M
1
2
3
4
1. Hinge-like motion of clavicle and first rib
2. Action of anterior scalene and subclavius to bring first rib and clavicle together
3. Effect of Hypertophy of anterior scalene and subclavius muscles
4. Combined compressive effects

Figure 23.1 Compressive elements in venous TOS. The compressive elements which underlie venous TOS. Drawing illustrates the (1) scissoring action of the clavicle and fist rib; (2) the force exerted by anterior scaleen and subclavius muscles to bring the clavicle and first rib toward each other; (3) the loss of space between the anterior scalene and subclavius muscle as these enlarge; (4) the combined effect of these elements.

Bones

Costo-Clavicular Space

The costo-clavicular space is the triangular space bound by the first rib, the clavicle and the anterior scalene muscle. Running along the undersurface of the clavicle is the subclavius muscle. Both the subclavius and anterior scalene muscles work to draw the clavicle and first rib toward each other.

The junction between the clavicle and first rib is mediated by the manubrium. The clavicular-manubrial junction is a synovial articulation, a joint which allows motion between the two. Extrinsic impingement on the subclavian vein is in part a function of the space between these bones. Abnormalities of bony anatomy may be present and lead to development of VTOS. These include cervical ribs, aberrant first ribs, fractures of the clavicle and fractures of the first rib. Abnormal growth of the first rib may also give rise to exostosis, which may impinge on the subclavian vein.

Muscles

The anterior scalene muscle arises from the cervical vertebrae (C3–6) and inserts onto the dorsal aspect of the first rib between the subclavian artery and the subclavian vein. The anterior scalene muscle functions as an accessory muscle of respiration, raising the first rib in conjunction with the respiratory cycle. The subclavius muscle runs along the inferior aspect of the clavicle and inserts onto the first rib. The anterior scalene and subclavius muscle draw the clavicle toward the first rib accentuating impingement between the bones. In a manner similar to the anterior scalene muscle, vigorous repeated exercise the subclavius muscle may hypertrophy dramatically, resulting in impingement on the subclavian vein. The space between the anterior scalene muscle and subclavius muscle is the venous channel through which the subclavian vein passes. The width of this space is directly related to the size of these muscles and the space between their insertions on the first rib (Figure 23.2).

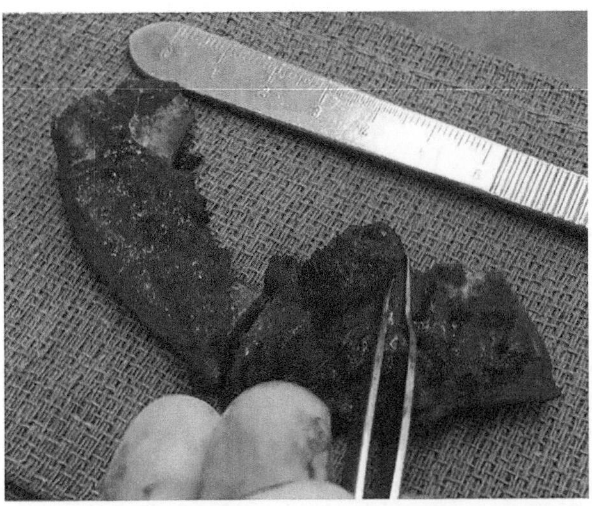

Figure 23.2 This is a photograph of a first rib from a patient with VTOS. Notice the reduced space between the anterior scalene and the subclavius muscles, which is being marked by the instrument. Normally this space should be about 8–10 mm; here it is about 2 mm. The reduced space is due to enlargement of the muscles.

NATURAL HISTORY OF PAGET-SCHROETTER SYNDROME

The natural history of Paget-Schroetter syndrome in our current time is difficult to ascertain as virtually all patients are provided with treatment of the DVT. From the mid-20th century there are reports of chronic congestion and disability from untreated Paget-Schroetter syndrome. In 1970, Edwards reported a series of 48 patients with spontaneous subclavian vein thrombosis managed with anticoagulation alone. These were followed over a period of 6.6 years. The authors noted recurrent thrombosis in 17%, persistent symptoms on 74% and chronic occlusion in 91% of patients treated with anticoagulation alone.[6]

CLINICAL DIAGNOSIS OF VTOS PSS

The diagnosis of Paget-Schroetter syndrome rests on a combination of history, symptoms, physical exam findings and appropriate testing. Presenting symptoms include swelling, discoloration and pain in the arm and hand. Most often these arise in young, active patients who are engaged in heavy labor, athletics or physical exercise. The exam on presentation typically demonstrates a swollen arm with congested veins and collateral veins seen across the shoulder and chest. Diagnostic testing most commonly involves ultrasonography. While this is often diagnostic, it may miss up to 25% of cases.[7] For this reason, cross-sectional imaging should be used in any patient with symptoms and exam findings consistent with PSS and a negative ultrasound.

INITIAL MEDICAL TREATMENT

Anticoagulation

The initial treatment at the time of presentation requires anticoagulation. This is done with the intention of stopping clot propagation and reducing the risk of PE. The mechanism of action of anticoagulation is halting thrombus propagation, but it does not directly offer removal of the thrombus from the vein.

Dissolution of the thrombus in patients treated with anticoagulation alone relies on intrinsic thrombolysis effected by proteins extruded from the endothelial cell wall. With sufficient time (months) the intrinsic thrombolysis will dissolve most the thrombus. Because of fibrous transformation of the blood clot, not all of the blood clots will be reliably dissolved with intrinsic thrombolysis. The consequence is that anticoagulation alone often results in chronic post-phlebitic changes to the vein wall, which in turn results in chronic venous insufficiency symptoms in the arm.

THROMBOLYSIS

A second approach to managing the acute DVT presentation is to augment anticoagulation with catheter-directed techniques (DCT) for removal of the blood clot from the subclavian vein. Catheter-directed therapy offers more rapid and reliable removal of thrombus from the subclavian vein. It has the advantage of rapid resolution of symptoms as well as reducing the time that there is thrombus within the vein in contact with the vein wall. This reduced vein wall inflammation and secondary post-thrombotic changes to the vein wall. Most significant is the ability to establish a conclusive diagnosis of VTOS.

The principal disadvantage is that a CDT procedure requires an interventional facility and is invasive. It may require hospitalization for a period of time. It does expose the patient to a small dose of radiation and to intravenous contrast. It exposes the patient to risk of bleeding, contrast allergy, exposure of and contrast nephrotoxicity. The risk of bleeding makes certain conditions contraindications for DVT: recent surgery, intracranial lesions, recent stroke, internal bleeding and hematological deficits. While effective in clearing the subclavian vein of thrombus on 90% of instances, catheter-directed therapy is not always successful. Finally, catheter-directed therapy requires more time, it costs more, and it is less convenient. Despite these concerns, evidence suggests that the advantages of CDT outweigh the risks. The benefit of a confirmed diagnosis of VTOS allows proceeding with surgical treatment with certainty and allows a sober weighing of risk and benefit in considering further care (Figure 23.3).

SURGICAL MANAGEMENT OF VTOS PSS

The surgical management of VTOS PSS involves two fundamental goals: decompression of the subclavian vein and restoration of the subclavian vein lumen.

Surgical Decompression

The first goal of surgery for VTOS is decompression of the costo-clavicular space. In order to accomplish effective decompression of the costo-clavicular space both bony elements and muscles need to be addressed. At the very least, bony decompression involves either removal

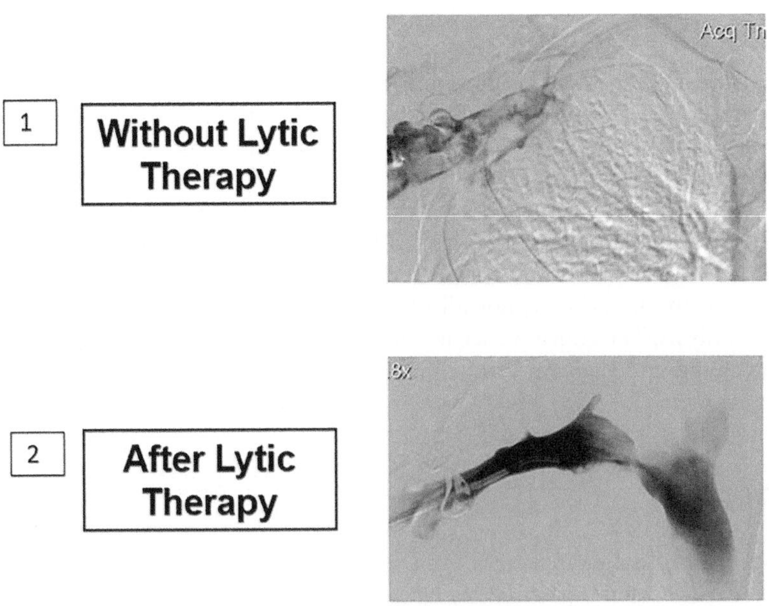

Figure 23.3 Venogram of patient with acute spontaneous subclavian vein thrombosis (Paget-Schroetter syndrome). (1) Venogram where contrast is injected into a thrombosed right subclavian vein. (2) A subclavian vein after the blood clot has been dissolved and removed.

of the anterior portion of the first rib or removal of the anterior portion of the clavicle. The muscular decompression requires division and partial resection of the subclavius and anterior scalene muscles. Muscular decompression is required in order to accomplish the bony decompression as the bone cannot be removed unless the attached muscles are divided.

Several alternative approaches have been demonstrated to be effective in achieving these goals. Medial claviculectomy, the removal of the medial portion of the clavicle, is the simplest approach to VTOS decompression.[8] In these operations an incision is made over the medial third to half of the clavicle, the clavicle is divided and the clavicular-manubrial joint is severed. The attachments of the subclavius muscle must be divided and then the medial clavicle is removed. Significant advantages of this operation are its simplicity, low risk of major nerve injury, and excellent exposure of the subclavian vein, which allows for open venous reconstruction. The principal disadvantage of medial claviculectomy is cosmetic. The resultant appearance of the chest wall is strikingly abnormal in slender patients. In heavy set patients it is not significantly noticeable.

First rib resection for VTOS decompression may be achieved via several approaches: transaxillary, praclavicular and infra-clavicular. It is important to note that a supraclavicular approach is inadequate for VTOS decompression. This approach is a partial rib resection that removes the posterior half of the first rib and does not decompression the costo-clavicular space.[9]

The transaxillary first rib resection has been used for VTOS decompression with great success. This operation allows for resection of the entire first rib from the cost-chondral junction to the articulation with the transverse process of T1.[10] The operation entails partial resection of the anterior scalene and subclavius muscles. Intraoperative video-endoscopy is helpful in assessing the efficacy of this resection.[11] This is an effective operation for VTOS as it removes the bony component of compression as well as the muscular components. The principal drawback of TAFR is that it does not allow direct intervention on the subclavian vein. Venous reconstructions such as open endovenolysis, patch angioplasty and venous interposition reconstruction are not possible via this approach. Should any of these procedures be required, a second incision in the supraclavicular or infraclavicular fossa would be necessary. The main advantage of TAFR is that it is a very effective operation with a well-established record of success. Cosmetically it is the most appealing approach as the incision is located beneath the arm. Functionally, there is no incapacitation resultant from this operation.

The para-clavicular approach to VTOS was developed in recognition that the supraclavicular approach alone is inadequate for VTOS decompression.[12] In the para-clavicular approach, the entire first rib is removed via two incisions: one above the clavicle (in a standard supraclavicular operation) and a second incision beneath the clavicle, which allows removal of the anterior portion of the firs rib. This is an effective operation for VTOS as it removes the bony component of compression as well as the muscular components. This approach also allows for direct interventions on the subclavian vein. The cosmetic impact of incisions for this operation is a limitation as these are located in highly visible portions of the chest.

The infraclavicular approach to first rib resection derives from the para-clavicular experience. The incision for this operation is below the clavicle on the anterior chest wall.[13] It allows for resection of the anterior portion of the first rib and so should be considered a partial rib resection. It is an operation designed specifically for VTOS decompression as it allows deconstruction of the costo-clavicular triangle along with resection of the subclavius and anterior scalene muscles. As it involves resection of the anterior portion of the first rib, the risk of injury to the brachial plexus and long thoracic nerves is minimal. Given the restricted exposure of the subclavian vein, venous interventions such as open endovenolysis, patch angioplasty and venous interposition reconstruction are not possible. The location of the incision on the anterior chest wall results in a noticeable scar. Potential concern revolves about resection the anterior portion of the first rib only. There is a possibility of re-growth of the first rib. Also, if insufficient length of rib is removed then the residual rib may still impinge on the subclavian vein.

Complications

A study of surgical errors in management of Paget-Schroetter syndrome indicates that the most common error is inadequate resection of the first rib.[14] This error may attend any of the approaches. It is always the case with patients who were managed with supraclavicular approaches. It occurs with patients undergoing transaxillary para-clavicular and infraclavicular approaches as well. The common denominator is failure to resect that portion of the FR that forms the costo-clavicular space.

Supraclavicular, para-clavicular and transaxillary first rib resections expose the patient to possible neurological complications such as brachial plexus, phrenic, long thoracic nerve injuries, dorsal scapular nerve injury and phrenic nerve injury. Fortunately, these nerve injuries are very uncommon.

The potential for lymphatic duct injury is uniquely elevated in all supraclavicular operations and is present in the para-clavicular approach; however this is not common in transaxillary or infraclavicular operations. Pneumothorax is a complication that attends all rib resections, however its significance overstated as air entry into the chest is most often due to a tear of pleura and not from a parenchymal pulmonary injury. In such cases contemporary management techniques make this 'complication' a minor one, on par with thrombophlebitis from an intravenous catheter.

VENOUS RESTORATION

Restoration of the subclavian vein to functional patency is a significant goal of surgical care of VTOS. This is based on the assumption that VTOS symptoms are consequent to loss of venous patency. Two general approaches are used for venous restoration: the open reconstruction and endovascular repair.

Open Reconstruction

Open reconstruction is accomplished by the three most common techniques: endovenolysis, patch angioplasty and interposition grafting. Endovenolysis refers to the technique where the subclavian vein is opened and any synechiae within the vein are removed. Frequently this technique is accompanied by patch angioplasty repair of the vein wall, where a patch of prosthetic material or vein is used to augment the diameter of the fibrotic subclavian vein.[15] Venous interposition reconstruction is reserved, for instance, where the subclavian vein is occluded. In these instances the occluded segment of subclavian vein is replaced with a graft.[16] The graft may be either prosthetic or native vein. Most common of the prosthesis include cadaveric veins or arteries. Adjunctive AV fistula in the ipsilateral arm has been used to maintain patency. Much like the other open techniques venous interposition reconstruction requires sufficient length of exposure to assure satisfactory inflow and outflow targets.

The open reconstruction techniques share several concerns: the requirement for proximal and distal control at points of uninvolved vein, the need to expose sufficient vein to allow for the reconstruction and the need for adequate inflow and outflow vessels. In some instances, if the axillary vein and brachial vein are occluded, then reconstruction is hampered by lack of adequate inflow. Similarly if the innominate vein were occluded the reconstruction may not be possible due to lack of adequate outflow.

Endovascular Approach

Endovascular restoration of subclavian vein patency relies on combining wire crossing of a venous stenosis or occlusion and then balloon angioplasty to restore the venous lumen to normal diameter. The idea behind this technique is that the subclavian vein once decompressed is able to be stretched back to normal diameter with a balloon angioplasty. Furthermore, if the subclavian vein is occluded it may be possible to traverse the occlusion with a guidewire and then use balloon angioplasty to restore the lumen.[17]

Stent reconstruction utilizes metal frames that are deployed using the balloon angioplasty technique. The metallic frames are used with the intention of preventing recoil narrowing of the vein wall. The use of stents in this location is contraindicated prior to surgical decompression. In the post-decompression setting, use of stents remains controversial as evidence for long-term success is not well established.

The decision for open versus endovascular restoration of subclavian vein lumen is controversial and unsettled. Much like with choice of surgical approach for decompression, the choice of which means to restore venous lumen tends to be based on a combination of experience and ability to manage a particular case with a given technique.

MANAGEMENT PROTOCOLS FOR PSS

Once all elements of care (diagnosis, thrombolysis, decompression, venous restoration) are appreciated they may be assembled into protocols of care. One of the first such protocols was developed by Dr Herbert Machleder at UCLA. First presented in 1987, the protocol revolved around thrombolysis to clear the acute thrombosis, anticoagulation to allow resolution of vein wall inflammation, reassessment of symptoms and venous patency to assure the need of surgery, transaxillary first rib resection for surgical decompression and then post-decompression venography to assess and restore venous lumen.[18] This protocol was employed in a prospective cohort of 50 patients and formed the basis of a publication in 1993. At the end of the project, about 70% of subclavian veins were patent, irregular or recanalized and 30% remained occluded. This represented a significant improvement in care of VTOS and sparked widespread interest in these techniques[19] (Figure 23.4).

Variations in this fundamental approach included introduction of novel thrombolytic agents, discovery of the optimal window for thrombolysis, adoption of early (during initial hospital stay) decompression as an alternative, use of intraoperative balloon angioplasty as part of the surgical decompression procedure and use of ultrasound scanning to assess postoperative patency.

Significant variations of this approach have been published from groups at Vancouver, Boston, Albany and Stanford.[20–23] The Stanford experience is significant in highlighting that not all patients who suffer Paget-Schroetter syndrome will require surgical

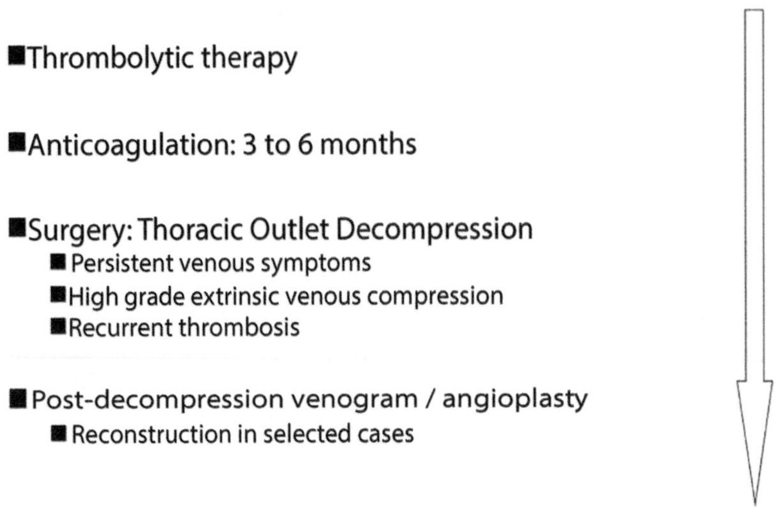

■Thrombolytic therapy
■Anticoagulation: 3 to 6 months
■Surgery: Thoracic Outlet Decompression
■ Persistent venous symptoms
■High grade extrinsic venous compression
■Recurrent thrombosis
■ Post-decompression venogram / angioplasty
■ Reconstruction in selected cases

Figure 23.4 Dr. Machleder's approach to Paget-Schroetter syndrome is illustrated with a flow diagram.

decompression. In their report, ultimately about 57% of their patients required surgical decompression.[24]

Current Protocol for Management of Paget-Schroetter Syndrome

The current approach to Paget-Schroetter syndrome relies on acute clearing of the subclavian vein with anticoagulation, thrombolysis and catheter clot aspiration as initial care. Surgical decompression is triaged according to severity of compression and patient preferences. If the compression is severe and we estimate a high chance of re-thrombosis on anticoagulation, then immediate surgical decompression is advised. If the stenosis is moderately severe but there is not a pressing concern for re-thrombosis, then patients are informed of their options: to have surgery immediately or at a later point in time. This decision may be affected by the patient's need to prepare for surgery. Some may find immediate surgery more convenient, and others may be better off delaying the surgery until personal matters can be organized. Anticoagulation is continued until after surgical decompression and after post-decompression imaging (Figure 23.5).

Post-decompression imaging (catheter venogram) is advised for all. We feel this is the most accurate assessment of the subclavian vein following surgery. In those instances where a residual stenosis of 50% or more is identified, then balloon angioplasty is performed. Anticoagulation is continued for 3–4 weeks post angioplasty. Repeat imaging (venogram) is reserved for those who may develop recurrent congestive symptoms.

In a retrospective analysis of 100 patients, those who underwent thrombolysis followed by first rib resection had better patency and reduced symptoms than those managed with anticoagulation alone and first rib resection. The final vein patency for those undergoing thrombolysis followed by FRR was 92%. The final vein patency for those managed with anticoagulation alone was 74%. Using standardized metrics, the thrombolysis group experience an 87% reduction in symptom severity versus only 20% reduction in those managed with anticoagulation alone.[25]

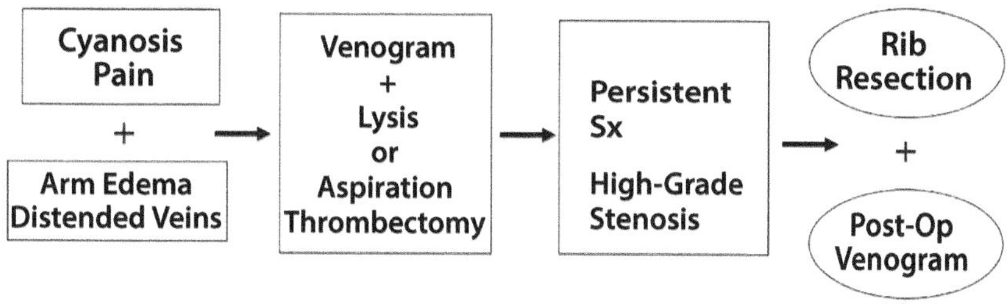

Figure 23.5 Flow diagram illustrating contemporary approach to Paget-Schroetter syndrome with acute presentation.

Chronic Paget-Schroetter Syndrome

The approach of immediate clearing of the thrombus in the subclavian vein by means of thrombolysis or thrombectomy has not been universally adopted. Many patients with spontaneous subclavian vein DVT are treated with anticoagulation and discharged from emergency rooms with instruction to seek consultation at a later time. As consequence, many patients present with 'chronic Paget-Schroetter syndrome', that is Paget-Schroetter syndrome presenting well beyond the 14 day window for thrombolysis. In these instances, the clearing of the thrombus within the subclavian vein is dependent on the endogenous thrombolytic process based on endothelial cell elaboration of tissue plasminogen activator. As noted, the efficacy of this process is variable, and so the patency of the subclavian vein is uncertain (Figure 23.6).

In such instances, a diagnostic venogram will provide information as to the condition of the subclavian vein. The decision to proceed with surgical decompression is based on the patient's symptoms and the condition of the subclavian vein. If the patient is symptomatic with congestion of the arm, particularly with use, then they may benefit from surgery. If the subclavian vein is patent but extrinsic compression is present, then surgical decompression would be indicated to prevent recurrent thrombosis. If the subclavian vein were occluded and the patient asymptomatic then no surgery would be needed as the risk of thrombosis is negligible and the patient has no significant symptoms.

Reports of surgical experience with chronic and subacute PSS presentations indicate that patients benefit from decompression and venoplasty. Freischlag and associates published a series indicating excellent patency and symptom resolution for these patients when managed with transaxillary first rib resection and post-decompression angioplasty.[26]

More recently, a comparison of patients treated with initial thrombolysis to those managed with anticoagulation alone indicated improved outcomes with thrombolysis but overall very good outcomes for those with chronic PSS presentations.[27]

The question of what care to offer patients with occluded subclavian veins remains unsettled. One reason to proceed with surgical decompression is to prevent recurrent thrombosis by decompressing a patent but compressed vein. If the vein is occluded, then it is not subject to recurrent thrombosis. Some such patients have significant symptoms of congestion and pain leading to considerable disability.

In those cases where the subclavian vein is occluded and the patient remains symptomatic, surgical decompression may be beneficial. In a cohort of 33 symptomatic patients with chronically occluded subclavian veins surgical decompression allowed restoration of subclavian vein lumen in 22 (66%). In the remaining 11, standardized measured indicate that even with persistent subclavian vein occlusion, the patients' symptoms were significantly alleviated following surgical decompression.[27]

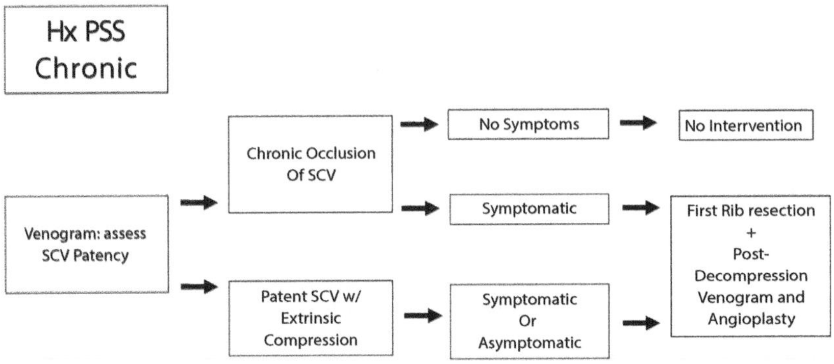

Figure 23.6 Flow diagram illustrating contemporary approach to Paget-Schroetter syndrome with chronic presentation.

CONCLUSIONS

Paget-Schroetter syndrome is a rare condition that presents with dramatic arm swelling, pain and discoloration. Unfortunately, due to the rarity of the condition many front line physicians are not familiar with optimal contemporary management. Appropriate initial treatment will alleviate the patient's symptoms and provide conclusive diagnosis. Surgical care has a very high success rate with restoration of function and relief of symptoms.

REFERENCES

1. Illig KA, Donahue D, Duncan A, Freischlag J, Gelabert H, Johansen K, Jordan S, Sanders R, Thompson R. Reporting standards of the Society for Vascular Surgery for thoracic outlet syndrome. J Vasc Surg. 2016 Sep;64(3):e23–35.
2. Sanders RL, Annest SJ. Chapter 5. Anatomy of the thoracic outlet and related structures, page 34. In Karl A. Illig, Robert W. Thompson, Julie Ann Freischlag, Dean M. Donahue, Sheldon E. Jordan, Ying Wei Lum, Hugh A. Gelabert (eds.), Thoracic Outlet Syndrome (2nd ed.), Springer Nature, Jan 25, 2021.
3. Illig KA, Rodriguez-Zoppi E. How common is thoracic outlet syndrome? Thorac Surg Clin. 2021 Feb;31(1):11–17.
4. Flinterman LE, Van Der Meer FJM, Rosendaal FR, Doggen CJM. Current perspective of venous thrombosis in the upper extremity. J Thromb Haemost. 2008 Aug;6(8):1262–66. doi:10.1111/j.1538-7836.2008.03017.x
5. George EL, Arya S, Rothenberg KA, Hernandez-Bouddard T, Ho VT, Stern JR, Gelabert HA, Lee FT. contemporary practices and complications of surgery for thoracic outlet syndrome in the United States. Ann Vasc Surg. 2021 Apr;72:147–158. doi:10.1016/j.avsg.2020.10.046
6. Tilney NL, Griffiths HJG, Edwards EA. Natural history of major venous thrombosis of the upper extremity. Arch Surg. 1970;101:792–96.
7. Brownie ER, Abuirqeba A, Ohman JW, Rubin BG, Thompson RW. False-negative upper extremity ultrasound in the initial evaluation of patients with suspected subclavian vein thrombosis due to thoracic outlet syndrome (Paget-Schroetter syndrome). J Vasc Surg Venous Lymphat Disord. 2020 Jan;8(1):118–26. doi:10.1016/j.jvsv.2019.08.011
8. Adams JT, McEvoy RK, DeWeese JA. Primary deep vein thrombosis of the upper extremity. Arch Surg. 1965;91:29–41

9. Thompson RW, Schnieder PA, Nelken NA, Skioldenrand CG, Stoney RJ. Circumferential venolysis and paraclavicular thoracic outlet decompression for "effort thrombosis" of the subclavian vein. J Vasc Surg. 1992 Nov;16(5):723–32.
10. Roos DB. Experience with first rib resection for thoracic outlet syndrome. Ann Surg. 1971 Mar;173(3):429–42.
11. Chan YC, Gelabert HA. High-definition video-assisted transaxillary first rib resection for thoracic outlet syndrome. J Vasc Surg. 2013 Apr;57(4):1155–58.
12. Thompson RW, Petrinec D, Toursarkissian B. Surgical treatment of thoracic outlet compression syndromes. II. Supraclavicular exploration and vascular reconstruction. Ann Vasc Surg. 1997 Jul;11(4):442–51. doi:10.1007/s100169900074
13. Siracuse, JJ, Johnsont PC, Jones DW, Gill HL, Connolly PH, Meltzer AJ, Schneider DB. Infraclavicular first rib resection for the treatment of acute venous thoracic outlet syndrome. J Vasc Surg Venous Lymphat Disord. 2015 Oct;3(4):397–400.
14. Archie MM, Rollo JC, Gelabert HA. Surgical missteps in the management of venous thoracic outlet syndrome which lead to reoperation. Ann Vasc Surg. 2018 May;49:261–67.
15. Molina JE, Hunter DW, Dietz CA. Paget-Schroetter syndrome treated with thrombolytics and immediate surgery. J Vasc Surg. 2007;45(2):328–34.
16. Vemuri C, Salehi P, Benarroch-Gampet J, McLaughlin LN, Thompson RW. Diagnosis and treatment of effort-induced thrombosis of the axillary subclavian vein due to venous thoracic outlet syndrome. J Vasc Surg Venous Lymphat Disord. 2016 Oct;4(4):485–500.
17. Chang KZ, Likes K, Demos J, Black JH, Freischlag JA. Routine venography following transaxillary first rib resection and scalenectomy (FRRS) for chronic subclavian vein thrombosis ensures excellent outcomes and vein patency. Vasc Endovascular Surg. 2012 Jan;46(1):15–20.
18. Kunkel JM, Machleder HI. Treatment of Paget-Schroetter syndrome. A staged, multidisciplinary approach. Arch Surg. 1989 Oct;124(10):1153–7; discussion 1157–8.
19. Machleder HI. Evaluation of a new treatment strategy for Paget-Schroetter syndrome: Spontaneous thrombosis of the axillary-subclavian vein. J Vasc Surg. 1993;17(2):305–15, discussion 316–7.
20. Lokanathan R, Salvian AJ, Chen JC, Morris C, Taylor DC, Hsiang YN. Outcome after thrombolysis and selective thoracic outlet decompression for primary axillary vein thrombosis. J Vasc Surg. 2001 Apr;33(4):783–88. doi:10.1067/mva.2001.112708
21. Lee MC. Grassi CJ, Belkin M, Mannick JA, Whittmore AD, Donaldson MC. Early operative intervention after thrombolytic therapy for primary subclavian vein thrombosis: An effective treatment approach. J Vasc Surg. 1998 Jun;27(6):1101–7; discussion 1107–8.
22. Kreienberg PB, Chang BB, Darling 3rd RC, Roddy SP, Paty PS, Lloyd WE, Cohen D, Stainken B, Shah DM. Long-term results in patients treated with thrombolysis, thoracic inlet decompression, and subclavian vein stenting for Paget-Schroetter syndrome. J Vasc Surg. 2001;33(2 Suppl):S100–5.
23. Lee WA, Hill BB, Harris Jr EJ, Semba CP, Olcott IV C. Surgical intervention is not required for all patients with subclavian vein thrombosis. J Vasc Surg. 2000;32(1):57–67.
24. Lee JT, Karwowski JK, Harris EJ, Haukoos JS, Olcott 4th C. Long-term thrombotic recurrence after nonoperative management of Paget-Schroetter syndrome. J Vasc Surg. 2006;43(6):1236–43.
25. Chun TT, O'Connell JB, Rigberg DA, DeRubertis BG, Jimenex JC, Farley SM, Baril DT, Gelabert HA. Preoperative thrombolysis is associated with improved vein patency and functional outcomes after first rib resection in acute Paget-Schroetter syndrome. J Vasc Surg. 2022 Sep;76(3):806–13.
26. Guzzo JL, Chang K, Demos J, Black JH, Freischlag JA. Preoperative thrombolysis and venoplasty affords no benefit in patency following first rib resection and scalenectomy for subacute and chronic subclavian vein thrombosis. J Vasc Surg. 2010;52(3):658–62, discussion 662–63.
27. Cheng MJ, Chun TT, Gelabert HA, Rollo JC, Ulloa JG. Surgical decompression among Paget-Schroetter patients with subacute and chronic venous occlusion. J Vasc Surg Venous Lymphat Disord. 2022 Nov;10(6):1245–50.

Index

Note: Page numbers in *italics* indicate a figure and page numbers in **bold** indicate a table on the corresponding page.

W

Y

For Product Safety Concerns and Information please contact our EU representative GPSR@taylorandfrancis.com Taylor & Francis Verlag GmbH, Kaufingerstraße 24, 80331 München, Germany

Printed and bound by CPI Group (UK) Ltd, Croydon, CR0 4YY
01/05/2025
01858540-0001